Detrimental Effects
of
Abortion

An Annotated Bibliography With Commentary

3rd Edition

Thomas W. Strahan

Detrimental Effects of Abortion: An Annotated Bibliography With Commentary

Copyright © 2001 Thomas W. Strahan

Published by Acorn Books

An imprint of Elliot Institute

P.O. Box 7348

Springfield, IL 62791-7348.

(217) 525-8202

www.afterabortion.org

First printing

ISBN 0-9648957-0-6

This title is also available in searchable electronic form.

Table of Contents

Introductory Material

Note On Corrections and Recommendations

This is an ongoing project. The editor welcomes any corrections or suggestions you may make. Recommendations regarding new or old studies that are not included in this bibliography, but should be, are also welcome. Corrections and recommendations should be sent to:

Thomas W. Strahan, Esq.
3740 Edmund Blvd.
Minneapolis, MN 55406
Phone: (612) 729-6765
email: strahan@pclink.com

Supplements and Updates

In order to keep the information in this bibliography as current as possible, the publishers will periodically (2 to 4 times a year) publish supplemental material in .PDF format on their web site.

The supplements will appear with the same numbering format as the original so new pages and sections can easily be added to the existing bibliography. Please visit the Elliot Institute/Acorn Books web site at www.afterabortion.org/bibliography for information on obtaining this publication and the supplements.

Notices of new supplement releases will also be sent to you if you sign up for the Elliot Institute email newslist at www.afterabortion.org.

Editor's Introduction

This annotated bibliography has now been retitled *Detrimental Effects of Abortion: An Annotated Bibliography with Commentary*. The earlier two versions were entitled *Major Articles and Books Concerning the Detrimental Effects of Induced Abortion*, the most recent of which was last published in 1996.

As in past versions, the citations contain key findings or conclusions of the authors as well as additional comments by myself which are designated as (Ed. Note). The findings and conclusions set forth represent only a portion of the research and interested persons are encouraged to consult the complete work.

In this version there has been an expansion of subjects relating to pregnancy decision making including sections on pregnancy as a crisis, responses to pregnancy, and personality changes shortly before abortion. In addition, there has been an attempt to separately categorize the various negative psychological responses such as ambivalence, denial, grief, guilt etc., and add other aspects such as dissociation and self-punishment. Various consequences of abortion have also been categorized which include psychiatric hospitalization or consultation, and deteriorating social and economic status with repeat abortion. In regard to physical and reproductive consequences, a section on endometritis has been added along with other sections relating to adverse consequences due to postabortion infections. Other additions include pregnancy-related mortality and homicide of pregnant women. Other subject areas have also been expanded. Many of the additional citations were located from search engines from the National Library of Medicine, including MEDLINE.

Most of the references are based upon studies of U.S. populations since abortion was legalized in 1973. Some references from Canada, England, Australia, Scandinavian countries are also included. References from third world countries were generally excluded. Virtually all citations are from studies of first-trimester abortion using the vacuum aspiration method which is, by far, the most common. Where other abortion methods are used the reference will so indicate. The listing of articles and books does not necessarily include all articles and books on a particular subject. Interested persons are encouraged to contact the author for possible additional references in specific subject areas of interest.

Pg 1

[Handwritten margin notes:]

Counselors are trained specifically at abortion service sites

↳ 16 hrs of medical training & techniques

• Constantly updating studies to tend w/ growing abortion patients

• Group therapy - if you can't afford individual

ɔ abortion which may be marked by anxiety, depression or
seeking abortion. Distress may arise from grief reactions which
ɔ terminate a pregnancy by abortion. This temporary depression,
ecision-making ability and the woman may be unable to fully
on risks or alternatives which interferes with the legal

with many adjustments needed. Reactions to pregnancy are
:motional and social support is an important factor as to whether
abortion takes place. Boyfriends or husbands frequently
ɡe or encourage abortion or act with indifference which is
tion for the prospective mother.

ly detrimental to male-female relationships. Casual or relatively
s are particularly likely to break up after the abortion. The
ɪppears to increase over time. Where couples do not break up
ɪblems and increased isolation are reported.

Repeat Abortion

If a woman has a first abortion, she is approximately 4 times more likely to repeat abortion compared with women who have not had a prior abortion. Presently, about 50% of the abortions in the United States are repeat abortions. Moral and social deterioration is increasingly evident as abortion is repeated. Women who repeat have increasingly less stable relationships, are more likely to be separated or divorced, are more likely to be on public welfare, are increasingly isolated, have more difficulty in getting along with others, are more likely to smoke or abuse alcohol or other drugs, are more likely to be hospitalized for psychiatric problems, are increasingly likely to suffer from anxiety disorders, have greater difficulty in sleeping and are more likely to attempt suicide.

Impact on Men

The impact on induced abortion on men has been greatly neglected and there is little available literature on the subject. However, some recent research has improved the situation to a degree. It appears from what is known that the reaction is one of guilt, sense of loss, regret, sadness, coldness or real or apparent indifference. Where abortion takes place despite the male objections, men may report a tremendous sense of helplessness. There is evidence that men may suppress their reactions to abortion to a greater degree than women.

Impact on Siblings

The impact of induced abortion on siblings in a family has been little studied. Small children are surprisingly aware of a pregnancy or abortion even when told nothing about it. Reactions of sibling to an abortion may be very severe. Fear of the mother, afraid of the world in general, self-blame, violent acting-out, despair and self-destructive behavior have been noted in various case studies.

Anxiety or Self-Punishing Behavior

There is growing evidence that women who have induced abortions will frequently exhibit a high level of anxiety, may fear they will be punished or deserve punishment, show paranoid behavior or fear of death. This may manifest itself in a number of contexts, such as fear of a dead child or deformed child in a subsequent pregnancy or self-destructive behavior such as drug or alcohol abuse or suicide attempts.

Cancer Risk

Whether or not induced abortion is an independent risk for breast cancer is controversial. Several recent studies have added to the existing research which concludes that an induced abortion increases the likelihood of breast cancer. This is of particular significance because approximately 44,000 women die each year from breast cancer in the U.S. Induced abortion, particularly of the first pregnancy, results in the loss of the protective effect against breast cancer because a pregnancy carried to term at an early age is protective against breast cancer. There is substantial evidence that induced abortion is an independent risk factor for breast cancer in women. Childbirth has been found to be protective against ovarian and endometrial cancer while induced abortion provides a lesser degree of protection or no protection. Induced abortion may be implicated in other types of cancer as well.

Substance Abuse

Women who have had abortions frequently report their first heavy use of alcohol or drugs to attempt to alleviate the stress related to abortion. Substance abuse in women following abortion may occur in an attempt to overcome nightmares or insomnia, as an attempt to reduce grief reactions and to attempt to repress the abortion experience itself.

Induced abortion contributes to fetal risk as women with prior abortions are significantly more likely to consume alcohol or drugs during subsequent pregnancies intended to be carried to term compared to women with other pregnancy outcomes.

Smoking

Postabortion women have a higher incidence of smoking than women with other reproductive outcomes. Some of the difference may be attributed to lifestyle, but there are at least three studies which implicate abortion directly as a factor in increased smoking in women. This has important health and social implications.

Suicide Attempts

Adolescents from dysfunctional homes or those who have run away from home have been found to have significantly elevated incidence of suicide attempts following induced abortion. Also, women who repeat abortion have a higher rate of suicide attempts than women with one abortion, according to a survey of women in a patient-led, post-abortion support group. A recent Finnish study has found that the incidence of suicide in women following induced abortion is six times higher than suicide following childbirth.

Maternal Death

This is an area which is currently the subject of interest to researchers. The definition of maternal death is very inadequate at present and reliance on death certificate information is very misleading. Research into pregnancy-associated deaths which have not been included as a pregnancy-related death but perhaps should be is underway. Additional research implicates induced abortion as substantially contributing to reproductive complications, low birth weight, risk of retardation or other serious illnesses in newborns, and increased risk of maternal death.

Thomas W. Strahan, Esq.
August 2001

Standard of Care for Abortion

1.1 Abortion Procedures - Standards and Guidelines

1.1.1   *Guidelines for Women's Health Care,*(Washington D.C.: The American College of Obstetricians and Gynecologists, 1996)

This publication provides comprehensive information on a wide range of ob/gyn subjects including abortion. The guidelines state that "properly performed abortion poses minimal risk to women." Further that "All legal requirements must be met, and clinicians who perform abortions should be aware of state statutes and regulations regarding abortion services."

1.1.2   "Medical Management of Abortion," ACOG Practice Bulletin. *Clinical Management Guidelines for Obstetricians-Gynecologists,* No. 26, April, 2001

Guidelines regarding use of Mifepristone, Methotrexate and Misoprostol for induced abortion.

1.1.3   "Antibiotic Prophylaxis for Gynecologic Procedures," . ACOG Practice Bulletin. *Clinical Management Guidelines for Obsterician-Gynecologists,* Number 23, January, 2001

Recommends tetracyclines and nitro-imidazoles for induced abortion and dilation and curettage.

1.1.4   *Abortion Practice*, Warren M. Hern M.D., Director, Boulder Abortion Clinic, (Boulder, Colorado: J.B. Lippincott Co., 1981, 1984, 1990).

An abortion service that provides no counseling at all is seriously deficient ... Training of counselors should include a minimum of 16 hours each of medical training and counseling techniques. Medical training should include reviews of reproductive anatomy and physiology, gynecologic diseases, venereal disease, breast and cervical cancer, sterilization, medical aspects of abortion, theory and case studies of oral contraceptives and intrauterine devices and conventional contraceptive methods. There should be a continuous inservice training program on the medical and psychological aspects of abortion. The Carkhuff method of empathy training is extremely helpful in abortion counseling. ... Individual counseling is time consuming and expensive, but it affords a better opportunity for patient evaluation and careful instruction. Group counseling is better than no counseling at all. To permit thorough questioning and full participation, groups should not exceed three or four patients ... There should be ample opportunity for those accompanying the patient to participate, with the patient's consent, during the portions of the counseling dealing with the abortion procedure and contraceptive methods. Arrangements for separate counseling should also be available.... Counseling should include the following: Social history relevant to the abortion, including feelings about pregnancy and abortion, brief explanation of reproductive anatomy and physiology, explanation of the abortion procedure and use of laminaria, discussion of birth control methods, presentation of the consent form for review by the patient.

1.1.5   "Standards for Obstetric-Gynecologic Services," The American College of Obstetricians and Gynecologists (Washington, D.C.: Committee on Professional Standards, 1981).

Policies covering abortions should be designed by the medical staff to guard the patient's health or improve the family life situation. Abortion is a surgical procedure. For its performance, adequate facilities, equipment and personnel are required to assure the highest standards of patient care. ... It is recognized that although an abortion may be requested by a patient or recommended by a physician, the final decision as to performing the abortion must be left to the medical judgment of the pregnant woman's attending physician, in consultation with the patient. No physician should be required to perform, nor should any patient be forced to accept an abortion. The usual informed consent, including operative permit, should be obtained. The same indications for consultation should apply to abortions as to other medico surgical procedures. Abortions should be performed only by physicians qualified to identify and manage complications that may arise from the procedure. pp. 64-65 (Most courts consider that the patient is "informed" if the following information is given: The processes contemplated by the physician as treatment, including whether the treatment is new or unusual; the risks and hazards of the treatment; the chances for recovery after treatment; the necessity of the treatment; the feasibility of alternative methods of treatment. There are two major exceptions to informed consent before treating a patient, i.e., emergency treatment and detriment to patient (therapeutic privilege). Therapeutic privilege can never be construed to allow a physician to misrepresent the facts and to state affirmatively that there is no danger when in fact great danger exists. The following reasons are not sufficient to justify failure to inform: [1] That the patient may prefer not to be told unpleasant possibilities regarding the treatment; [2] Full disclosure might suggest infinite dangers to a patient with an active imagination thereby causing her to refuse treatment; [3] That the patient, on learning the risks involved, might rationally decline treatment. The right to decline is the specific fundamental right protected by the informed consent doctrine. (It is advisable to get a written consent. In addition, it is suggested that a physician make a written notation on the patient's record indicating the information communicated.) pp-66-67

1.1.6   *Standards for Obstetric-Gynecologic Services 7th Edition,* The American College of Obstetricians and Gynecologists, College of Obstetricians and Gynecologists, 409 12th St. S.W. Washington D.C. 20024-2188 (1989).

This publication includes detailed standards for ambulatory care for obstetrics and gynecology and specifically states "Ambulatory care facilities should meet the same standards of care for abortion facilities as for other surgical procedures." p. 68.

1.1.7   *Ambulatory Maternal Health Care and Family Planning Services Policies. Principles. Practices,* ed. Florence E.F. Barnes, Committee on Maternal Health Care and Family Planning, Maternal and Child Health Association, American Public Health Association, Interdisciplinary Books and Periodicals For the Professional and the Layman (1978).

Community efforts are needed to assure that abortion services meet high standards. Prospective abortion patients usually want greater confidentiality for this procedure than for most other medical services. Thus the woman is in a peculiarly vulnerable position because she may be reluctant to complain to any authority concerning the quality of service received. Since a woman will probably require this service only once in her life, she has no option to change providers as a result of her experience. In addition, she has a very limited time to find appropriate services and to learn anything about the quality of providers before her pregnancy advances to a state where the risks, costs, and psychological impact of abortion are substantially increased. p. 45

The basic principles of abortion counseling are [1] counseling should be entered into freely; [2] it should be supportive and non-judgmental regardless of the circumstances of the pregnancy, and [3] it should be an educational experience. The aims of abortion counseling are [1] to aid the woman in reaching a decision considering such factors as relationships to family and others, the future of the infant if she were to carry it to term, the impact of the pregnancy and a child on her own educational and vocational goals and economic situation; [2] to help her implement whatever decision she makes; and [3] to offer assistance in controlling future pregnancies.

There should be written criteria to serve as a guide in the counseling process for caution, postponement, or rejection of a patient in an ambulatory facility. Counseling should be so timed and arranged that it need not be cut short in order for the physician to proceed with the abortion. It is recommended that counseling take place the day before, or if possible, two to three days before the scheduled operative time so that an ambivalent patient may have time to assimilate new information, talk with family or partner, if appropriate, and reflect on her decision. Overall content of counseling in the facility should cover: [1] Financial arrangements. [2] Alternative arrangements of handling the pregnancy. [3] Reproductive and contraceptive history by interview or self taken history. [4] Relevant medical history by interview or self-taken history. [5] Relevant social history by interview or self-taken history. [6] Discussion and information on sexuality and sexual behavior as appropriate. [7] Information and instructions regarding the examination, abortion, postoperative care, symptoms of trouble, where to call for post procedure help. [8] Informed consent process. [9] Contraceptive counseling and information.

1.1.8   "Administrative. Counseling and Medical Practices in National Abortion Federation Facilities," U. Landy and S. Lewit, Family Planning Perspectives 14(5): 257-262, Sept/Oct 1982.

Summarizes the counseling standards of National Abortion Federation facilities. Reported that 70% of the women came to NAF facilities without referral from a doctor.

1.1.9   "Standards For Abortion Care," National Abortion Federation, 900 Pennsylvania Ave. S.E. Washington D.C. 20003. (Revised November 1986).

Procedural and substantive standards for members of the National Abortion Federation. These standards are now out of date and have been replaced by NAF clinical policy guidelines.

1.1.10   Obstetrical Decision Making, Second Edition, Eds. Emanuel A. Friedman, David B. Acker, Benjamin P. Sachs, (Philadelphia: B.C. Decker, 1987).

The editors of this text are on the staff of Beth Israel Hospital and Professors or Assistant Professors at Harvard Medical School. It also includes a series of articles written by other authors. "Induced Abortion," Max Borten M.D. "It is essential for the gravida to be fully informed about alternative resources and options and about the safety and risks of the procedure. Psycho-social assessment and counseling are done at the very first step. In addition to the medical history, an in depth social history including relationships with others, attitudes about abortion, and support systems must be obtained at this time. Pre-abortion counseling should be open and understanding. No decision should be made by the gravida in haste, under duress, or without adequate time and information. Special attention should be given to feelings of ambivalence, guilt, anger, shame, sadness, and sense of loss. Family supports, if available, should be mobilized. Postoperative contraception must be emphasized. Counseling should also be done prior to the procedure and again during the follow-up visit." p. 44. A valuable flow chart is included. See also "Psycho-social Assessment," Patricia S. Stewart, M.S., M.S.W., describing the basic elements of psycho-social assessment, p. 301.

1.1.11 "Ethical Issues in Clinical Obstetrics and Gynecology," Benjamin Freedman, *Current Problems in Obstetrics, Gynecology and Fertility,* ed. John M. Leventhal, 8(3): 1-47, (Chicago: Year Book Medical Publishers, 1985).

Extended ethical discussion of important topics, including physician's authority, goals of treatment, information and truth telling, counseling, duties to others, family, physician autonomy.

1.1.12 "The Hippocratic Oath," trans. W.H.S. Jones, *Child and Family Quarterly* 2(2) (1972)

See also Declaration of Geneva, adopted by the World Medical Association in 1948, which attempted to update the Hippocratic Oath, pp. 98-99. For comment on the Hippocratic Oath, see *Child and Family Quarterly*, 10(1):2-3 (1971) and *Linacre Quarterly* 45(2): 106 (May 1978).

1.1.13 "The Hippocratic Oath: A Code for Physicians, not a Pythagorean Manifesto," P. Prioreschi, *Medical Hypotheses* 44: 447-462, 1995

The Hippocratic Oath is to be considered a code of conduct for all physicians and not a Pythagorean Manifesto. Many of the principles upheld by the Oath are found in other documents unrelated to the Pythagoreans.

1.2   Informed Consent

1.2.1 "Informed Consent in Crisis Pregnancy and Abortion," W Brett and A Brett, *Journal of Christian Health Care* 5(1): 3-10, March, 1992.

Discusses autonomy, veracity, justice, beneficence and non-maleficence. During pregnancy and perinatal medicine, issues of consent may be especially difficult and complex, particularly when the pregnancy produces a life crisis or when induced abortion is considered.

1.2.2 "Ethical Dimensions of Informed Consent," American College of Obstetricians and Gynecologists, *Women's Health Issues* 3(1): 1-10, Spring, 1993

Comprehensive statement on the various aspects of informed consent with commentary.

1.2.3   "Misrepresentation or Ignorance of Fetal Development as a Factor in Psychological Injury Following Induced Abortion," Thomas Strahan, *Association for Interdisciplinary Research in Values and Social Change* 9(4):1-8, May/June 1996

Accurate information on fetal development is relevant and material to informed consent prior to induced abortion.

1.2.4   "Lack of Individualized Counseling Regarding Risk Factors For Induced Abortion: A Violation of Informed Consent," Thomas Strahan, *Association for Interdisciplinary Research in Values and Social Change* 10(1): 1-8 July/August 1996

The likelihood of post-abortion infections, perforation of the uterus, or missed abortion varies greatly among individual women obtaining induced abortion.

1.2.5   "Lack of Individualized Counseling Regarding Risk Factors For Induced Abortion: A Violation of Informed Consent. Part 2," Thomas Strahan, *Association for Interdisciplinary Research in Values and Social Change* 10(2): 1-8, Sept/Oct, 1996

The incidence of incomplete abortion, cervical injury, bleeding or hemorrhage, pain, adverse reproductive effects and psychological problems following induced abortion varies greatly among individual women obtaining induced abortions.

1.2.6   "Akron v. Akron Center for Reproductive Health," 462 U.S. 416, 445(1983).

"A state may require that a physician make certain that his patient understands the emotional and physical implications of having an abortion."

1.2.7   "Planned Parenthood of Central Missouri v. Danforth," 428 U.S. 52, 67(1976).

A state may require informed consent even in the first trimester.

1.2.8   "Planned Parenthood of S.E. Pa. v. Casey," 505 U.S. 112 S. Ct. 2791 (1992)

Upheld a state statute requiring disclosure of the nature of the abortion procedure, the risks of the procedure, the alternatives to the procedure, the gestational age of the unborn child and the medical risks of carrying to term. If a woman so requests, she must be given a state department of health brochure describing fetal development and a list of agencies offering alternatives to abortion.

1.2.9   "Abortion and Informed Consent: A Cause of Action," Joseph Stuart, Ohio Northern Univ. *Law Review,* 14(I): 1-20, (1987)

The right to decide to have an abortion in consultation with a physician is one that can be truly exercised only if the pregnant woman has full knowledge of the abortion procedure, its risks and alternatives, as well as a description of who or what is to be aborted.

1.2.10   "Informed Consent: 1. II. III," Jeslie J. Miller, *Journal of the American Medical Association* 244

(18): 2100, Nov. 7, 1980; *JAMA* 244 (20): 2347, Nov. 21, 1980: *JAMA* 244(22): 2556, Dec. 5, 1980

Good overview of the law of informed consent.

1.2.11   "Counseling, consulting and abortion," Mary Anne Wood and W. Cole Durham, Jr. *Brigham Young University Law Review* 1978, 783-845

States may wish to pay greater attention to civil remedies that would provide compliance incentives in the area of informed consent.

1.2.12   "Informed Consent to Abortion: A Refinement," T.L. Jipping, *Case Western Reserve Law Review* 38:329-386 (1987/88)

Reviews inconsistencies in the U.S. Supreme Court decisions involving informed consent. Suggests that informed consent law should focus on the woman, not the doctor, that the reasonable patient model should be followed, and that a definition of health should be used consistent with the breadth given to health when the abortion right was established.

1.2.13   "Informed Consent and the Danger of Bias in the Formation of Medical Disclosure Practices," Schneyer, *Wisconsin Law Review* 124 (1976)

Good general summary; no specific mention of abortion.

1.2.14   "Current Opinions of the Council on Ethical and Judicial Affairs of the American Medical Association," (1988), *Informed Consent* (8.08)

Informed consent is a basic social policy for which exceptions are permitted (1) When the patient is unconscious or otherwise incapable of consenting and harm from failure to treat is imminent, or (2) When risk disclosure poses such a serious psychological threat of detriment to the patient as to be medically contraindicated. Social policy does not accept the paternalistic view that the physician may remain silent because divulgence might prompt the patient to forgo needed therapy. Rational, informed patients should not be expected to act uniformly even under similar circumstances in agreeing to or refusing treatment.

1.2.15   "Uninformed Consent and Terms Without Definitions," Joseph E. Hardison, *American Journal of Medicine* 74:932-933, June, 1983

During the time of denial, turmoil and intense personal loss and grief, it is understandable that many patients may give uninformed consent. Forcing the patient to face reality may precipitate panic, psychosis or suicide. We must give time to help them adjust to what is wrong before consent is meaningfully and truly informed.

1.2.16   "Abortion Legislation After Webster v. Reproductive Health Services: Model Statutes and Commentaries," David M. Smolin, *Cumberland Law Review* 20:71, 141, (1989-90)

In an investigation of abortion facilities a Miami Herald reporter posing as a potential client in a

Florida abortion clinic said "What about the baby. I'm worried about hurting the baby." "What baby', answered the clinic owner. There's just two periods there that will be cleared out." "You mean I'm not pregnant?" Oh, you're pregnant. But there is no baby there... two periods and some water. If you don't terminate, then it will become a fetus, and after birth it will become a baby." Quoting Sontag, "An Abortion," *Miami Herald*, Sept 17, 1989, Tropic at pg. 14 "The Woman's Right to Know: A Model Approach to the Informed Consent of Abortion," S.A. Oliver, R. Shaheen, M. Hegarty, *Loyola University of Chicago Law Journal* 22(2): 409, Winter, 1991

1.2.17   "Informed Consent Civil Actions for Post Abortion Psychological Trauma," Thomas E. Eller, *Notre Dame Law Review* 639, 1996

1.2.18   "The link between the elements for an informed consent cause of action and the scientific evidence linking induced abortion with increased breast cancer risk," J Kindley, *Wisconsin Law Review* 1595-1644, 1998

1.2.19   "Fetal Development Information: An Essential Aspect of Informed Consent," Monte Liebman, *Association for Interdisciplinary Research Newsletter* 3(1): 1-2, Spring, 1990

If people were informed that the life of a human individual is eliminated by abortion, then many would freely choose to forego the abortion) (It is not irrational to be fearful of terminating another's life, that is human.

1.2.20   *Aborted Women: Silent No More,* David C. Reardon, (Chicago: Loyola Univ. Press, 1987)

In every one of the thousands of cases documented by Women Exploited by Abortion, a full explanation of the possible risks and complications was not given by the abortion provider. Even when direct questions were asked, answers about risks are understated, construed or avoided. Rather than risks, alternatives or fetal development, abortion counseling is generally devoted to discussing birth control techniques.

1.2.21   "A New Problem in Adolescent Gynecology," M. Bulfin, *Southern Medical Journal* 72 (8):967-968, August 1979.

Fifty-Four teenage patients were seen with significant complications after legal abortion. None felt they had been afforded any meaningful information about the potential dangers of the abortion operation. Perforation of the uterus, peritonitis, pelvic pain, pelvic abscesses, bleeding and cramping, cervical lacerations, severe hemorrhage and adverse psychological and psychiatric sequelae were noted in various case reports.

1.2.22   "Physical and Psychological Injury in Women Following Abortion: Akron Pregnancy Services Survey," L.H. Gsellman *Association for Interdisciplinary Research Newsletter,* 5(4):1-8, Sept/Oct 1993.

In a retrospective study of post-abortional women at an Ohio pregnancy services center only about one-half said they had been adequately informed about fetal development or possible psychological and/or physical complications.

1.2.23   "Regulating Abortion Services," (letter), Virginia P. Riggs, *New England Journal of Medicine,* February 7, 1980, p. 350.

A description of the fetus is relevant to a woman's decision about abortion... To claim that this information does not pertain directly to the abortion procedure is to deny any possibility that a second being is involved. Women deserve to know exactly what would be removed before they make a decision. The doctor who protects them from the facts to preserve them from anxiety and guilt has made a moral decision on their behalf.

1.2.24   "Crisis and Informed Consent: Analysis of a Law-Medical Malocclusion," Fran Camerie, *American Journal of Law and Medicine* 12:54-97, 1986

People in crisis states undergo psychological and cognitive changes which temporarily impede their ability to render an informed and rational decision, yet do not render them incompetent.

1.2.25   "The "Exceptions" to the Informed Consent Doctrine: Striking a Balance Between Competing Values in Medical Decision-Making," Alan Meisel, *Wisconsin Law Review,* 413, 1979

Discusses the interests of the individual, family and friends, society, the professions, the nature of the decision, waiver, voluntariness, incompetency, therapeutic privilege, and decision-making by others; critical of therapeutic privilege.

1.2.26   "Wilson v. Scoll," 412 SW2d 299(1967)

Disclosure to patient is required if there is a 1% risk of hearing loss.

1.2.27   "Cobbs v. Grant," 8 Cal 3rd 229, 502 P2d 1(1972)

Good general discussion of disclosure requirements.

1.2.28   "Reynier v. Delta Women's Clinic," 359 So2d 733 (La. App. 1978)

An abortionist was not liable on a theory of lack of informed consent as there was no showing that the plaintiff would not have obtained the abortion if the risk were known.

2   **Abortion Decision-Making**

2.1   General Background Studies

2.1.1   "Abortion Counseling," M Kahn-Edrington, *The Counseling Psychologist* 8(1): 37-38, 1979

The following knowledge is recommended for effective abortion counseling: (1) Aware of the definition, prevalence, myths, types of procedures, risks and sequels of abortion. (2) aware of alternatives to problem pregnancy: abortion, adoption, marriage. (3) Have information about sexuality, contraception, and community resources. (4) Have knowledge of value systems of other cultures and religions. Counselors should have crisis intervention and problem solving skills. (Ed Note: This model lacks any recognition of the fetus as a patient, treats abortion and childbirth as moral equivalents , concentrates on the technique of abortion or contraception, and views the counselors role as no more than a facilitator.)

2.1.2   "Differential Impact on Abortion on Adolescents and Adults," W Franz and D Reardon, *Adolescence* 105:162-172, 1992

Women who aborted as teenagers compared to women who aborted at 20 years of age or older, were less satisfied with services at the time of the abortion, were more likely to feel forced by circumstances to have the abortion, were more likely to report being misinformed, more often reported severs psychological distress, and more often wanted to give birth and keep the baby.

2.1.3   "Interview Follow-up of Abortion Applicant Dropouts," M Swiger et al, *Social Psychiatry* 11:135-143, 1976

Women who originally sought abortion and then elected to carry to term were studied. Factors most important in influencing the decision were religious or moral objections; partner desires baby; fear of abortion procedure; abortion equated with loss of part of self; single, getting married; and response to family's push for abortion.

2.1.4   "Emergence and Resolution of Ambivalence in Expectant Mothers," P Trad, *Am J Psychotherapy* 44(4): 577-589, Oct 1990

Therapists should help the expectant mother work through her ambivalent feelings toward her infant in order that a more adapting and accepting attitude is achieved.

2.1.5   "Unwanted Pregnancy-A Neurotic Attempt of Conflict-Solving? An Analysis of the Conflict Situations of 228 Women Immediately Before Legal Abortion," P Goebel, *Zscr. Psychosom Med* 28:280-299, 1982

A German study of women seeking abortion evaluated the psycho-social situation at the time of conception. Several conflict situations were determined in which the "unwanted pregnancy" was an attempt to overcome actual neurotic needs.

2.1.6   "Partnership and Pregnancy Conflict," H Roeder et al, *Psychother Psychosom Med Psychol* 44(5): 153-158, 1994

A German study found that whether or not a child is aborted depends on the general commitment of the man involved with the relationship, the compatibility of a child with the professional situation of the pregnant woman, and their relationship with their own mother. The relationship with their mother is combined with the pregnant woman's trust in her own motherly competence.

2.1.7   "Abortion, adoption, or motherhood: An empirical study of decision-making during pregnancy,"

MB Bracken et al, *Am J Obstet Gynecol* 130(3): 251, Feb 1978

Women delivering were in significantly longer relationships with partners who had also been less cooperative about contraception. Discussion with significant others occurred more often in decisions to deliver and greater support was received for that option. For many women, the abortion decision, and to a lesser degree, the decision to deliver, was conflictual, options evenly balanced, and considerable indecision reported.

2.1.8   "Psychological Factors Involved in Request for Elective Abortion," M Blumenfield, *The Journal of Clinical Psychiatry,* 1978 pp. 17-25

Contraceptive failure in women seeking a first or repeat abortion was not because women did not have access to adequate contraception, but occurred because of underlying psychological conflicts in the female and sometimes the male. Frequent depression in women at the time of pregnancy was noted. Many males had a strong wish to father a child. In many cases, women attributed the failure to use contraceptives on medical factors, but such a factor was used as a form of rationalization to abandon contraception when the woman had an emotional need to become pregnant. The request for repeat abortion indicates that the ambivalence has persisted, and is acted out once again or a new circumstance has awakened underlying conflicts.

2.1.9   "Outcome and Management of Crisis Pregnancy Counseling," A Brett, W. Brett, *New Zealand Medical Journal* 105:7, 1992.

Counseling in a New Zealand crisis pregnancy center consisted of 1.5 hours of personal interviews separated in time and location from the abortion procedure, providing visual material on the development of the fetus and a waiting period of I to 2 weeks for reflection on the decision. Among 18 women who had planned to continue their pregnancies, 2 elected to terminate their pregnancies after the counseling. Among 72 women who had originally decided to terminate their pregnancies, 14 decided to continue their pregnancy after the counseling. Among 49 women regarded as ambivalent, 9 chose to terminate their pregnancies and 35 elected to continue their pregnancies. The study concluded that such counseling clearly affects the original decision about the continuation or termination in a substantial proportion of women in a "crisis" pregnancy.

2.1.10   "Abortion Counseling - A New Component of Medical Care," Uta Landy, *Clinics in Obstetrics and Gynecology* 13 (l):33, March, 1986.

This article by the former national director of the National Abortion Federation describes conflicts with partner, ambivalence, guilt, anger, fear of pain and concern about suitable birth control as major themes which consistently appear in counseling. (Ed Note: This article is frank and revealing.)

2.1.11   "Abortions: Predicting the Complexity of the Decision-Making Process," M.L. Friedlander, T.J. Kaul and C.A .Stirnel, *Women and Health* 9(l):43-54. Spring, 1984.

Existing beliefs about oneself and morality tend to be inadequate guide for decision-making in the face of an abortion dilemma, and in order to overcome this disequilibrium often will require the woman to develop new cognitive constructions of the situation. Citing the writings of Carol Gilligan.

2.2 Crisis Theory

2.2.1 *Crisis Counseling,* Howard W. Stone, (Minneapolis: Fortress Press, 1976).

Comments by author:

One of the worst things a person can do who is in crisis is to become isolated. Isolation often leads to bouts of depression and self-pity.

Crisis behavior includes tiredness and exhaustion, lethargy, feelings of helplessness and inadequacy, sense of confusion, anxiety, disorganization and poor functioning in work relationship, possible anger or hostility.

People in crisis are often less in touch with reality and are more vulnerable to change than they are in non-crisis periods.

Irrespective of how the client depicts the problem, all crises are religious at their core: they involve ultimate issues with which one must come to terms if one's life is to be fulfilling.

One of the most important things a person can offer an individual in a crisis is a relationship through which is communicated the sense that life has meaning, purpose and hope.

The more seriously threatening an individual's appraisal of an event, the more primitive or regressive his or her coping resources will likely be. A result of this regression to primitive coping methods is increased suggestibility and diminished trust, leading to what is referred to as "heightened psychological accessibility." This is probably the most unique and important concept within the theory of crisis intervention.

2.2.2 *Principles of Preventive Psychiatry,* Gerald Caplan, (New York: Basic Books, 1964).

Heightened psychological accessibility has obvious and important implications when it comes to counseling a person in crisis. The author states: "A relatively minor force, acting for a relatively short time, can switch the whole balance to one side or to the other- to the side of mental health or to the side of ill-health."

2.2.3 "Crisis Theory: A Definitional Study," Howard Halpern, *Community Mental Health Journal*, 9(4): 342, 349, Winter, 1973.

The author has verified this heightened psychological accessibility in his research on the defensiveness of people in crisis. He found that they tend to protect themselves less than other people and are more open to outside help and assistance toward change.

2.2.4 "Theory of Crisis Intervention," Wilbur E. Morley, *Pastoral Psychology* 21:203 (April 1970), p. 16.

A person in crisis is in a state of "upsetness" or cognitive dissonance. Much less of the personality is firmly planted on the line between stability and instability. The individual wants to reestablish stability, and is therefore very susceptible to any influence from the inside or outside which will aid in resolving the crisis. With a minimal effort on the part of the minister, mental health professional, or family member, a maximum amount of leverage may be exerted upon the individual.

2.3 Pregnancy as a Crisis

2.3.1 "Some Considerations of the Psychological Processes in Pregnancy," Grete L. Bibring, *Psychoanalytic Study of the Child*, 14:113-121, (1959)

Comments by author: Pregnancy, like puberty or menopause, is a period of crisis involving profound psychological as well as somatic changes.

These crises are equally the testing ground of psychological health, and we find that under unfavorable conditions they tend toward more or less severe neurotic solutions.

Stress is inherent in all areas: in the endocrinological changes, in the activation of unconscious psychological conflicts pertaining to the factors involved in pregnancy, and in the intra-psychic reorganization of becoming a mother. A new organization of all forces must be made, and this necessity leads to the crisis of pregnancy. Within this crisis, of course, individual problems and neurotic conflicts of significance are highlighted.

As the modern family becomes isolated, and as other important group memberships break down, the individual must rely increasingly on the nuclear family, especially on the marital relationship, and this unit is rarely equipped to replace all these figures in their varied supportive functions.

The enormous improvement in medical management, (and) in lessening the physical dangers of pregnancy, has contributed to a waning concern with the concomitant psychological changes on the part of society in general. This waning concern stands in marked contrast to the unchanged, conservative, inner psychological processes and anxieties, especially of the primigravida.

What was once a crisis with carefully worked out traditional customs of giving support to the woman passing through this crisis period , has become at this time a crisis with no mechanisms within the society for helping the woman involved in this profound change of conflict solutions and adjustive tasks.

2.3.2 "A Study of the Psychological Processes in Pregnancy and of the Earliest Mother-Child Relationship," G. Bibring, T. Dwyer, D. Huntington, and A. Valenstein, *Psychoanalytic Study of the Child* 16:9 (1961).

An example of a young pregnant woman whose family did not initially support her pregnancy and her subsequent ambivalence; whereas a social worker's simple appreciation of her role as an expectant mother dramatically changed her attitude toward her pregnancy – this is a good example of how an apparent minor comment makes a big difference to someone in a crisis situation. Any

12

normal girl, though she might have intense wishes for a child and though she might love the man who is the father of the child, still must make a major developmental move in becoming a mother. At any point along this line of integration and adjustment complications may arise; be it from relation to the husband, or men in general; be it from the modes of receiving, retaining or releasing which the woman has established as a result of her own infantile development and her leading libidinal positions; be it from the emotional change of her object relationship which may be prevalently positive or ambivalent or destructively hostile; be it from her relationship to herself as compared or contrasted with that to the external world and its objects. All these will be reflected in the signs of crisis.

2.3.3   "Outcome and management of crisis pregnancy counseling," A Brett and W Brett, *New Zealand Medical Journal* 105:7-9, 1992

A study of women in crisis pregnancy situations informed women about the physical and emotional effects of pregnancy, normal fetal development, and options that were available over about a 1.5 hour period. Overall, 47% of the women changed an initial decision or reached a final decision regarding their pregnancy, and 46% ultimately continued with their pregnancies. The authors concluded that the study provided support for considering the crisis pregnancy as an obstetric emergency.

2.3.4   "Informed Consent in Crisis Pregnancy and Abortion," W Brett and A Brett, *Journal of Christian Health Care* 5(1) : 3-10, March, 1992.

This article reviewed the ethical basis of informed consent during pregnancy where the doctor has an ethical duty to both the woman and the fetus. Principles of autonomy, veracity, beneficience, non-maleficience, and justice were discussed. The authors concluded that, "disturbingly and quite inappropriately, the ethical responsibilities implicit in the doctor-fetus relationship may also be neglected in the crisis pregnancy."

2.3.5   "The Spectrum of Fetal Abuse in Pregnant Women," JT Condon, *The Journal of Nervous and Mental Disease* 174(9):509, Sept, 1986.

The fetus, whose intrapsychic representation is a curious admixture of fantasy and reality, is a recipient "par excellence" for projection and displacement.

2.3.6   "Pregnancy, Miscarriage and Abortion," Dinora Pines, *International Journal of Psychoanalysis* 71:301, 1990

For some women, the fetus is not represented as a baby in fantasy, dreams, or reality, but rather as an aspect of the bad self or as a bad internal object that must be expelled. Analysis of such patients reveals an early relationship with the mother which is suffused with frustration, rage, disappointment, and guilt. Loss of the fetus is experienced as a relief rather than a loss, as if the continuing internal bad mother had not given permission to become a mother herself.

2.3.7   "Therapeutic Abortion Clinical Aspects," Edward Senay, *Archives of General Psychiatry*, 23:408-415, November 1970

Even brief exposure to this population should serve to convince the skeptic that the frequent reports of insomnia, somatic complaints, intense anxiety, depressive feelings, suicide ideation and intense preoccupation with the problem of getting rid of the unwanted pregnancy define a population of people in crisis.

2.3.8 "The experiences of women who face abortions "V Slonim-Nevo, *Health Care for Women International* 12(3): 283-292, 1991

Israeli women who were about to have abortions were interviewed and found to be in crisis as evidenced by intense emotions of sadness, ambivalence, confusion, and fear. The women were dependent upon the professional counselor for technical and emotional support.

2.3.9 "Paternalistic vs. egalitarian physician styles: the treatment of patients in crisis," S LeBaron, J Reyher, JM Stack, *Journal of Family Practice* 21(1)): 56-62, July, 1985.

Among women who had elective abortions, those who were treated in a paternalistic manner had significantly higher responsiveness to suggestibility compared to those treated in an egalitarian interpersonal style.) (Ed Note: This study demonstrates how individuals in crisis are susceptible to influence from others.

2.3.10 "Emotional Crises of School-Age Girls During Pregnancy and Early Motherhood," Maurine LaBarre, *Journal of the American Academy of Child Psychiatry* 11(3): 537-557 (1972).

The theoretical concepts we have found most useful in studying and working with pregnant girls are those of "crisis." These young girls are experiencing concurrently a triple crisis of maturational or developmental phases of feminine life. They have not yet completed adolescent development when they are experiencing their first pregnancy, and they are struggling with adjustments to new roles as wives or mothers-to-be. In some cases the discovery of the pregnancy or other life events precipitates an acute episode of shock, stress, and anxiety, disrupting the previous adjustment and requiring the reorganization or development of new coping methods to deal with the trauma.

2.3.11 "Life Situation Associated with the Onset of Pregnancy," N. Greenberg, J. Loesch and M. Lakin, *Psychosomatic Medicine* 21:296(1959).

In approximately two thirds of the cases studied, loss of a meaningful relationship or separation from a loved person occurred within six months of the onset of the woman's pregnancy.

2.3.12 "Unwed Mothers: A Study of 100 Girls in Melbourne. Australia N," Shanmugan and C. Wood, *Australian and New Zealand Journal of Sociology* 6:51(1970).

More than a quarter of the girls had lost fathers by death or divorce, and only 10 percent of all girls felt they were very close to either parent.

2.4   Pregnancy Reactions/Unwanted Pregnancy

2.4.1   "Psycho-Social Aspect of Induced Abortion," B Raphael, *Medical Journal of Australia* 2:35-40, July 1, 1972

Tremendous variation exists in motivations for becoming pregnant, and influences may range from the mature and natural fulfillment of an adult, loving and involved marital relationship to the neurotic, repeatedly illegitimate pregnancies of the immature teenager. Self-punishment or self-destructive tendencies may operate so that either the pregnancy itself or the abortion represents a way of punishing herself for unrecognized feelings of guilt. Guilt may derive from earlier events in the woman's life, e.g. a previous abortion, a sadistic or rejecting act, or it may be related to deep-seated conflict concerning her sexuality which she may perceive as being bad, sinful, dirty or uncomfortable. Women may become pregnant while they are depressed. Passivity and failure to care may make them casual in their contraceptive practice. Or they may unconsciously believe that a pregnancy may make them feel better, filling the emptiness inside or giving them the sense of worth and fulfillment they so desperately need in their depressive mood. A second or third undesired conception may represent a rather pathetic attempt to undo previous failure-to relive the situation of the last abortion, the previous pregnancy, more satisfactorily. But the woman driven by deep neurotic motives rarely achieves such reparation even if she carries to term, and instead repeats once more her abnormal patterns of behavior, reinforcing again her guilt, anxiety and conflict. It is vitally important for any doctor dealing with a woman who may come to him seeking termination of pregnancy to recognize the possibility of such influencing factors. Only in this way can he help her deal with the crisis that continuing the pregnancy or terminating it may mean to her.

2.4.2   "Elective Abortion: Woman in Crisis," Naomi Leiter, *New York State Journal of Medicine* 2908-2910, December 1, 1972.

A woman may have an unwanted pregnancy because of (1) an acting out against and in defiance of the parent and a wish to get away from home, (2) loneliness and a desire to get closer to a man and have a baby to love as the person wishes to be loved, and (3) loss or threatened loss of a significant person in one's life. his loss or threat of loss may be real or fantasied.

2.4.3   "The Mental Health of Women 6 Months After They Gave Birth to an Unwanted Baby: A Longitudinal Study," JM Najman et al, *Social Science Med* 32(3):241-247, 1991

An Australian study found that mothers proceeding with an unwanted pregnancy, on the whole, manifest few subsequent mental health problems.

2.4.4   "Unwanted Conceptions.Research on undesirable consequences," E. Pohlman, *Eugenics Quarterly* 14:143, 1967.

We think, not in terms of dichotomies such as 'wanted' and 'unwanted', but of a continuum of feelings ranging from total rejection to to nearly total acceptance." Conscious rejection may (1) continue and remain conscious; (2) continue but become repressed and unconscious; (3) decrease in intensity as positive aspects become more apparent-with resulting ambivalence; (4) become submerged by positive feelings, even at the unconscious level; (5) be only a superficial façade, perhaps in order to conform to social ideas. In this last instance, the pregnancy fills needs and is not rejected: here it is the acceptance of pregnancy that is repressed and concealed beneath a conscious façade of rejection.

2.4.5   "Children Born to Women Denied Abortion," Z Dytrych et al, *Family Planning Perspectives* 7(4): 165, July/Aug 1975; "Follow-up Study of Children Born to Women Denied Abortion," Z Matejek et al, *Ciba Foundation Symposium* 115, 1985, 136,148.

A Czech study of children born where their mothers were twice refused a request for abortion reported that " by and large the mothers did move from initial rejection to ultimate acceptance in the 9 year interval" since the birth. Thirty-eight percent of the mothers subsequently denied ever seeking an abortion; some said they hated the commission for refusing their request; others said they were now very grateful the commission had refused; fourteen percent of the mothers refused induced abortion reported a spontaneous abortion (early miscarriage).

2.4.6   "The effect of pregnancy intention on child development," TJ Joyce et al, *Demography* 37(1): 83-94, Feb 2000.

Based on data from the National Longitudinal Survey of Youth it was found that unwanted pregnancy is associated with prenatal and postpartum behaviors that adversely affect infant and child health, but that unwanted pregnancy has little effect with birth weight and child cognitive outcomes. Estimates of the association between unwanted pregnancy and maternal behaviors were greatly reduced after controls for unmeasured family background were included in the model. There were also no significant differences in maternal berhaviors or child outcomes between mistimed and wanted pregnancies.

2.4.7   "Defining dimensions of pregnancy intendedness," JB Stanford et al, *Maternal Child Health Journal* 4(3): 183-189, Sept 2000.

Women indicated that their partners had a strong influence on preconception and postconception desire for pregnancy.

2.4.8   "Pregnancy Resolution Decisions: What If Abortions Were Banned?" J Murphy, B Symington, S Jacobson, *The Journal of Reproductive Medicine* 28(11): 789-797, 1983.

The availability of another person to help with an unplanned child was most closely associated with the decision to carry the baby to term or abort it.

2.4.9   "Life Events and Acceptance of Pregnancy," MM Helper et al, *Journal of Psychosomatic Research* 12:183-188, 1968.

This study determined what life events are judged by women to impose difficulties in adjustment to pregnancy.

2.4.10 "L'interruption volontaire de grossesse a repetition," I Tamian-Kunegel, *Gynecol Obstet Fertil* 28:137-140, 2000.

Repetitive abortions reveal an ambivalence towards contraception. The desire for pregnancy does not always go along with a desire for motherhood. It is a neurotic expression full of guilt that shows that these women did not overcome a childish rivalry with their mothers, and remain within a symbiotic relationship with them.

2.4.11 "The effects of termination of pregnancy: A follow-up study of psychiatric patients," R Schmidt and RG Priest, *Br J Medical Psychology* 54:267-276, 1981.

In a British study of women seeking abortion for mental health reasons, many women described considerable difficulties in current relationships at the time of their abortion request. Some women had used the pregnancy in the hope that the men would remain with them. Many had unresolved conflicts in their family of origin. It was concluded that the unwanted pregnancy may represent for women a vehicle for the restorative and reparative wishes as well as for their destructive wishes.

2.4.12 "Abortion-Pain or Pleasure," Howard W. Fisher in *The Psychological Aspects of Abortion*, Ed. D Mall and W Watts, (Washington, D.C.: University Publications of America, 1979) 39-51.

Confusion of sexual identity (can) lead to attempts to "prove" femininity with sexual acting out and resultant pregnancy. This is why contraception 'fails'. Actually, the pregnancy is not totally 'unwanted' The author concludes that abortion has both masochistic and sadistic components.

2.4.13 Personality Changes Shortly Before Abortion

Very pronounced psychological, psychiatric , and cognitive changes occur in a majority of women shortly before they undergo an induced abortion. The following studies are illustrative.

2.4.14 "Coping with Abortion," L Cohen and S Roth, *Journal of Human Stress* 140, Fall, 1984.

A generalized stress response syndrome was found in women upon arrival at an abortion facility similar to responses of bereaved populations.

2.4.15 "Grief and Elective Abortions:Breaking the Emotional Bond?" Larry Peppers, *Omega* 18(1): 1, 1987-88.

An intense grief response was found in women at a pre-abortion counseling session. A wide range of responses was observed.

2.4.16 "The Effects of Termination of Pregnancy: A Follow-up Study of Psychiatric Referrals," R Schmidt and Priest, *Br J Medical Psychology* 54:267, 1981.

Prior to abortion, the mean score on hostility (predominately self-criticism and guilt) was about two standard deviations above the normal mean which is similar to psychiatric populations.

2.4.17 "Psychiatric Morbidity and Acceptability Following Medical and Surgical Methods of Induced Abortion," DR Urquhart and AA Templeton, *Br J Obstetrics and Gynecology* 98:396, 1991

Two days before the abortion, 60% of women had high scores for anxiety and depression which was compatible with psychiatric morbidity.

2.4.18 "Testing a Model of the Psychological Consequences of Abortion," Warren B Miller, David J Pasta, Catherine L Dean in *The New Civil War. The Psychology, Culture and Politics of Abortion,* Ed. Linda J. Beckman and S Marie Harvey, (Washington, D.C.:American Psychological Association, 1998) 235-267

Women who participated in a clinical trial of Mifepristone abortion exhibited acute pre-abortion stress which was dominated by high avoidance, intrusion, and anxiety. The authors concluded that, "what appears to be happening is that the women are trying to control their response to the unwanted pregnancy/abortion by avoiding thinking about it."

2.4.19 "Psychological consequences of induced abortion," L Schleiss et al, *Ugeskr Laeger* 159(23):3603-3606, 1997

Fifty-two percent of Danish women were psychologically influenced before the abortion to an extent which indicated severe crisis or actual psychiatric illness.

2.4.20 "Family Relationships and Depressive Symptoms Preceding Induced Abortion, D Bluestein and CM Rutledge," *Family Practice Research Journal* 13(2): 149, 1993

Women about to undergo induced abortion had depressive symptoms which were moderate to severe in intensity which were strongly associated with unsatisfactory family relationships. Depressive symptoms increased as dissatisfaction with choosing abortion increased.

2.4.21 *The Ambivalence of Abortion,* Linda Bird Francke. (New York: Random House, 1978) 93.

The author cites a Canadian study of married couples which found in many cases that the wife exhibited "great stress" and underwent a temporary personality change. The effect of the unwanted pregnancy was sufficiently great to swamp whatever personality similarities the women had previously shared with their husbands.

2.4.22 "Counselling of Patients Requesting an Abortion," Joyce Dunlop, *The Practitioner* 220:847-851, June, 1978

This article quotes a psychiatric counselor who said, "the 24 hour period prior to the woman obtaining an abortion is a period of intense anxiety and ambivalence."

2.5 Characteristics of Women Having Induced Abortion

2.5.1 "Abortion Surveillance-United States. 1992," L.M. Koonin et. al., *MMWR* 45, No, 55-3:1, May 3 1996

For 1992, 1,359,145 legal abortions were reported to CDC, representing a 2.1% decline overall, from the number reported for 1991. 45.8% of women were repeating abortion with 26.9% reporting a second abortion, 10.8% (third), and 6.4% having four or more abortions. The abortion ratio was more than nine times greater for unmarried women than for married women. The abortion rate for white women was 15 per 1000 white women compared to 41 per 1000 black women and 32 per 1000 Hispanic women.

2.5.2   *The Long Term Psychological Effects of Abortion,* Catherine A. Barnard, (Portsmouth N.H. : Institute For Pregnancy Loss, 1990) see also "Stress Reactions in Women Related to Induced Abortion," *Association For Interdisciplinary Research Newsletter* 3(4):1-3, Winter 1991

A study of 80 women (3-5 years post abortion) who had abortions at a Baltimore area clinic in 1984-86 using the Millon clinical Multi-Axial Inventory (MCMI) found that women had significantly higher scores in areas of histrionic, narcissistic and anti-social characteristics compared to the sample on which the test had been normed. They also exhibited higher levels of anxiety and paranoia.

2.5.3   "Abortion and Subsequent Pregnancy," C. Bradley, *Canadian Journal of Psychiatry* 29: 494, Oct. 1984.

A Canadian study on married women who had recently given birth to a child found that women with a history of induced abortion were more likely to describe themselves as self-reliant, independent, rebellious and to enjoy being unattached and not tied to people, places or things, they were also much more likely to work outside the home following the birth of their baby.

2.5.4   "The Characteristics and Prior Contraceptive Use of U.S. Abortion patients," S. Henshaw and Silverman, *Family Planning Perspectives* 20(4): 158-168, July/Aug. 1988.

In a 1987 survey of 9480 women at 103 hospitals, clinics and doctors offices women undergoing abortion were more likely to be non-white than women generally, be eligible for medical assistance, be enrolled in school, never married, cohabitating, divorced or supported and with lower family income. 42.9% reportedly were repeating abortion.

2.5.5   "Gestation, Birth-Weight, and Spontaneous Abortion in Pregnancy After Induced Abortion," Report of Collaborative Study by World Health Organization Task Force on Sequelae of Abortion, *The Lancet,* January 20, 1979, pp. 142-145.

Women who have had an induced abortion are not a random sample of the population, but the degree to which they deviate from the norm varies with the attitude of their society. In general, the study suggests that they were more likely to smoke, to have had failed contraception, and to be uncertain of menstrual dates when compared with primigravidae of similar age or with women who had a previous spontaneous abortion. See also *Bulletin World Health Organization,* S. Harlap, A. Davies, 52(149) 1975.

2.5.6   "Motivational Factors in Abortion Patients," F.J. Kane, P. Lachenbruch, M. Lipton, and D. Baram, *American Journal of Psychiatry,* 130(3): 290-293, March, 1973.

Forty percent were found to have motivational factors that may have influenced the outcome of the pregnancy, such as guilt over the use of contraception, a severe acting out of a character disorder, or a reaction to loss.

2.5.7 "Prospective Study of Spontaneous Fetal Losses After Induced Abortions," S. Harlap, P. Shiono, S. Ramcharan, *New England Journal of Medicine*, 301(13): 677-681, September 27, 1979.

Women with previous induced abortions were more likely to be unmarried, black, regular drinkers and smokers.

2.6   Abortion Decision Making - Role of Males

2.6.1 *Passage Through Abortion,* Mary K. Zimmerman (New York: Praeger Publishers, 1977).

In an in-depth study of 40 U.S. women undergoing abortion in 1973 The male partner played a central role in the abortion experience for 38 out of 40 women. In 20% of the cases resulting in abortion the woman initially wanted to have the baby, but the man was opposed. In addition, 16 males stated they agreed with the decision of abortion while 8 disagreed with the decision of abortion. Opposition by the male was disruptive for the woman. Fifty percent terminated their relationship with the man involved in the pregnancy. Abortion appeared to assist in a decision for marriage in 3 cases. Six women reported no change in their relationships.

Women overwhelmingly denied their own responsibility in having the abortion in an attempt to view themselves as "moral" persons. Two out of 3 said they had "no choice" in the matter of abortion or were "forced" to have an abortion.

2.6.2 "The Relationship of Social Support and Social Networks to Anxiety During Pregnancy," Joan Jurich, Ph.D. Dissertation, Purdue University, 1986, *Dissertation Abstracts International* 48(1), July 1987, Order No. DA 8709818.

In a study of 65 women receiving prenatal care from Methodist Hospital of Indiana, the most consistent predictors of anxiety at each point of inquiry throughout pregnancy were the woman's need for emotional support and their satisfaction with their relationship with their partner. Informational support was found to be relevant to anxiety only at the outset. Material support was not significantly related to anxiety at any point during pregnancy.

2.6.3 "Psychologic and Emotional Consequences of Elective Abortion: A Review," G.S. Walter, *Obstetrics and Gynecology* 36(3):482-491, September 1970.

It is known that women seeking abortion may do so at the insistence of partners whose neurotic behavior is being acted out upon their wives. Citing several studies.

2.6.4 "Why Do Women Have Abortions?," Aida Torres and Jacqueline Forrest, *Family Planning Perspectives* 20(4): 169-176, July/August 1988.

In a survey by the Alan Guttmacher Institute in 1987 of women at abortion facilities, lifestyle change, can't afford baby now, problems with relationships-or avoidance of single parenthood or not ready for responsibility, doesn't want others to know she has had sex or is pregnant or thought she is not mature enough to have a child were the primary reasons cited by the self-report of the women based upon the questions posed.

2.6.5   *A Study of Abortion in Primitive Societies,* George Deveraux, (New York: The Julian Press, 1955), p. 136.

Anthropologist George Deveraux, in his study of abortion in primitive societies, observed that female attitudes toward maternity appear to be largely determined by masculine attitude toward paternity. He found that the romanticization of the maternal role the Madonna complex is conspicuously absent in primitive societies, even where children are ardently desired and where fertile women are much esteemed ... and even when women abort of their own free will, and including instances where they abort from spite or as a result of a domestic quarrel, they do so under the impact of a genuine or expected masculine attitude.

2.6.6   "Life Events and Acceptance of Pregnancy," M. Helper, R. Cohen, E. Beitenman and L. Eaton, *Journal of Psychosomatic Research* 12:183-188(1968).

The attitude of the father is an important factor in the degree of stress related to a pregnancy. In a study at the University of Nebraska on women from wide ranging backgrounds, it was found that the most stressful events occurring during pregnancy were, "The woman is pregnant out of wedlock and receives no help from the father of the baby, " and "The husband doesn't want the baby she is carrying.")

2.6.7   *Men and Abortion. Lessons. Losses and Love,* Arthur Shostak and Gary McLouth, (New York: Praeger, 1984).

Sociologist Arthur Shostak, in his study of 1, 000 U.S. men interviewed at abortion clinics, found that a sizable bloc (45%) recalled urging abortion (37% of the married men, 48% of the unwed males). The vast majority were pro-choice with only 9% favoring a law to outlaw abortion (83% were opposed). Men emphasized their belief that pregnancy was a distinct trauma for their sex partner and one that required and justified the location of 51% or more of the decision making power in their hands alone.

2.6.8   "Husbands of Abortion Applicants: A Comparison With Husbands of Women Who Complete Their Pregnancies," F. Lieh-Mak., Y. Tam and S. Ng, *Social Psychiatry* 14:59- 64(1979).

In a Hong Kong study of 130 husbands of women seeking abortions, 44% of the husbands instigated the abortion with economic reasons being predominant. Characteristics of husbands of women seeking abortion were compared to husbands of women who delivered. More abortion husbands reported poor relationships with either or both parents. 27% of the abortion husbands reported psychiatric illness in the family compared to 8% of the controls; abortion husbands had a higher prevalence of alcoholism, drug dependency, neurosis and compulsive gambling compared to controls. An unhappy childhood was reported by 20% of abortion husbands versus 5% for controls. 70% of the abortion husbands reported they used contraception compared to 35% for controls. Abortion husbands tended to use unreliable contraceptive methods such as withdrawal (18% vs. 6%) or reliance upon a "safe" period (12% vs. 4%). The authors concluded, "Our study has served to emphasize the important role that the husband plays in abortion seeking and fertility regulation behavior. It is high time we should give substance to the shadowy figure that we call the male partner."

2.6.9   *Aborted Women: Silent No More,* David C. Reardon, (Chicago: Loyola Press, 1987).

In a study of 252 women members of Women Exploited by Abortion, 51% reported they were encouraged to have an abortion by a husband or boyfriend.

2.6.10   "Psychosis in Males Related Parenthood," R. Towne and J. Afterman, *Bulletin of the Menninger Clinic* (1955), pp. 19-26.

The child may be seen as a rival by the father and a target for unconscious aggressive feelings.

2.6.11   "Abortion in Relationship Context," Vincent M. Rue, *International Review of Natural Family Planning* 9:95-121, Summer 1985

Abortion serves well the erotically compulsive male or one with such tendencies, who strives to maintain his self-esteem and to gratify narcissistic needs through sexual achievement. Typically, this Don Juan male is minimally involved in the personality of his partner since his capacity to love is sharply limited. His sexual activity is invested in countering feelings of inferiority by proving erotic successes. After such a conquest he loses interest in the chosen woman and reacts with hostility towards her, since he devalues her after the successful conquest. Abortion is a handy passport for such adventure.

2.6.12   "Husband's Attitudes Towards Abortion and Canadian Abortion Law," Osborn and Silkey, *Journal of Biosocial Science* 12:21-30(1980).

This study found that religious affiliation is strongly related to male opinions about abortion. Permissive attitude toward abortion was associated with the use of highly effective contraceptive methods and with prior use of abortion.

2.6.13   *Expectant Fathers,* S Bittman and S. Zalk, (New York: Hawthorn, 1978, 1980).

A man may have guilt feelings or anger during his wife's pregnancy which may occur if his wife has had a previous miscarriage or abortion. The male may feel somehow responsible and if so there is a good chance that he will resent the baby and his wife that much more. The authors state, "[This is] not an auspicious way to begin family life.") p. 134 (After the first pregnancy and childbirth experience, many fears of the man dissipate on the second pregnancy. pp. 148-149

2.6.14   "Attitudes of Adolescent Males Toward Pregnancy and Fatherhood," Marcia A. Redmond, Family Relations, *Journal of Applied Family and Child Studies* 34(3):337-341, July 1985.

In a study of 74 adolescent males in Ontario, Canada of their attitudes toward adolescent pregnancy and fatherhood, all males wished to be told if a pregnancy occurred, whether or not they were in a casual or serious dating relationship. Male attitudes toward abortion were markedly different depending on the type of relationship. Some 32% of the casual daters believed the desired pregnancy outcome should be abortion compared to only 13% of the serious daters. Most males wished to be included in the decision-making process and receive emotional and social support during this time. When not included they felt confused and neglected. Males were a factor in the decision-making process even when ignored by professionals. The study concluded, "In regard to teenage pregnancy, it seems appropriate for professionals to recognize the male sexual partner as part of the problem as well as part of the solution."

2.7   Adoption as An Option

2.7.1   "Hispanic Adolescent Pregnancy Testers: A Comparative Analysis of Negative Testers, Childbearers and Aborters," DK Berger, *Adolescence* 26(104): 951 (1991)

In a sample of pregnant Hispanic adolescents, none chose adoption.

2.7.2   "Abortion, adoption, or motherhood: An empirical study of decision-making during pregnancy," MB Bracken and LV Klerman, *Am J Obstet Gynecol* 130(3):251 (1978)

Adoption was not considered among population of pregnant young black women.

2.7.3   "The Adoption Alternative for Pregnany Adolescents: Decision Making, Consequences, and Policy Implications," MP Sobol and KJ Daly, *Journal of Social Issues* 48(3):143 (1992)

The authors estimated that only 3% of U.S. adolescents who carry to term place their infant for adoption and that there an estimated 50,000 unrelated adoptions each year in the U.S. Among adolescents who placed for adoption, parents were more likely to have been involved in the decision.

2.7.4   "Adoption as an Option for Unmarried Pregnant Teens," Marcia Custer, *Adolescence* 29(112): 891 (1993)

Societal sanctions, low level of knowledge, anticipated psychological discomfort, and lack of support from helping professions were found to be barriers to adoption.

2.7.5   "Physician's Preferences for Adoption, Abortion and Keeping a Child Among Adolescents," V Powell, et al *Research in the Sociology of Health Care* 9:33 (1991)

Physicians were generally supportive of adoption

2.7.6   "Adoption, Adoption Seeking, and Relinquishment for Adoption in the United States," Advance Data, No. 306, Centers for Disease Control, May 11, 1999

This study found that 232,000 ever married U.S. women were currently taking active steps toward adoption in 1995.

3   **Psychological Effects of Abortion**

3.1   Validity of Studies

3.1.1   "The Psychological Complications of Therapeutic Abortion," G Zolese and CVR Blacker, *Br J Psychiatry* 160: 724, 1992

Women who choose abortion are not amenable to endless questions on how they feel, are less likely to return for follow-up, and baseline assessments before they become pregnant are impossible. Most psychological studies were conducted when standardized psychiatric instruments were not available or used self-devised queastionnaires without proven reliability.

3.1.2   "Emotional Sequelae of Elective Abortion," I Kent et al, *British Columbia Medical Journal* 20:118, 1978

Sharp discrepancies were noted between data derived from a questionnaire survey administered through a general practice with the responses of women in a therapy group with deep and painful feelings not emerging in a questionnaire survey.

3.1.3   *Aborted Women: Silent No More,* David C Reardon, (Chicago: Loyola University Press, 1987

In a survey of long-term effects of abortion on women, over 70% reported there was a time when they would have denied the existence of any reactions from their abortion. For some, denial lasted only a few months; for others it lasted over 10-15 years. Subsequently, they were able to share the severe adverse effects of abortion on their lives.

3.1.4   "Underreporting Sensitive Behaviors: The Case of Young Women's Willingness to Report Abortion," LB Smith et al, *Health Psychology* 18(1): 37, 1999

U.S. young women were likely not to disclose prior induced abortion when interviewed. They were more likely to disclose smoking habits than abortion history.

3.1.5   "Some Problems Caused by Not Having a Conceptual Foundation for Health Research: An Illustration From Studies of the Psychological Effects of Abortion," EJ Posavac and TQ Miller, *Psychology and Health* 5:13, 1990

The authors reviewed 24 empirical studies and concluded that psychological research was of poor quality, failed to state the basis of the theory to be tested, failed to track women over time, and made superficial assessments.

3.1.6   "Psychological Impact of Abortion: Methodological and Outcomes Summary of Emperical Research Between 1966 and 1988," JL Rogers et al, *Health Care for Women Int'l* 10:347,1989.

Concludes that the literature on the psychological sequelae is seriously flawed and makes suggestions for critique of the literature. The authors conclude that both advocates and opponents of abortion can prove their points by judiciously referring only to articles supporting their political agenda.

3.1.7   "Mental Health and Abortions: Review and Analysis," Philip G. Ney and A. Wickett, *Psychiatric Univ. Ottawa* 14(4): 506-516, (1989)

A review of the literature shows a need for more long-term, in-depth studies; there's no satisfactory evidence that abortion improves the psychological state of those not mentally ill; mental ill-health is worsened by abortion; there is an alarming rate of post-abortion complications such as pelvic inflammatory disease and subsequent infertility.

3.1.8   "Psychiatric Aspects of Therapeutic Abortion," B. Doane and B. Quigley, *CMA Journal* 125:427-432, September 1, 1981

Concludes that a search of the literature on the psychiatric aspects of abortion reveal poor study design, lack of clear criteria for decisions for or against abortion, poor definition of psychologic symptoms experienced by patients, absence of control groups in clinical studies, indecisiveness and uncritical attitudes in writers from various disciplines. The study also concludes that "there is little evidence that differences in abortion legislation account for significant differences in the psychologic reactions of patients to abortion."

3.1.9   "Psychological and Social Aspects of Induced Abortion," J.A. Handy, *British Journal of Clinical Psychology,* February 21, 1982, Part I, pp. 29-41

A good summary of prior studies on the effects of abortion; states that a variety of methodological faults makes the results of many studies difficult to interpret.

3.1.10   "Interpreting Literature on Abortion," (letter), WL Larimore, DB Larson, KA Sherrill, *American Family Physician* 46(3):665-666, Sept 1992

Various review articles on abortion share few of the same references, interpretation of the same article differs between reviewers.

3.1.11   "Abortion: A Social-Psychological Perspective," Nancy Adler, *Journal of Social Issues* 35(1): 100-119 (1979)

Concludes there is a need for continuing research on the negative effects of abortion and for intervention designed to diminish those negative effects for all concerned.

3.1.12   "Psychiatric Sequelae of Induced Abortion," Mary Gibbons, *Journal of the Royal College of General Practitioners* 34:146-150(1984)

Observes that many studies concluding that few psychiatric problems follow induced abortion were deficient in methodology, material or length of follow-up. It concludes that a large amount of the previously reported research on the psychiatric indications of abortion may be unreliable.

3.2   Risk Factors for Adverse Emotional Consequences of Abortion

3.2.1   "Complicated Mourning: Dynamics of Impacted Pre and Post-Abortion Grief," Anne Speckland, Vincent Rue, *Pre and Perinatal Psychology Journal* 8(81):5, Fall, 1993.

Emotional harm from abortion is more likely when one or more of the following risk factors are present: prior history of mental illness; immature interpersonal relationships; unstable, conflicted relationship with one's partner; history of negative relationship with one's mother; ambivalence regarding abortion; religious and cultural background hostile to abortion; single status especially if no born children; adolescent; second-trimester abortion; abortion for genetic reason; pressure and coercion to abort; prior abortion; prior children; maternal orientation.

3.2.2   "Adolescent Abortion Option," G. Zakus, S. Wilday, *Social Work in Health Care,* 12(4):77, Summer, 1987.

Certain categories of women are much more likely to have post-abortion problems sometimes many months or years later. These include: being forced or coerced into abortion; women who place great emphasis on future fertility plans; women with pre-existing psychiatric problems; women suffering from unresolved grief reactions or women with a history of sexual abuse, including incest, molestation or rape.

3.2.3   "Outcome Following Therapeutic Abortion," R.C. Payne, A.R. Kravitz, M.T. Notman, J.V. Anderson, *Arch. Gen. Psychiatry* 33:725, June, 1976.

This study measured short- term outcomes of anxiety, depression, anger, guilt and shame following abortion. The authors concluded that women who are most vulnerable to difficulty are those who are single and nulliparous, those with previous history of serious emotional problems, conflicted relationships to lovers, past negative relationships to mother, ambivalence toward abortion or negative religious or cultural attitudes about abortion.

3.2.4   "The Decision-Making Process and the Outcome of Therapeutic Abortion, C," Friedman, R. Greenspan and F. Mittleman, *American Journal of Psychiatry* 131(12): 1332-1337, December 1974.

There is high risk for post-abortion psychiatric illness when there is (1) Strong ambivalence; (2) Coercion; (3) Medical indication; (4) Concomitant psychiatric illness and (5) A woman feeling the decision was not her own.

3.3   Post-Abortion Stress/Trauma/Post-Abortion Syndrome

3.3.1   "Post-Abortion Perceptions: A Comparison of Self-Identified Distressed and Non-distressed Populations," G. Kam Congleton, L.G. Calhoun. *The Int'l J. Social Psychiatry* 39(4): 255-265, 1993

Women reporting distress were more often currently affilliated with conservative churches and reported a lower degree of social support and confidence in the abortion decision. They were also more likely to recall experiencing feelings of loss immediately postabortion.

3.3.2   "Post-Trauma Sequelae Following Abortion and Other Traumatic Events," J.O. Brende, *Association for Interdisciplinary Research in Values and Social Change* 7(1): 1-8, July/August 1994

Case studies include a lonely woman with a history of multiple traumas, including sexual assault. After a divorce, she moved in with a man who promised to take care of her but eventually began to abuse her. When she became pregnant, he abandoned her, and she had an abortion. Severely depressed, she began to rely heavily on sleeping pills and alcohol to sleep because of nightmares and a repetitive dream about reaching for an infant that floated beyond her reach. One night, she overdosed on her pills but telephoned a friend who called for help. Her suicide was prevented and she was admitted to a psychiatric hospital for treatment. It was during this hospitalization that she received help, the first step toward breaking her victimization cycle.

A second case study involved a 21- year old woman who visited an abortion facility to obtain an abortion. However, the abortion was incomplete and she had bleeding, cramping and a low grade fever. She was admitted to a hospital where an intact fetus was observed on ultrasound. An abortion was performed and fetal parts were removed. Predisposing factors for trauma included her impulsive decision to have the abortion and poor treatment by the doctor at the abortion facility. She sought counseling 3 ½ months after the abortion, after six months, and again 9 ½ months after the abortion when her depression worsened and she overdosed on medications. She then had six counseling sessions and was diagnosed with Post-Traumatic Stress Disorder. After 2 ½ years she had intrusive images, flashbacks, and reliving experiences; anger at the doctor and others; grief; distractibility; selective concentration; vivid memory of the abortion; numbing and detachment; startle reactions; fear of men and of having sex ; physical symptoms including abdominal and stomach pain.

3.3.3   "Fragmentation of the Personality Associated with Post-Abortion Trauma," J.O. Brende, *Association for Interdisciplinary Research in Values and Social Change* 8(3): 1-8, July/August 1995

People enduring extreme stress often suffer profound rupture in the very fabric of the self. Severity of fragmentation is dependent upon several variables (1) the degree to which the trauma is experienced as a violation, (2) the presence or absence of support, (3) the presence of shame or self-blame, and (4) the loss of idealism and purpose.

3.3.4   *The Long-Term Psycho-social Effects of Abortion,* Catherine A. Barnard (Portsmouth, N.H.: Institute For Pregnancy Loss, 1990).

Some 18.8% of women who had undergone induced abortion 3-5 years previously reported all Post Traumatic Stress Syndrome criteria (DSM-III R). Some 39-45% of women still had sleep disorders, hyper-vigilance and flashbacks of the abortion experience. Some 16.9% had high intrusion scores and 23.4% had high avoidance scores on the Impact of Events Scale. Women showed elevated scores on the MCMI test in areas of histrionic, anti-social narcissism, paranoid personality disorder and elevated anxiety compared with the sample on which the test had been normed.

3.3.5   "Post Abortion Syndrome. An Emerging Public Health Concern," Anne C. Speckhard and Vincent M. Rue, *Journal of Social Issues*, Vol. 48(3):95-119, 1992.

Concludes that post abortion syndrome is a type of Post Traumatic Stress Disorder composed of the following basic components (a) exposure to or participation in an abortion experience, which is perceived as the traumatic and intentional destruction of one's unborn child; (b) uncontrolled negative re-experiencing of the abortion event; (c) unsuccessful attempts to avoid or deny painful abortion recollections, resulting in reduced responsiveness; and (d) experiencing associated symptoms not present before the abortion, including guilt and surviving.

3.3.6   "Methodological considerations in empirical research on abortion," RL Anderson et al in *Post-Abortion Syndrome: Its Wide Ramifications*, Ed Peter Doherty, (Portland: Four Courts Press, 1995) 103-115

A study at an psychiatric outpatient service, compared women who presented with a history of elective abortion and sought psychiatric services in response to negative adjustment to abortion, with women with a history of elective abortion who presented seeking outpatient services for reasons that were not abortion-related. A second control group consisted of women who sought outpatient services but denied any abortion history. 73% of the abortion- distressed group met the criteria for DSM-IIIR. Abortion distressed women reported more frequently that they believed abortion to be morally wrong and had fewer recent adverse life events than abortion non-distressed women.

3.3.7   "Psychological Responses of Women After First-Trimester Abortion," B Major et al, *Arch Gen Psychiatry* 57:777, 2000.

This study reported that 6 of 442 women (1.36%) reported PTSD two years postabortion according to DSM-IV criteria. An increasing number of women had negative emotional reactions with the passage of time. In this study it appears that the standard for identifying a case of abortion-related PTSD was set to exceptionally high level. First, women were required to the cause of each symptom as having been directly related to the abortion. Nightmares that they did not associate to their abortion, for example, would not have been included as an intrusive symptom. In addition, it appears that only women who rated the degree of the reaction at the highest level, for every PTSD symptom, were included. Women with a moderate level of distress in one symptom area, for example, were not counted as having PTSD. This high standard is useful for verifying with a high degree of certainty that abortion is the direct cause of PTSD in at least some cases. On the other hand, because the standard appears to be set higher than is normally the case in population studies of PTSD, the findings may under represent the actual incidence rate.

3.3.8   *Psycho-Social Stress Following Induced Abortion,* Anne Speckhard, (Kansas City: Sheed and Ward, 1987).

A study of 30 women who reported stress following their abortion found grief reactions, fear and anxiety, changes in sexual relationships, unresolved fertility issues, increased drug and alcohol use, changes in eating behaviors, increased isolation, lowered self-worth and suicide ideation and attempts.

3.3.9   *Post-Abortion Trauma: 9 Steps to Recovery,* Jeanette Vought, (Grand Rapids: Zondervan, 1991)

Experiences of men and women in a religiously-based postabortion recovery group.

3.3.10   "The Conception of the Repetition-Compulsion," E. Bibring, *Psychoanalytic Quarterly* 12:486-519(1943).

Repetition-compulsion is a regulating mechanism with the task of discharging tensions caused by traumatic experiences after they have been bound in fractional amounts.

3.3.11   "Two cases of post-abortion psychosis," W. Pasini and H. Stockhammer, *Annales Medico Psichologiques* [Paris] 128(4): 555-564 (1973).

Two cases of post-abortion psychosis are presented. One resulted in suicide while the other thought a nurse was attempting to poison her. One abortion was illegal, the other legal. A possible neurological basis for post-abortion psychological problems was presented. (French)

3.3.12   "Abortion Trauma: Application of a Conflict Model," R.C. Erikson, *Pre and Perinatal Psychology Journal* 8(1): 33. Fall, 1993.

Elective abortion is a potentially traumatizing event. Clinic experience indicates the symptoms and development of post traumatic stress disorder following abortion. A conflict model of trauma is presented with the woman as both victim and aggressor.

3.3.13   "Iatrogenic Post-Traumatic Stress Disorder," (letter), R. Fisch and O. Tadmor, *The Lancet,* December 9, 1989, p. 1397.

PTSD following induced abortion with post-abortion complications was reported. Soon after the abortion the patient exhibited severe anxiety, depression, recurrent intrusive thoughts and images related to the abortion, insomnia, recurrent nightmares, avoidance behavior along with other social problems continuing over two and a half years without much remission.

3.3.14   "Obsessive-Compulsive Disorder Apparently Related to Abortion," Ronald K. McGraw, *American Journal of Psychotherapy* 43(2):269-276, April 1989.

A married woman with a history of three abortions was obsessed with the idea she would become pregnant by someone other than her husband although she was not sexually active outside her marriage, and she compulsively underwent repeated pregnancy tests although there was no sign of pregnancy. If she became pregnant she thought she would die in childbirth. It was concluded that the obsessive-compulsive disorder was precipitated by routine medical tests that brought back memories of the prior abortions with associated guilt and fear of punishment.

3.3.15 "Incidence of complicated grief and post-traumatic stress in a post-abortion population," Leslie M. Butterfield, Ph.D. Dissertation, Virginia Commonwealth University (1988), *Dissertation Abstracts International* 49(8): 3431-B, February 1989, Order No. DA 8813540.

Stress responses were found in 55% of women six months following first trimester abortion. Posttraumatic stress was heightened by loss of partner and wishful thinking. Social support seeking and problem-focused coping was negatively associate with post-traumatic stress and grief. Women consistently showed death anxiety on the Grief Experience Inventory (GEI).

3.3.16 "Past trauma and Present Functioning of Patients Attending a Women's Psychiatric Clinic," EFM Borins, PJ Forsythe, *Am J Psychiatry* 142(4) :460, 1985

In a Canadian study, abortion correlated significantly with three or more trauma factors.

3.3.17 "Post Traumatic Stress Disorders in Women Following Abortion: Some Considerations and Implications for Martial/Couple Therapy," D Bagarozzi, *Int'l Journal of Family and Marriage* (Delhi, India) 1 (2): 51, 1993

Clinical examples of abortion related post traumatic stress disorder.

3.3.18 *The Mourning After Help for Post Abortion Syndrome,* Terry L. Selby with Marc Bockman (Grand Rapids: Baker Book House, 1990).

Designed for the clinical counselor. It has valuable chapters on subjects such as grief, denial the importance of faith and detailed case histories which provide valuable insights.

3.3.19 *Diagnostic and Statistical Manual of Mental Disorders-Revised,* DSM-III-R 309.89 (Post Traumatic Stress Disorder), (Washington, D.C.: American Psychiatric Press, 1987), pp. 20, 250. (Abortion is included as a possible psychosocial stressor under physical injury or illness. (Ed Note: Abortion as a possible psychosocial stressor was not included in DSM-IV manual)

Grief and Loss

3.4 General Background Studies (Grief and Loss)

3.4.1 *Living Through Personal Crisis,* Ann Kaiser Stearns, (New York: Ballantine Books, 1984).

Ed Note: Inexpensive paperback available in local bookstore; the author states that "grief is profoundly misunderstood in American society." She attempts to deal with grief and loss in theoretical terms as well as practical examples, including abortion. The author states that the failure to understand grief, has distorted the literature on the effects of induced abortion.

3.4.2 *Attachment and Loss,* J. Bowlby, (London: Hogarth Press, 1980)

Ed Note: This work as well as other writings on the subject by John Bowlby, are considered to be the classic works on the subject.

3.4.3 "Absence of Grief," Helene Deutsch, *Psychoanalytic Quarterly* 6:12-22 (1937)
Comments by the author:

The work of mourning does not always follow a normal course. It may be excessively intense, even violent, or the process may be unduly prolonged to the point of chronicity when the clinical picture suggests melancholia.

If the work of mourning is excessive or delayed, one might expect to find that the binding force of the positive ties to the lost object had been very great. My experience corroborates Freud's finding *that the degree of persisting ambivalence is a more important factor than the intensity of the positive ties*, (emphasis added)

Guilt feelings toward the lost object, as well as ambivalence, may disturb the normal course of mourning. In such cases, the reaction to death is greatly intensified, assuming a brooding, neurotically compulsive, even melancholic character. Indeed, the reaction may be so extreme as to culminate in suicide. Every unresolved grief is given expression in some form or another.

3.4.4 "Typical Findings in Pathological Grief," Varnik Volkan, *Psychiatric Quarterly* 44: 231-250 (1970). Comments by the author:

People who suffer from pathological grief reactions are either caught in this struggle of loss and restitution without coming to a solution or have achieved restitution which is symptomatic.

Funeral rites and religious rituals are attempts to deal with common psychological components of grief-aggression for one. Therefore the mourner should be allowed to fully indulge in mourning rituals.

(Delayed Grief) Often the patients' first reaction to the death of the lost one is not enough to be prophylactic, and the grief must be delayed until a future time. These patients are symptomatic prior to the appearance of these symptoms on a clinical level, but the symptoms are hidden. The turning point in acknowledging the symptoms is often an *anniversary* of the death. Sometimes the factor which produces acute symptoms in relation to the important loss, is *another real or fantasized loss*.

The patient suffering from pathological grief reactions has a history of repeating dreams in which the dead person is alive, and *usually appears undisguised*.

The persistent seeking of reunion with the lost object appears to be the main motivation present in pathological mourning although it appears in forms which, because of repression and splitting, have become disguised and distorted.

3.4.5 "Traumatic Grief as a Risk Factor for Mental and Physical Morbidity," G Prigerson et al, *Am J Psychiatry* 154(5): 616-623, May, 1997

Symptoms of traumatic grief are predictors of future physical and mental health problems.

3.4.6 "Symptomatology and Management of Acute Grief, Erich," Lindemann, *American Journal of*

Psychiatry, 101:141-148(1944)

Discusses normal grief, morbid grief reactions, anticipatory grief reactions. (Ed Note: This is considered to be an important foundational article.)

3.4.7   "Loss and Restitution," G. Rochlin, *Psychoanalytic Study of the Child* 8:288. (1953).

Humans cannot be without an object, and when loss occurs the object must be restored, although they may be forced to modify it.

3.4.8   "Mourning and the Prevention of Melancholia," Beverley Raphael, *British Journal Medical Psychology* 51: 303-310 (1978).

Freud considered the disturbance of self-regard which occurred in melancholia to be absent in mourning; in melancholia the relation to the object is no simple one; it is complicated by the conflict due to ambivalence...hate and love contend with each other. Preventive support at the time of the crisis may be helpful in lessening pathological effects. In some bereavements ambivalence may predispose the mourning to melancholia. Crisis support which facilitates the working through of this ambivalence may prevent or lessen the melancholia.

3.4.9   "Delinquency as a Manifestation of the Mourning Process," M. Shoor and M. Speed, *Psychiatric Quarterly,* 37: 540-558. (1963).

Delinquent behavior in a previously conforming adolescent may be a manifestation of a mourning process-a substitute pathologic grief reaction. Recognition of this etiologic factor may be crucial to proper management in such cases. Sexual promiscuity and mourning complicated by guilt are included as examples.

3.4.10   "Normal Adolescent Mourning," Max Sugar, *American Journal of Psychotherapy* 32: 258- 269 (1968)

Cites examples of normal and abnormal behavior of adolescents. The author states, "One of the tasks of adolescence is to learn the control of impulses."

3.4.11   "Treatment of the Adolescent with Borderline Syndrome," James Masterson, *Bulletin of the Menninger Clinic* 35: 5-18 (1971)

The adolescent with a Borderline Syndrome is defending himself against an abandonment depression...he or she wants reunion, not consolation for the loss. Their first unspoken question (to the therapist) will be: "How do I know you are any different? Prove to me that you have the capacity to understand me. Nobody else ever has. Prove to me you will not abandon me.") (Ed. Note: Families with this dynamic appear to be at risk for adolescent pregnancy and pressure for abortion by the mother of the adolescent.

"The mother of a patient with Borderline Syndrome often suffers form a Borderline Syndrome herself. The mother's pathologic needs impel her not to support and encourage the patient's separation and individuation, but rather cling to the child to prevent separation, discouraging moves toward individuation by withdrawing her support... Parents never having been mothered cannot mother, and never having been fathered cannot father. They perceive their children as parents, objects or peers.... They cling to the children to defend themselves against their own feelings of abandonment and cannot respond to the child's unfolding individuality. The child is subjected to scapegoating of the most extreme sort. Fathers, passive, inadequate men, dominated by and dependent upon their wives, play little parental role. The mothers are controlling women who need and vigorously battle to maintain the symbiotic tie with the child. These families communicate mostly by acts not words. Consequently, the adolescent expresses their need for help by an act-a plea for help- expresses as exactly and poignantly as any words, the blind, helpless, trapped crying out for succor and aid."

3.4.12   "On the Process of Mourning," Jeanne Lampl-De Groot, *Psychanalytic Study of the Child,* 38:9-13(1983)

Latency children, adolescents, and adults know intellectually that a dead person never returns; emotionally they all more or less deny this fact. In pathological cases, the denial cannot be corrected. Various inner and outer factors determine whether a mourning process will lead to a "normal" or to a "disturbed" mental life: a person's ability to master his unconscious guilt feelings and his need for punishment due to repressed infantile death wishes toward the deceased parent or sibling; the overcoming of his unconscious triumph over the deceased: "You are dead, I am alive"- the survivor guilt; the capability to sublimated destructive impulses into constructive activities.

3.4.13   "The "Replacement Child": A Saga of Unresolved Parental Grief," Elva Orlow Poznanski, *The Journal of Pediatrics,* 81(6): 1190-1193, Dee, 1972.

Replacing a child with another allows the parents partially to deny the first child's death. The replacement child then acts as a barrier to the parental acknowledgment of death, since a real child exists who is a substitute. Thus the first stages of bereavement are prematurely arrested and the process of mourning continues indefinitely with the replacement child acting as the continuing vehicle of parental grief.

3.4.14   "The Management of Stillbirth - Coping With an Unreality," Emanuel Lewis, *The Lancet,* September 18, 1976, pp. 619-620.

Mourning stillbirth is difficult because although there is a sense of loss, there is little sense of having lost somebody. The difficulty of grieving someone "missing believed killed" is well known; a death without a body seen by anyone seems unreal. There is an added sense of unreality with stillbirth as there are no experiences with the baby to remember. Looking at and holding the dead baby, giving the baby a name, arranging the certification, attending the funeral, and seeing the baby's grave help make stillbirth a reality to the family. With these activities, memories are created which aid the recovery processes of mourning.

3.4.15   "On Replacing a Child," A. Cain and B. Cain, *Journal of the American Academy of Child Psychiatry,* 3: 443-456 (1964).

Discusses the cases of disturbed children who were conceived shortly after the death of another child. Mothers had suffered a surprising number of family losses in their own childhood. The parents had an intense narcissistic investment in the child who had died. The authors state: "We hope our conservative application of these findings will serve as a counterbalance to the stunning casualness found in some pediatric quarters in recommending the 'replacement' of dead children to grieving parents."

3.4.16   "The Effects of Sibling Death on the Surviving Child: A Family Perspective," R. Krell and L. Rabkin, *Family Process,* 18: 471-477 (1979)

Surviving siblings frequently become the focus of maneuvers unconsciously designed to alleviate guilt and control fate through silence and efforts to maintain silence, through substitution for the lost child and through endowing the survivor-child with qualities of the deceased. In a young family of childbearing age, a decision may be taken to produce a replacement-in the face of an earlier painful resolve to remain barren, whether out of fear or in payment of some guilt-ridden debt to the lost child. The new offspring is intended to fill the family void. The newcomer is perceived as a replacement, dealt with as a reincarnation, and hemmed in by diffuse conscious and unconscious expectations.

3.4.17   "The Inhibition of Mourning by Pregnancy," E. Lewis, *Bulletin British Psychoanal. Soc.* 10:24-26 (1977)

3.5   Grief and Loss Following Abortion

Many people will experience grief and loss both before and after abortion. Others may not experience grief or loss. These articles demonstrate some of the situations where grief and loss are manifested.

3.5.1   "Induced Abortion," Betty Glenn Harris in *Parental Loss of a Child,* Ed Therese A Rando (Champaign, IL: Research Press Co., 1986)

3.5.2   "I Killed My Baby- The Emotional Aftermath of Abortion" in *Helping People Through Grief,When a Friend Needs You,* Delores Kuenning (Minneapolis: Bethany House Publishers, 1987)

3.5.3   "The Hidden Grief of Abortion," Julia Upton, *Pastoral Psychology* 31(1): 19-25, 1982

3.5.4   "Grief and Elective Abortion: Implications for the Counselor," Larry G Peppers in *Disenfranchised Grief. Recognizing Hidden Sorrow,* Ed. Kenneth J Doka (1989)135-146 see also "Grief and Elective Abortion:Breaking the Emotional Bond", Larry G Peppers, *Omega* 18(1): 1-12 ,1987-88

Anticipatory grief prior to the abortion was found. High pre-abortion grief scores were found among women having a D&E abortion, those indicating frequent church attendance, indicated infrequent sexual activity, had discussed their decision with a minister, had a family member who opposed the abortion, the relationship with their partner had ended, sought abortion for financial reasons, had several weeks to consider the abortion, black women, and those with less than a high school education.

High grief reactions 6 weeks post-abortion included Catholic women, those with less than a high school education, women with a prior live birth, women with multiple abortions, women with previous miscarriages, those seeking abortion because of financial reasons or age, and those with no one to talk to prior to the abortion. The author concluded that grief associated with elective abortion is symptomatically similar to that following involuntary infant/fetal loss. (Ed Note: An important finding in the Peppers study was that substantially different groups of women had high pre-abortion grief scores as compared to the groups with high post-abortion grief scores. This demonstrates the wide range and diversity of grief responses.)

3.5.5   "Induced Elective Abortion and Perinatal Grief," Gail B Williams, *Dissertation Abstracts Int'l* 53(3): 1296-B, 1992.

A wide range of long term grief responses on the Grief Experience Inventory was found among women with only one induced abortion and no other self-reported prenatal losses within five years, or previous psychiatric history. The author concluded that some women will have grief responses for many years following their abortion.

3.5.6   "Psychological Aspects of Abortion," Edna Ortof in *Psychological Aspects of Pregnancy, Birthing and Bonding* ed. Barbara L. Blum, (New York: Human Science Press, 1980).

Describes post-abortion dreams in several women. For example, one woman dreamt two months after her abortion, "I was passing shops with an urgency to get somewhere. I walked down steps into a grocery. I came to a shelf of small jars of baby food. I put loads in the basket. Someone said. You can't have those. I left them and had a feeling of panic and ran out of the store." The therapist stated in response: "women who abort after having children seem to suffer greater discomfort than women who have not borne children. The sense of loss, when present, frequently is related to whatever hopes and fantasies the pregnancy represents, i.e., the loss of possibility of a child, the loss of a lover, the loss of hope of a marriage and motherhood, the loss of fantasy of one's importance to a lover."

3.5.7   "Ritual Mourning for Unresolved Grief After Abortion," K McAll and W Wilson, *Southern Medical Journal* 80(7): 817-821, July, 1987

Case studies taken from over 400 spontaneous or induced abortion experiences described a woman of strong religious belief who developed anorexia nervosa as a reaction to accompanying her friend who obtained an abortion; depression in a woman following abortion; repressed grief at a mother's miscarriage; sexual promiscuity in a 26 year old woman traceable to her mother's abortion; adverse reaction of children to abortion. Spiritual intervention was successfully utilized to resolve the grief.

3.5.8   "Psychological Adjustment to First Trimester Abortion," Janice Muhr, *Dissertation Abstracts Int'l, Psychology, Clinical* 4054-B ,1979

Pre and post abortion interviews found that among women who experienced abortion as a loss, mourning processes were blocked because of the volitional and moral nature of the decision. An affective cycle of guilt and loss was identified which did not resolve itself over time.

3.5.9   "Emotional Responses of Women Following Therapeutic Abortion," Nancy Adler, *American Journal Orthopsychiatry* 45(3): 446-454, April, 1975

Post-abortion women may feel a sense of loss precipitated by either internally based emotions or socially based emotions.

Guilt

3.6   Guilt —General Background Studies

Guilt is much understood in contemporary society. Some believe that guilt is only relative to the culture, while others believe that results from violation of some basic value intrinsic in human nature.

3.6.1   "The Psychophysiology of Confession: Linking Inhibitory and Psychosomatic Processes," J.W. Pennebaker et al, *J. Personality and Social Psychology* 52(4): 781, 1987.

Failure to confide traumatic events was found to be stressful and associated with long-term health problems.

3.6.2   "Sin, The Lesser of Two Evils," O. Hobart Mowrer, *American Psychologist,* May, 1960, pp. 301-304.

Comments by the author:

For several decades we psychologists looked upon the whole matter of sin and moral accountability as a great incubus and acclaimed our liberation from it as epochmaking.... In reconsidering the possibility that sin must, after all, be taken seriously, many psychologists seem perplexed as to what attitude one should take toward the sinner. Non-judgmental, nondirective, warm accepting, ethically neutral are words generally used.... We have reasoned the way to get the neurotic to accept and love himself is for us to love and accept him, an inference which flows equally from the Freudian assumption that the patient is not really guilty or sinful but only fancies himself so and from the view of Rogers that we are all inherently good and are corrupted by our experiences with the external, everyday world.

But what is here generally overlooked, it seems, is that recovery (constructive change, redemption) is most assuredly attained, not by helping a person reject and rise above his sins, but by helping him *accept them.* This is the paradox which we have not at all understood and which is the very crux of the problem. Just so long as a person lives under the shadow of real, unacknowledged, and unexcited guilt, he *cannot* (if he has any character at all) "accept himself"; and all our efforts to reassure him and accept him will avail nothing. He will continue to hate

36

himself and to suffer the inevitable consequences of self-hatred. But the moment he (with or without "assistance") begins to accept his guilt and his sinfulness, the possibility of radical reformation opens up; and with this, the individual may, legitimately, though not without pain and effort, pass from deep, pervasive self-rejection and self-torture to a new freedom of self-respect and peace.

3.6.3   "The Myth of Mental illness," Thomas Szasz, *American Psychologist* 15:113-118 (1960).

"The notion of mental illness has outlived whatever usefulness it might have had and..-now functions merely as a convenient myth...mental illness is a myth whose function is to disguise and thus render more palatable the bitter pill of moral conflicts in human relations."

3.6.4   "The Theology of Therapy: The Breach of the First Amendment through the Medicalization of Morals," Thomas Szasz, N.Y.U. *Review of Law and Social Change* (1975); also. "The Control of Conduct: The Ethics of Helping People," Szasz, Crim. *Law Bulletin II,* pp. 617-622, September-October 1975.

"In the Therapeutic State many medical acts are considered scientific when, in fact, they are moral, and many psychiatric acts are considered medical, when, in fact, they are religious."

Szasz observes a close parallel between church and state relations 200 years ago and between medicine and state relations today. He notes that "in each case (church or medicine) we are faced with a social institution to which men and women turn to for protection when they feel most endangered. Hence, they want their protector to be as powerful as possible. [But] protection from injuries and diseases requires knowledge and skills, not power; protection from guilt and shame requires honesty and courage, not power; power is necessary to oppose the external enemies of freedom but not the internal enemies of freedom."

3.6.5   "Guilt and Guilt Feelings," Martin Buber, *Proceedings of the International Conference on Medical Psychotherapy, Vol. Ill, International Conference of Mental Health, London, 1948.* (New York: Columbia University Press, 1948).

Comments by the author:

As a result of the teachings of Freud, who presented the naturalism of the enlightenment with a scientific system.. .guilt was simply not allowed to acquire an ontic character; it had to be derived from the transgression against ancient and modern taboos, against parental and social tribunals. The feeling of guilt was now to be understood as essentially only the consequence of dread of punishment and censure by this tribunal. (p. 115)

Guilt does not exist because a taboo exists to which one fails to give obedience, but rather that taboo and the placing of taboo have been made possible only through the fact that the leaders of early communities knew and made use of a primal fact of man as man-the fact that man can become guilty and know it. (pp-116-117)

The psychotherapist is no pastor of souls and no substitute for one. It is never his task to mediate a salvation; his task is only to further a healing, (p. 119)

The therapist in order to do this must recognize one thing steadfastly and recognize it ever again: There exists real guilt, fundamentally different from all the anxiety induced bugbears that are generated in the cavern of the unconscious. Personal guilt, whose reality some schools of psychoanalysis contest and others ignore, does not permit itself to be reduced to the trespass against a powerful taboo, (pp. 119-120)

Each man stands in an objective relationship to others; the totality of this relationship constitutes his life as one that factually participates in the being of the world. It is this relationship, in fact, that first makes it at all possible for him to expand his environment into a world. It is his share in the human order of being, the share for which he bears responsibility.

Injuring a relationship means that at this place the human order of being is injured. No one other than he who inflicted the wound can heal it. *He who knows the fact of this guilt and is a helper can help him try to heal the wound* (p. 120).

The doctor is not concerned with whether or not the demand of the society is right or not. This does not concern the doctor as doctor; he is incompetent here.. .nor can faith be his affair. Here the action commences within the relation between the guilty man and his God and remains therein. The therapist may lead up to conscience but no farther. Conscience means to us the capacity and tendency of man radically to distinguish between those of his past and future actions which should be approved and those which should be disapproved. Conscience only rarely fully coincides with a standard received from the society or community. Self-illumination, perseverance and reconciliation is required. (pp. 120-121)

3.6.6 *Toward a Psychology of Being,* Abraham Maslow (Princeton: F. Van Nostrand Co., 1962)

"Intrinsic conscience" is the necessity of being true to one's inner self, and not denying it our of weakness or for special advantage.

3.6.7 *Conscience and Guilt,* Tames A. Knight, (New York: Appleton-Century-Crofts, 1969).

The bond between the principle and the act is conscience. There is something wrong with psychology's emphasis on "adjustment", rather than "goodness." Real guilt follows in the wake of wrongdoing, seen and accepted as such by the doer, who seeks expiation and makes restitution.

3.7 Abortion-Related Guilt/Regret/Violation of Conscience or Belief

By adopting a pragmatic approach to abortion-decision making, higher ethical, moral or religious standards are frequently violated as the following studies demonstrate.

3.7.1 "Many in Survey Who Had Abortion Cite Guilt Feelings," George Skelton, *Los Angeles Times,* March 19, 1989 p.28

In a national U.S. telephone survey by the Los Angeles Times in March, 1989, 56% of women who admitted to at least one abortion expressed a sense of guilt and 26% said they now mostly regretted their abortion.

3.7.2   "Abortion Counselling. A New Component of Medical Care," Uta Landy, *Clinics in Obstetrics and Gynecology* 13(1):33, 1986

An article by the former executive director of the National Abortion Federation based on observations of its members stated that women obtaining abortions will make the decision by a "spontaneous" response without much thought, engage in denial or procrastination, be overly rational, or allow others to make the decision for them thus making it more likely that the women will have later regrets.

3.7.3   "Testing a Model of the Psychological Consequences of Abortion," WB Miller et al in *The New Civil War. The Psychology, Culture, and Politics of Abortion,* Ed. LJ Beckman and SM Harvey, (Washington, D.C.:American Psychological Association, 1998) 235

Women about to undergo abortion with Mifepristone exhibited acute stress and appeared to be trying to control their response to the unwanted pregnancy/abortion situation by not thinking about it The researchers concluded that there is a broad, multidimensional affective response.At two weeks postabortion 29.7% of the women expressed some guilt. At 6-8 months 35.9% of postabortion women expressed some guilt. The authors concluded that long term studies should be undertaken to ascertain the psychological effects of abortion.

3.7.4   "Physical and Psychological Injury in Women Following Abortion:Akron Pregnancy Services Study," L Gsellman, *Association for Interdisciplinary Research in Values and Social Change Newsletter* 5(4):1-8, 1993

In a questionnaire survey of postabortion women receiving a variety of services at a pregnancy services center, 66% expressed guilt and 54% expressed remorse or regret approximately 6 years postabortion.

3.7.5   "Induced Abortion as a Violation of Conscience of the Woman," Thomas Strahan, *Life and Learning VI.. Proceedings of the Sixth University Faculty for Life Conference. (*June, 1996, ed. Joseph W. Koterski

A majority of U.S. women appear to violate their conscience by obtaining an induced abortion. Among the reasons are a belief that if it is legal it must be all right; encouragement of her male partner or others, including abortion facility workers to obtain an abortion, lack of respect for the moral or religious beliefs of the woman, and a frequent crisis situation where the woman may be easily influenced by others or use primitive coping methods.

3.7.6   "Objective Versus Subjective Responses to Abortion," James M Robbins, *Journal of Counsulting and Clinical Psychology* 47(5): 994-995, 1979

In a study of medically indigent unmarried black women who had abortions, deep regret was reported by 14.6%, some regret by 34.1%, a little regret by 19.5%, and no regret by 31.7% one year postabortion.

3.7.7   "Obsessive-Compulsive Neurosis After Viewing the Fetus During Therapeutic Abortion," S

Lipper and W Feigenbaum, *Am J Psychotherapy* 30:666-674, 1976

Following her abortion, a woman was preoccupied with thoughts of being " dirty" and washed her hands 30-40 times a day.

3.7.8 "Unsafe Abortions: Methods Used and Characteristics of Patients Attending Hospitals in Nairobi, Lima, and Manila," A Ankomah et al, *Health Care for Women* Int'l 18:43, 1997

The beliefs of women regarding when abortion is justified conflicted with their actions in a study of postabortion women in Kenya, Peru and the Philippines. The authors concluded, " it can be seen that abortion is not an acceptable option even for those who resort to it , and that it is employed as the final option."

3.8 Ambivalence or Inner Conflict

Ambivalence is common both pre and postabortion. It appears to be acceptable at one level of consciousness, but unacceptable at a different level.

3.8.1 "The Ambivalence of Abortion," Linda Bird Francke (1978).

Interviews with various people involved in abortion. Demonstrates ambivalence as well as many other emotions and considerable confused thought. For an extensive discussion of this book see *Rachael Weeping*, James T. Burtchaell (1982,1984)

3.8.2 "Abortion: Subjective Attitudes and Feelings," Ellen Freeman, *Family Planning Perspectives* 10:150-155, 1978.

This article concludes that feelings of ambivalence, both before and after the abortion, are common..

3.8.3 "The Psychological Reaction of Patients to Legalized Abortion," J Osofsky and H Osofsky, *American Journal Orthopsychiatry* 42(1): 48-60, January, 1972.

A leading early study on the effects of abortion, often cited. Psychological evaluation of 250 postaborted women reported 24% experiencing guilt (much or moderate); 47% reported the decision was either considerably difficult (28%) or mildly difficult (19.5%). Some 32.5% expressed the desire for the child as the reason for difficulty. 45%-48% expressed happiness or much relief following abortion.

3.8.4 "Pregnancy Decision Making as A Significant Life Event: A Commitment Approach," J Lydon et al, *Journal of Personality and Social Psychology* 71(1): 141-151, 1996.

Initial commitment to the pregnancy predicted subsequent depression, guilt and hostility among those who had abortions. Women who previously had at least one prior abortion reported more commitment to the pregnancy than women with no prior abortion history.

3.8.5   Fragmentation of the Personality Associated with Post-Abortion Trauma , Joel O Brende, *Association for Interdisciplinary Research in Values and Social Change Newsletter* 8(3): 1-8. July/Aug 1995.

People enduring extreme stress often suffer profound rupture in the very fabric of the self. Factors which are likely to produce dissociation, memory lapses, and evidence of self-fragmentation, include (1) the severity of the violation, (2) lack of support from others, (3) subsequent self-blame and shame, (4) loss of idealism and purpose. Fragmentation predisposes to unstable and destructive relationships.

3.8.6   "Post-Abortion Syndrome as a Variant of Post Traumatic Stress Syndrome," Robert C Erikson, *Association for Interdisciplinary Research in Values and Social Change Newsletter* 3(4):5-6, Winter, 1991.

Conflict between incompatible goals of attachment and destruction leads to the experience of stress.

3.9   Anxiety

These studies demonstrate that different types of anxiety manifest themselves in postabortion women.

3.9.1   *The Long Term Psychological Effects of Abortion,* Catherine A Barnard. (Portsmouth, NH: Institute for Pregnancy Loss, 1990).

47.5% of women exhibited an elevated level of anxiety on the Millon Clinical-Multi-Axial Inventory 3-5 years postabortion.

3.9.2   "Emotional Distress Patterns Among Women Having First or Repeat Abortions," EW Freeman, *Obstetrics and Gynecology* 55(5):630, 1980.

Phobic anxiety was identified as a postabortion reaction and was higher among women repeating abortion compared to women with one abortion.

3.9.3   "Incidence of complicated grief and post-traumatic stress in a post-abortion population," LM Butterfield, *Dissertation Abstracts Int'l* 49(8): 3431-B, 1988.

Postabortion women consistently showed death anxiety on the Grief Experience Inventory.

3.9.4   "Psychological Responses Following Medical Abortion (using Mifepristone and Gemepost) and Surgical Vacuum Aspiration," R Henshaw et al, *Acta Obstet Gynecol Scand* 73:812, 1994.

A Scottish study found that postabortion anxiety correlated with cigarette smoking with the most anxious women having the heaviest smoking habits.

3.10 Intrusion/Avoidance/Dreams/Nightmares

This section demonstrates that it is easier to physically remove the aborted child from the body of the mother than remove the image from the mind of the mother.

3.10.1   *Introduction to Psychodynamics: A New Synthesis,* MJ Horowitz (New York: Basic Books, 1988) 48

Four stages of grief are identified (1) outcry, (2) denial, (3) intrusion, and (4) working through. When the intrusion phase is prolonged, the bereaved person may be troubled by recurring thoughts or images including nightmares and flashback experiences which may interfere with sleep and daytimes activities for months and years beyond the time expected for normal grieving.

3.10.2   "Postabortion Syndrome: An Emerging Public Health Concern," AC Speckhard and VM Rue, *Journal of Social Issues* 48(3):95, 1992.

Intrusive nightmares of postabortion women fall into three general categories: horrors about how the fetal child dies, fearful symbols of judgment and penalty, and searching for something precious that cannot be found.

3.10.3   The Negative Impact of Abortion on Women and Families, E Joanne Angelo in *Post-Abortion Aftermath,* ed. Michael T Mannion (Kansas City, MO: Sheed&Ward, 1994) 50.

Clinical psychiatrist E Joanne Angelo has observed: " the woman has often formed a mental image of her child which haunts her day and night- an image of an infant being torn to pieces, sucked down a tube, crying out in pain, or reaching out to her for help. She may have named her baby and have regularly occurring conversations with him or her in mind begging forgiveness for what she has done."

3.10.4   *Experiencing Abortion,* Eve Kushner (New York: Harrington Park Press, 1997) 166.

One 22 year old woman, the night after her abortion said, " I felt my baby's spirit come to visit me." She adds that the spirit "found its body gone. Then it disappeared. I was positive that's what happened and I cried like I never had before, sobbing and sobbing. The world seemed so empty, with nothing left to live for."

3.10.5   *Abortion. Loss and Renewal in the Search for Identity,* Eva Pattis Zoja (English Trans. Henry Martin (New York: Routladge, 1997) 91-94

This book describes a woman's dream 5 days before her abortion: " We've only got five more days. Then you will have to go. It's going to be horrible and I'm the one who has made that decision. For now, we're still together, we've still got a little time, I'll be with you, up until the end." The night before the abortion, this same woman had this dream: " It was the morning of the abortion. I knew I had to go to the hospital. My partner and two little boys had given me gifts; it seemed like my birthday. My younger sister was also there; there was a family atmosphere. Everybody was ready to accompany me. It made it easy to enter the hospital."

Seven months later, at precisely the time when the baby was due, this same woman had the following dream: " I was in the bathroom at the home of my parents. I was sitting on the toilet, and I thought that I was having my period. I realized that a tiny baby had fallen out into the water, where it was moving about like a sea horse. I saw that it was alive, but the front of its head seemed squashed, as though it had no brain. It was a spontaneous miscarriage. I felt very sorry for it. I knew that the child couldn't survive; it would die as soon as I lifted it out of the water. I took it out of the water and held it in my hand. I didn't want it to die alone. There were people around me, and I found that very disturbing. I looked for a place in which to be alone, and found the room I had had as a little girl. Then Maria entered, an aunt of whom I was very fond. Finally alone and quiet, I saw that the child had died in the palm of my hand. I knew that I was supposed to burn the body. Now it looked like a sheet of paper, and I set fire to one of its corners. It burned and burned, but didn't turn to ashes; it took on a series of very bright colors, like the colors of a figure in enamel. It had turned into a Christ child, and was alive and smiling."

3.10.6   *The Long Term Psychological Effects of Abortion,* Catherine A Barnard, (Portsmouth NH: Institute for Pregnancy Loss, 1990.)

In a study of women 3-5 years postabortion, 23% had recurrent and distressing dreams of the event, 45% had a sense of reliving the experience, 29% had recurrent and intrusive recollections of the event, 45% had hypervigilance, 35% made efforts to avoid feelings associated with the event, and 11% made efforts to avoid activities associated with the event.

3.10.7   "Abortion in Adolescence," NB Campbell et al, *Adolescence Vol XXIII* No.92: 813, 1988

Women in a postabortion support group who had abortions as teenagers were more likely to have nightmares after abortion (80%) compared to women who had abortions as adults (43%)

3.10.8   "Therapeutic Abortion During Adolescence: Psychiatric Observations," P Barglow and S Weinstein, *Journal of Youth and Adolescence* 2(4): 331, 1973

This article describes numerous dreams and nightmares of adolescents, both pre and postabortion. The authors stated," almost all adolescent subjects experienced the abortion procedure as frightening, dangerous, and punitive, and often as temporarily overwhelming." Dreams represented the fetus as a baby, child, or animal such as a worm, frog, parakeet, cat or even a dinosaur. The abortion procedure, hospital, or doctor appeared without disguise in 95% of the dreams." Examples of the content of these dreams include a 16 year old girl with a Black Muslim mother. The girl wept and screamed in terror during the abortion procedure. Her preabortion dream: " I dreamed the devil performed the abortion. He just reached up his black hand, pulled it out, and then danced around me with it in his hands while laughing and yelling";Another who had a conflict with her mother dreamt following her abortion " My mother and four men chased me into a white garage. The men held me and my mother made a cut in my vagina while I screamed"; A 16 year old who underwent a second abortion who was evaluated for severe depression and suicidal preoccupation after her abortion had the following dream before her abortion. "I had a nightmare that there was an atomic war and that I alone was left in the world."

3.10.9 "Prolonged Grieving After Abortion: A Descriptive Study," D Brown et al, *The Journal of Clinical Ethics* 4(2):118, 1993

Postabortion women frequently fantasized about the aborted fetus and had other intrusive thoughts when reminded of pregnancy or childbirth.

3.10.10 "A consideration of ketamine dreams," P Hejja, S Galloon, *Can Anaesth Soc J* 22(1): 100-105, Jan, 1975

This study used ketamine anesthesia to attempt to reduce the incidence of unpleasant dreams at the time of abortion.

3.10.11 "Induced Elective Abortion and Perinatal Grief," GB Williams, *Dissertation Abstracts Int'l* 53(3): 1296-B, 1992.

Inability to control overt emotional responses had the highest scores in a Grief Experience Inventory 11 years postabortion.

3.11 Denial

3.11.1 *The People of the Lie,* M. Scott Peck, (New York: Simon and Schuster, 1983).

Ed Note: This is a popular book that deals extensively with the problem of deception.

3.11.2 "Doctor-Patient Relationships in Fetal/Infant Death Encounters," Larry G. Peppers and Ronald J. Knapp, *Journal of Medical Education* 54:776-780, October 1979

Many physicians thought less about death than control group subjects, patients and other nonprofessionals but they were more afraid of death.

3.11.3 "Psychological Treatment for Anxiety Disorders: A Review," MG Gelder, *Journal of the Royal Society of Medicine* 79:230-233, April 1986

There is now wide agreement that the best psychological treatment for cases of phobic avoidance is exposure to situations that have been avoided, presumably because avoidance interferes with the natural processes by which anxiety reactions are terminated.; citing Mathews, Gelder, Johnston, *Agora-Phobia: Nature and Treatment.* London: Tavistock Publications (1981).

3.11.4 *Aborted Women: Silent No More,* David C. Reardon, (Chicago: Loyola Press, 1987).

In a survey of 252 women who had abortions and later became members of Women Exploited by Abortion, over 70 percent reported there was a time when they would have denied the existence of any reactions after their abortions. For some this denial stage lasted only a few months, for others it lasted over ten or fifteen years.

3.11.5 "Abortion and the Techniques of Neutralization," W. C. Brennan, *Journal of Health and Social*

44

Behavior 15:358 (1974).

The author examines various techniques of rationalization whereby aborters alleviate guilt, depression and anxiety, including denial of personal responsibility for the pregnancy; denial that the unborn is a victim by referring to it as a piece of tissue or characterizing it as an aggressor; portrayal of and-abortion activists as hypocritical, chauvinistic or morally arrogant; appealing to feminist or Protestant church groups for justification.

3.11.6   *The Anatomy of Bereavement,* B. Raphael, (New York: Basic Books, 1983), p. 238.

A woman may have required a high level of defensive denial of her tender feelings for the baby to allow her to make the decision for termination. This denial often carries her throughout the procedure and the hours immediately afterward, so that she seems cheerful, accepting, but unwilling to talk at that time when supportive counseling may be offered by the clinic.

3.11.7   "Testing a Model of the Psychological Consequences of Abortion," Warren B Miller, David J Pasta, Catherine L Dean in *The New Civil War. The Psychology, Culture and Politics of Abortion,* Ed. Linda J Beckman, S Marie Harvey, (Washington, D.C.:American Psychological Association, 1998) 235-267

Women who participated in a clinical trial of Mifepristone abortion exhibited acute pre-abortion stress which was dominated by high avoidance, intrusion, and anxiety. The authors concluded that, "what appears to be happening is that the women are trying to control their response to the unwanted pregnancy/abortion situation by avoiding thinking about it.")

3.11.8   "Current Status and Trends in the Development of Post Abortion Healing," Sr. Paula Vandegaer, *Healing Visions Conference, Part II, Center for Continuing Education, University of Notre Dame,* July 1987.

Denial can be overcome by confronting the individual factually and helping the woman talk about her abortion. Defense mechanisms such as rationalization, suppression, repression, compensation and reaction formation are some of the defense mechanisms used.

3.11.9   "Coping with Abortion," Larry Cohen and Susan Roth, *Journal of Human Stress,* 10:140- 145, Fall, 1984,

This study found a wide range of responses to the abortion procedure. A generalized stress response syndrome was reported. Groups designated as "avoiders" expressed more distress than "non-avoiders"; approachers decreased in stress over time while non-approachers did not.

3.11.10 "Family Relationships and Depressive Symptoms Preceding Induced Abortion," D Bluestein and CM Rutledge, *Family Practice Research Journal* 13(2): 149, 1993

Depression scores of women immediately before undergoing an abortion increased as denial increased.

3.11.11 "Understanding Adolescent Pregnancy and Abortion," Sherry Hatcher, *Primary Care* 3(3): 407-

425, September 1976,

The early adolescent tends to deny any responsibility for her pregnancy; she has used no contraceptive measures and employs defensive denial as much as possible throughout her pregnancy experience.

3.11.12 "Psychophysiologic Aspects of Denial in Pregnancy: Case Report," K. Milstein and P. Milstein, *J. Clin. Psychiatry* 44(5): 189-190, May, 1983.

Denial is defined as "a defense mechanism, operating unconsciously, used to resolve emotional conflict and allay anxiety by disavowing thoughts, feelings, wishes, needs or external reality factors that are consciously intolerable." Despite intense denial, the patient was functioning adequately in all observable areas of her life. (Ed Note: This case illustrates that denial may be related to a violation of moral or religious standards.)

3.11.13 "Denial of Pregnancy and Childbirth," P. Finnegan, E. McKinstry and G.E. Robinson Canadian *Journal of Psychiatry,* 27: 672, 74, December 1982.

Anxiety associated with psychological conflicts may threaten to overwhelm the pregnant woman's ability to cope in an adaptive fashion and may result in the denial of the pregnancy as a defense. Denial and rationalization of symptoms and denial of pregnancy may result in inadequate behavioral responses at the time of childbirth and may result in the death of the newborn.

3.11.14 "Uninformed Consent and Terms without Definitions," Joseph E. Hardison, *American Journal of Medicine,* 74:932-933, June, 1983.

During the time of denial, turmoil and intense personal loss and grief, it is understandable that many patients may give uninformed consent. Forcing the patient to face reality may precipitate panic, psychosis or suicide. We must give patients time and help them adjust to what is wrong, before consent is meaningfully and truly formed.

3.11.15 "Religious Conversion. An Experimental Model for Affecting Alcohol Denial," Marc Galanter, *Currents in Alcoholism* 6:69-78(1979),

Ed Note: This raises an important aspect of denial in the abortion context, as many women who have come forward to tell their story of the trauma following abortion have undergone religious conversions.

3.11.16 "Denial of Pregnancy in Single Women," Burns, *Health and Social Work* 7(4): 314-319, November 1982,

Describes a small group of single women who conceal pregnancy, obtain no prenatal care and place the child for adoption.

3.11.17 "Denial: Are Sharper Definitions Needed?," Norman Cousins, *Journal of the American Medical Association* 248(2): 210-212, July 9,1982,

Use of the term "denial" may be inappropriate and misleading in cases where a physician makes a superficial determination. Denial can sometimes be channeled into a higher level of cooperation.

3.11.18 "Early Object Deprivation and Transference Phenomena: The Working Alliance." T Fleming, *Psychoanalytic Quarterly*, (1972) pp. 23-49.

Delayed grief and mourning due to denial created an inability to manage developmental tasks.

3.11.19 "Denial and Repression," Edith Jacobson, *Journal of American Psychoanalytic Association*, Vol. V: 6192 (1957),

In general, patients who deny show a propensity for acting out. Therapy must be directed essentially against denial and distortion of reality.

3.11.20 "The Longitudinal Course of Para-Natal Emotional Disturbance, N," Uddenberg, and L. Nilsson, *Acta Psychiatrica Scandinavica*, 52:160-169. (1975)

Ninety-five nulliparous women were interviewed during pregnancy and four months postpartum. The possibility of predicting mental disturbance postpartum was studied. When the woman was mentally disturbed during pregnancy, the prognosis was better in the case of a poor social situation, or lack of support from the father of the child should be regarded as favorable prognosis for her mental health postpartum. In contrast, repudiation of the mother as well as a negative attitude toward future child bearing seems to indicate a poor prognosis. When the woman appears well adapted during pregnancy it may be more difficult to predict mental adaptation postpartum. A tendency to keep the pregnancy experience out of the consciousness should be regarded as a warning. Denial of the pregnancy prevents the woman from gradually working through any difficulties connected with her new situation and impairs her possibilities for a gradual adaptation to motherhood. Such a gradual adaptation is probably important in preventing mental breakdown during the first period postpartum. Citing two studies.

3.11.21 "Early Object Loss and Denial," R. Stolorow and F. Lachmann, *Psychoanalytic Quarterly*, 44 (4): 596-611 (1975).

Description of the psychoanalytic treatment of a young woman whose father had been killed in a concentration camp when she was four years old. It illustrates the defensive use of denial in lieu of mourning. The ability of the surviving parent to counter the process of denial of loss, to serve as a model in the mourning process and as a necessary adjunct to the child for the eventual termination of mourning, plays a decisive role. Ed. Note: The literature contains few examples of the impact of loss of a father on a girl. Yet this seems to be of importance in the case of adolescent pregnancy. See, for example, Kane, "Motivation Factors in Pregnant Adolescents," *Diseases of the Nervous System* 35:131-134(1974).

3.11.22 "Abortion as Fatherhood Glimpsed. Clinic Waiting Room Males as (Former) Expectant Fathers," Arthur Shostak, Presented at Eastern Sociological Society Meeting, March, 1985, Philadelphia, PA.

Thoughts about fatherhood shaped an unusual grieving process as many males mourned the loss of paternity in a hidden and denied fashion. Most males put on a show of fortitude and relief consistent with a macho role. Authentic and overt grieving got short shrift as energy focused instead on demonstrating a capacity to "take it" and keep going.

3.11.23   "On the Reclaiming of Denied Affects in Family Therapy," David A. Berkowitz, *Family Process* 16(4); 495-501, December 1977.

A central developmental task of the family is to help its members develop the capacity to cope with the grief attendant on separation and loss. In order to work through such feelings, each member must be first able to acknowledge the affect as present, internal and belonging to the self. Depending upon the degree of intra-psychic differentiation, and the degree of abandonment, family members may seek to avoid awareness of such feelings within themselves. The disclaimed emotions remain powerful unconscious motivators of behavior, exerting their influence despite their denial. Hidden intense grief stays unresolved as long as it remains unrecognized. It is an important task for the therapist to facilitate the grieving process. Quoting Paul, "The Role of Mourning and Empathy in Conjoint Marital Therapy," in Zuk and Boszormenyi-Nagy, eds, *Family Therapy and Disturbed Families,* (Palo Alto: Science and Behavior Books, 1967).

3.11.24   "Development of a Quantitative Rating Scale to Assess Denial," T. P. Hackett and N.H. Cassem, *Journal of Psychosomatic Research* 18:93-100 (1974).

Denial is defined as "the conscious or unconscious repudiation of part or all of the total available meaning of an event to allay fear, anxiety or other unpleasant effects." Major deniers shared certain characteristics. They verbally denied fear, tended to minimize or displace symptoms to other organ systems, downplayed danger, displaced the threat to other objects (e.g., finances), projected their fear, displayed a jovial, hearty manner, regularly debunked worry and used cliches whenever asked about death.A rating scale of 31 items was developed).

3.11.25   "Denial and Affirmation in fullness and Health," Arnold R. Beisser, *American Journal of Psychiatry* 136(8): 1026-1030. August, 1978.

"Positive" attitudes about health may have a powerful effect on patients. For the most part, these attitudes have been based in religious faiths. Physicians and behavioral scientists have frequently taken the role of adversary to these faith and faith healing perspectives as they have observed how patients are sometimes influenced to ignore symptoms and fail to obtain medical care with disastrous consequences. There is a new recognition that there are states of consciousness and awareness which are inadequately explained by concepts of illness and its absence and that these states may produce higher levels of functioning and health (i.e., the holistic health movement). The patient and the physician find different meanings in the situation. The physician is concerned with the "reality" of the patient's illness; the patient is concerned with the "reality" of what makes life worth living. Behavioral scientists have come to regard denial as a primitive defense and to view its presence as a signal of serious underlying psychopathology. (Ed. note-This author at times seems to be talking about hope rather than denial, although he uses the word denial.)

3.11.26 "The Relationship Between an Avoidance of Existential Confrontation and Neuroticism: A Psychometric Test, P," Thauberger, and D. Sydiaha-Symor, *Journal Humanistic Psychology,* 17(1): 89-91, Winter 1977.

A positive correlation was found between avoidance of existential confrontations and neuroticism using previously developed scales. Sources of existential anxiety indude death, fate, guilt, emptiness, meaninglessness, loneliness and isolation. Existential anxiety cannot be avoided except through the distortion of reality. Such distortion breeds neurotic anxiety-the distress produced by yielding to the illusory hopes of overcoming contingency and finiteness. Alternately, confronting existential anxiety means to acknowledge its presence and incorporate it into one's being. Neuroticism may give rise to avoidance tactics which at least temporarily serve the well-being of the individual by sparing him or her from existential stresses which would be overwhelming and self-defeating. Quoting J. F. Bugenthal, *The Search for Authenticity* New York: Holt, Rinehart and Winston (1965).

3.12 Dissociation

3.12.1 "Mediation of Abusive Childhood Experiences: Dissociation and Negative Life Outcomes," E Becker-Lausen, *Am J Orthopsychiatry* 65(4): 560, 1995

Dissociation was significantly related to reports by females of previously becoming pregnant and having an abortion in high school. The author stated that individuals who detach from reality by dissociation may disregard clues that may otherwise warn them of danger and become "sitting ducks" for later abuse.

3.12.2 "Partial Dissociation as Encountered in the Borderline Patient," Paul Dince, *Journal of the American Academy of Psychoanalysis* 5(3): 327-345, 1977

Partial dissociation occurs as a consequence of the patient's need to bring about an altered state of consciousness in order to shut out or expel a danger-laden piece of psychic reality. Patients can engage in purposeful, deliberate and initially conscious triggering of dissociated ego states which gradually slip further and further from the individual's control until they take over and run their course. Dissociative capacities of the borderline patient, which are at times consciously (volitionally) set in motion and which at times constitute semi-automated responses to highly charged aggressive or sexual-aggressive effect, are fueled and maintained by the chronic, persistent reliance upon denial as the main mechanism of defense. The dissociated self, the not-me has to be triggered and take over in order to do that which would evoke fearful guilt and shame in the original hated self.

3.12.3 "Fragmentation of the Personality Associated with Post-Abortion Trauma," Joel O Brende, *Association for Interdisciplinary Research in Values and Social Change Newsletter* 8(3):1-8, July/August, 1995.

Splitting and dissociative mechanisms are used as one of the defenses to keeping unwanted traumatic memories, shame, and undesirable emotions out of awareness and hiding the internal pain by using ego defenses which may appear adaptable but are potentially unstable and destructive.

3.12.4 "Childhood trauma, dissociation and self-harming behaviour: a pilot study," G Low et al , *Br J Med Psychol* 73(Pt 2) 269-278, 2000.

A British study reported a strong association between high levels of dissociation and an increasing frequency of self-harming behaviour.

3.13 Narcissism

For many, abortion is looked upon as a "quick fix" to a problem pregnancy. This is the primary reason why those supporting abortion emphasize " relief" following abortion, even if there are other negative consequences.

3.13.1 *The Culture of Narcissism,* American Life in an Age of Diminishing Expectations, Christopher Lasch, (New York: W.W. Norton, 1979)

The contemporary climate is therapeutic, not religious. People today hunger not for personal salvation, let alone for the restoration of an earlier golden age, but for the feeling, the momentary illusion of personal well-being, health, and psychic security.

3.13.2 "Narcissistic Personality Disorder: Clinical Features," V. Siomopoulos, *Am. J. Psychotherapy,* Vol. XLII, No. 2:240-253, April, 1981)

Excellent over-view of the subject and review of the writings of H. Kohut and 0. Kernberg. Narcissistic individuals are dominated by *rage and shame.*

3.13.3 *Aborted Women: Silent No More,* David C. Reardon, (Chicago: Loyola Press, 1987) p. 23.

In a survey of 252 post-abortion women, "many of those surveyed reported that their abortion left them feeling extreme and chronic 'anger' or "rage' at others. Anger, resentment and even hatred was directed at husbands or boyfriends who had been involved in the abortion. "Postabortion anger is often directed against the abortionists or abortion counselors who "didn't give me the other side of the picture.")

3.13.4 "Outcome Following Therapeutic Abortion," R. Payne, A. Kravitz, M. Notman and J. Anderson, *Archives General Psychiatry* 33:725, June 1976.

In a study of 102 women up to six months following abortion, it was found that Catholics exhibited more guilt and shame than Protestants and Protestants more than Jews. Women who had previously borne children experienced significantly less guilt and shame than did a woman who never had a child. Women with a negative or ambivalent relationship with their children experienced greater depression and shame. Women who became pregnant using the rhythm method, foam or no contraceptive had more guilt and shame (p=.048) than did women using a diaphragm, IUD or contraceptive pills.

3.13.5   *The Long-Term Psychological Effects of Abortion,* C. Barnard, (Portsmouth, N.H.: Institute for Pregnancy Loss, 1990).

An elevated narcissistic response, in post-abortion women, nearly 3 times greater than the sample on which the test had been normed, was found on the Millon Clinical Multiaxial Inventory (MCMI) in a sample of 80 women 3-5 years post-abortion. (32.5 vs. 11.0, Chi-Square - 42.02, P= .01) (60% were found to have given the wrong phone number to the abortion clinic).

3.13.6   "Women who seek Therapeutic Abortion: A Comparison with Women who Complete Their Pregnancies," C. Ford, P. Castelnuovo - Tedesco, and K. Long, *Am. J. Psychiatry* 129(5): 546-552, Nov, 1972.

Women obtaining abortions tend to be narcissistic and regard the fetus as a competitor for the succorance and dependent care they themselves need.

3.13.7   "The Abortion Clinic: What Goes On," Susan Reed, *People Magazine* 24(9): 103-106, August 26, 1985.

Women at a Phoenix, Arizona abortion clinic have an appointment to return in two weeks. The counselor stresses, "It's important to come back. We need to check for possible infection and to see that your cervix has healed properly." However, it is reported that two-thirds of them will never be heard from again. "We'll call the number they've listed, and it will be non-existent, explains the counselor." (Ed Note: There is evidence that many of these women were ashamed at having an abortion.

3.14   Self-Image

3.14.1   "Characteristics of women with cosmetic breast augmentation surgery compared with breast reduction surgery and women in the general population of Sweden," JP Fryzek et al, *Ann Plast Surg* 45(4): 349-356, 2000.

Women with cosmetic implants were significantly more likely to be current smokers, have had a prematurely terminated pregnancy (induced abortion or miscarriage), and have fewer live births compared to women who had breast reduction or women in the general population.

3.14.2   "Characteristics of Women With and Without Breast Augmentation," KS Cook et al, *JAMA* 277:1612-1617, 1997

A population based study of U.S. white women found that women with breast implants were twice as likely to have had a history of termination of pregnancy than other women.

3.14.3   "Motivation of Surrogate Mothers: Initial Findings," Philip J Parker, *Am J Psychiatry* 140(1): 117, January, 1983.

51

In a sample of 125 women who applied to be surrogate mothers, 44 (35%) either had had a voluntary abortion (26%) or had relinquished a child for adoption. Most women admitted that they would experience some feelings of loss and sadness but minimized them by saying, " It would be their baby, not mine"; " I'm only an incubator"; " I'd be nest watching"; and "I'll attach myself in a different way-hoping it's healthy."

3.14.4   "Psychodynamic Aspects of Delayed Abortion Decisions," J Cancelmo et al, *British J Medical Psychology* 65:333, 1992.

A study of New York city women who were primarily women of color found that abortion at later gestational ages was significantly associated with a greater disturbance of the basic sense of self due to gender/sexual conflict and lower levels of internalized striving or ambition.

3.15   Self-Punishment (Masochism) or Punishment of Others (Sadism)

3.15.1   "Abortion-Pain or Pleasure?" Howard W. Fisher in *The Psychological Effects of Abortion*, ed. D Mall and WF Watts (Washington, D.C.: University Publications of America, 1979) 39-52

A sample of postabortion women who had abortions between 1971-78 was described by a psychiatrist as being ill medically and psychiatrically, low in achievement, and prone to act out in destructive ways. The author described their view of pregnancy as " outside" the psychological self, but inside the physical self... As long as the pregnancy is indistinguishable from the inner-self, the woman can be "unaware" of it and logically abort "it" as though it was not there. Because of incomplete separation-individuation, these women have difficulty conceiving of the fetus as separate because of problems with self-object discrimination. This is a basic problem in reality testing. In a sense, the fetus is like an inner feeling that is denied, something these women did regularly with all their feelings, especially angry ones.

Since pregnancy is viewed as a punishment visited on the self, abortion is a "logical" attempt to rid the self of painful responsibility, a form of expiation. But psychologically, abortion is further self-punishment which occurs because the "thing" that is sacrificed is felt to be a portion of the self. It is a though the self seeks the pleasure of conception and the pain of loss in one unconscious moment, making abortion truly masochistic... It is interesting that women who need self-punishment do not abort themselves more often... the projection of responsibility to an external punishing agent (physician) accomplishes a lessening of guilt. Abortion is done "to" the woman, with her as only a passive participant. This is a further indication of masochism.

3.15.2   "Psychosocial Aspects of Induced Abortion.Its Implications for the Woman, Her Family and Her Doctor," : Part 1, Beverley Raphael, *The Medical Journal of Australia,* July 1, 1972 pp.35-42.

Self-punishment or self-destructive influences may operate so that either the pregnancy itself or the abortion represents a way of punishing herself for unrecognized feelings of guilt. This guilt may derive from earlier events in the woman's life (a previous abortion, a sadistic or rejecting act, etc) or may be related to deep-seated conflict concerning her sexuality, which she may perceive as being bad, sinful, dirty or uncontrollable...The pregnancy and its disturbance of the woman's life represent the punishment which may be timed so that school or career patterns are disrupted, shame is publically displayed, or a relationship which promised intimacy and security is broken. The abortion may represent the punishment of the loss of a longed-for child. Some women appear to harbour deep masochistic needs which lead them to repeated illegitimate pregnancies or repeated illegal abortions, and their self-destructiveness may be so intense that they may have personality characteristics in common with those who attempt suicide.

3.15.3   "Psychiatric Illness Following Therapeutic Abortion," N Simon, AG Senturia and D Rothman, *Am J Psychiat* 124 (1): 97-103, 1967

Therapeutic abortion offers an optimal circumstance for acting out sadomasochistic fantasies and impulses, both in terms of interaction between the patient and the physician and also by the actual physical circumstances of the abortion itself. Pregnancy in many ways fulfills the role of gratifying the woman's unconscious masochistic wish, while the abortion gratifies the sadistic impulse (directed against the fetus) as well as the masochistic wish (assault on the self).

3.15.4   "Fragmentation of the Personality Associated with Post-Abortion Trauma," Joel O Brende, *Association for Interdisciplinary Research In Values and Social Change Newsletter* 8(3): 1-8 July/Aug 1995

People who have endured extreme stress often suffer profound rupture in the very fabric of the self. Fragmentation predisposes to unstable and destructive relationships including sadistic, masochistic, abusive, and battering relationships.

Depression

3.16   General Background Studies

3.16.1   "Depressive symptoms during pregnancy: Relationship to poor health behaviors," B. Zuckerman et al.. *Am. J. Obstet. Gynecol.* 160: 1107-1111, 1989.

In a study of 1014 women of mostly poor and minority status at Boston City Hospital between 1984-1987, depressive symptoms during pregnancy were associated with increased life stress, decreased social support, poor weight gain, and use of cigarettes, alcohol and cocaine.

3.16.2   "Increasing Rates of Depression," . G.L. Klerman, M.M. Weissman, *JAMA* 261 (15):2229-2235, April 21, 1989.

Several studies have observed important changes in rates of depression among those born after W.W.II including a decrease in the age of onset with an increase in the late teenage and early adult years; an increase between 1960 and 1975 in the rates of depression for all ages; the risk of depression is consistently 2 to 3 times higher among women than men of all ages.

3.16.3   "Continuing Female Predominance In Depressive Illness, A.C," Leon, G.L. Klerman, P.

Wickramaratne, *Am.J. Public Health* 83 (5): 754, May, 1993.

Women continued to show higher rates of depression than men. Regardless of sex or period of time, subjects seemed to be at greatest risk of a first major depressive episode between ages 16-25.

3.16.4   "Social Adjustment and Depression: A Longitudinal Study," E. S. Paykel and M. Weissman, *Archives of General Psychiatry* 28: 659-663 (1973).

Depressed women showed residual dysfunctions in the areas of interpersonal friction and inhibited communication that remained relatively unchanged even when other symptoms of depression and sodal maladjustment dissipated.

3.16.5   "Interpersonal Consequences to Depression," C. L. Hammen, and S.D. Peters, *Journal of Abnormal Psychology* 87: 322-332 (1978).

Depressed persons elicit more negative reactions from others than non-depressed.

3.16.6   "Irrational Beliefs in Depression," R.E. Nelson, *J. of Consulting and Clinical Psychology* 45: 1190-1191 (1977).

The strongest correlates of depression are general irrationality, a need to excel in all endeavors, a need to feel worthwhile as a person, a feeling that things are terrible when they are not like one wants, obsessive worry, and a belief that it is impossible to overcome one's past.

3.16.7   "Life Events and Depressive Order Reviewed," I and II, C. Lloyd, *Archives of General Psychiatry* 37: 529-535 May, 1980.

Loss of parents may double or triple the depressive factor.

3.16.8   "Epidemiology of Affective Disorders," Robert Hirschfield and C.K. Grass, *Archives of General Psychiatry* 39(1): 35 (1982).

A good summary of the literature.

3.16.9   "Hostility and Depression," E.S. Gershon, M. Cromer and G.L. Klerman, *Psychiatry* 31: 224-235 (1968).

Hostility may have separate mechanisms both for its initiation and its defensive alterations. The expression of hostility may drain off the awareness of depression. It may express a "great despairing cry for love."

3.16.10 "Life Events and Depression: A Controlled Study," E.S. Paykel, J.K. Myers, M. Dienelt, *Archives of General Psychiatry* 21: 753-760 (1969).

Study noted an excessive number of stressful life events prior to depression.

3.16.11 "Masked Depression in Children and Adolescents," Kurt Glaser, *American Journal of Psychotherapy* 566-574 (1966).

Behavior problems and delinquent behavior such as temper tantrums, disobedience, truancy, running away from home, failure to achieve in school may indicate depressive feelings.

3.16.12 "Sex Differences and the Epidemiology of Depression," Myron Weissman and Gerald Klerman, *Archives of General Psychiatry* 34: 98-111 (January 1977).

Authors review various studies and conclude that women predominate among depressives; psycho-social explanations include social status hypothesis of social discrimination against women. It is hypothesized that inequities lead to legal and economic helplessness, dependency on others, chronically low self-esteem, low aspirations and ultimately clinical depression. The learned helplessness theory proposes that socially conditioned, stereotypical images produce in women a cognitive set against assertion which is reinforced by societal expectations. Learned helplessness is characteristic of depression.

3.16.13 "Toward a Comprehensive Theory of Depression: A Cross Disciplinary Appraisal of Objects. Games and Meaning," Ernest Becker, *Journal of Nervous and Mental Disease* 135: 26-35 (1962). Comments by the author:

Until Edward Bibring's theory, self-directed aggression was considered a primary mechanism in depression. Bibring signaled a radical departure from previous theory when he postulated that self-directed aggression was *secondary* to an undermining of self-esteem. Thereby, he delivered an apparently telling blow to formulations around the concepts of morality and aggression.

In the classical psychoanalytic formulation of depression, mourning and melancholic states, loss of a loved object was considered to be a crucial dynamic. The ego which (theoretically) grows by ideationally gathering objects into itself, was thought to sometimes massive trauma when loved objects had to be relinquished. The loss of an object in the real world meant a corresponding depletion of the ego.

The sociological view has stressed not object depletion in the ego as the motivation for funeral and mourning rites, but rather the social dramatization of solidarity at the loss of one of society's performance members. Ceremonies of mourning serve as a reaffirmation of social cohesiveness even though single performers drop out of the plot.

To lose an object is to lose someone to whom one has made appeal for self-validation.

It was formerly thought that depression was rare among the "simpler peoples for several reasons-- it was thought that the accumulation of guilt so prominent in the depressive syndrome-there was also the lingering myth of the happy savage.

The most difficult realization for man is the possibility that life has no meaning.

"Acknowledgment of personal sin or confession of guilt may sometimes be a defense against the possibility that there may be no meaning in the world....

Guilt in oneself is easier to face than lack of meaning in life." (quoted from *On Shame and Search for Identity* Helen Merrell Lynd, Harcourt-Brace [1958] p. 58)

The more people to whom one can make appeal for his identity, the easier it is to sustain life-meaning. Object loss hits hardest when self-justification is limited to a few objects.

3.16.14 "The Mechanism of Depression," E. Bibring, in Greenacre, P., Ed., *Affective Disorders,* (New York: International Universities Press, 1953) pp. 13-48.

3.16.15 *Depression,* A.T. Beck, (New York: Hoeber, 1967)

Ed Note: This is an important work on depression.

3.17 Abortion-Related Depression

3.17.1 "A Developmental Approach to Post-Abortion Depression," Frederick M. Burkle, *The Practitioner* 218:217, February 1977.

If the loss is valued depression will occur. To resolve the depression a process of mourning must occur.

3.17.2 "Reproductive Factors Affecting the Course of Affective Illness in Women," B.L. Parry, *Psychiatric Clinics of North America* 12(1): 207, March, 1989

Major depressive disorders are increasing with time, the age of onset is becoming earlier, and women continue to show an increased incidence of the disorder. Women are vulnerable to depressions associated with abortion.

3.17.3 "Testing a Model of the Psychological Consequences of Abortion," WB Miller et al in *The New Civil War. The Psychology, Culture, and Politics of Abortion,* ed. Linda J. Beckman and S Marie Harvey. (Washington, D.C.: American Psychological Association, 1998)

A multi-dimensional study of the psychological effects of induced abortion using mifepristone/misoprostol concluded that studies which emphasize unitary responses to abortion such as feelings of shame or guilt, loss or depression, and relief may be missing an important broader picture as what appears to happen following abortion involves not so much a unitary as a broad, multidimensional affective response. Findings suggest that during the first few days or weeks following an abortion, many women's reactions are incomplete and not necessarily representative of subsequent reactions. It is also very likely that different kinds of women follow a different time course. More studies are needed that examine the short-term consequences using sequential "snap shots" and there is more need for more postabortion longitudinal research.

3.17.4 "Personality and Self-Efficacy as Predictors of Coping with Abortion," C Cozzarelli, *Journal of Personality and Social Psychology* 65(6): 1224-1236, 1993

A wide range of depression scores was obtained on women immediately following abortion and at three weeks post-abortion.

3.18 Depression Shortly Prior to Abortion

3.18.1 "Family Relationships and Depressive Symptoms Preceding Induced Abortion," D Bluestein and CM Rutledge, *Family Practice Research Journal* 13(2): 149-156, 1993

Moderate to severe depression was found in women seeking abortion. Depression symptoms increased as measures of denial, difficulties with communicating with male partner, pregnancy symptoms, contraceptive use and dissatisfaction with abortion increased.

3.18.2 "Postabortion Psychological Adjustment: Are Minors at Increased Risk?" LM Pope et al, *Journal of Adolescent Health* 29:2-11, 2001

Thirty-five percent of young women aged 14-21 exhibited moderate to severe depression on the Beck Depression Inventory shortly prior to abortion.

3.18.3 "Psychological Factors that predict reaction to abortion," D.T. Moseley, D.R. Follingstad, H. Harley, R.V. Heckel, *J. of Clinical Psychology* 37(2):276,1981

A University of South Carolina study on women who elected abortion in an urban southern area administered the Multiple Affective Adjective Check List (MAACL) to women when they entered the clinic and a post-test in the recovery room prior to discharge following their abortion. Pre-abortion depression was much higher than the MAACL norms previously reported. Significant decreases in anxiety and depression were noted following abortion but not with respect to hostility. A woman's relationship with her partner was a crucial factor in post-abortion adjustment. Women with negative feelings toward their partners had higher levels of pre-abortion depression and post-abortion depression compared to women who were assisted in the decision by their sexual partners.

3.18.4 "Coping with Abortion," L. Cohen and S. Roth, *Journal of Human Stress,* Fall, 1984, pp. 140-145.

Researchers at Duke University of 55 women presenting for abortion a private clinic in Raleigh, NC evaluated symptoms of intrusion, avoidance, depression and anxiety upon their arrival at the clinic and in the recovery room after their abortion. The level of anxiety and depression was measured by the Symptom Checklist-90 (SCL-90). The mean level of depression decreased from 24.1 initially to 18.4 following abortion. Women exhibiting high avoidance had significantly higher level of depression both before and after their abortion compared to women exhibiting low avoidance.

3.18.5 "Psychological Factors Involved in Request for Elective Abortion, M," Blumenfield. *The Journal of Clinical Psychiatry*, Jan. 1978, pp. 17-25.

A study of 13 women requesting a first abortion and 13 women requesting a repeat abortion was undertaken at Kings County Hospital Clinic in New York utilizing a largely open-ended interview. The purpose was to determine the surrounding circumstances which gave rise to the request for abortion. It was found that the failure of contraception was not due to lack of access to adequate contraception. In 9 of 26 cases there was evidence of underlying psychological conflicts in the woman. These women were frequently lonely and/or depressed frequently because of isolation, loss of support, loss or separation from loved ones, or due to conflicts with partners. The data suggested that many of the male partners had a strong wish to father a child. The author stated "a pregnancy which leads to a request for an abortion usually reflects an underlying unresolved conflict which is being acted out through the pregnancy--a request for a repeat abortion would seem to indicate that the ambivalence has persisted and is being acted out through pregnancy once again or that a new circumstance has reawakened underlying conflicts.")

3.19   Depression During Subsequent Pregnancies

3.19.1   "Abortion and Subsequent Pregnancy," C.F. Bradley, *Canadian Journal Psychiatry* 29:494, Oct-1984.

A study of 254 pregnant women in Victoria, B.C. were followed from the second trimester of their pregnancy until 12 months post-partum. Twenty-eight women had a prior induced abortion and 216 had no prior induced abortion. Women who had a prior abortion had significantly higher levels of depressive effect in the third trimester of pregnancy (35 weeks gestation) and also at intervals of I month, 6 months and 12 months in the post-partum period. A Depressive Adjective Checklist developed by other researchers was used as the evaluation tool. Women with prior abortions also described themselves as less well-adjusted during the prenatal period and had lower self-esteem in the post-partum period than those without any abortion history. The author suggested that it may have been those factors which were related to their depressive mood.

3.19.2   "The Relationship Between Previous Elective Abortions and Postpartum," Depressive Reactions. N.E. Devore, *Journal of Obstetric Gynecologic and Neonatal Nursing*, July/August 1979, pp-237-240

In a study of 73 women among the obstetrical population at the Hospital of Albert Einstein College during 1975-76, 25 pregnant women who had one abortion and 48 women who were pregnant for the first time were interviewed 6-8 weeks postpartum. Seventy-one percent of the women with abortion history reported they were depressed at the time of the abortion, yet only 12% reported that they had received emotional counseling at the time of the abortion. The range of time from the earlier abortion to the current pregnancy was 2-8 years, mean 3.9 years. Using the Beck Depression Inventory, the study found postpartum moderate depression in 16% of women with a prior abortion compared to 12% of the women without any abortion. Eighty percent of the women with abortion history compared to 56% without abortion history reported the "baby blues." The study suggested that a few women who have had a previous elective abortion will still experience feelings of guilt or depression in connection with it. Spontaneous comment from the women with abortion history suggested that anxiety during pregnancy concurring the infants health was a greater source of discomfort than was post-partum depression.

3.19.3   "Previous induced abortion and ante-natal depression in primipare: preliminary report of a survey of mental health in pregnancy," R. Kumar, K. Robson, *Psychological Medicine* 8:711-715, 1978

A British study of 119 pregnant women found an association between a previous abortion (legal or illegal) and depression and anxiety in an early subsequent pregnancy. An intensification of fears of fetal abnormality was noted in women having had a prior abortion. The study concluded that "unresolved feelings of guilt, grief and loss may remain dormant long after an abortion until they are apparently re-awakened by another pregnancy. Normal anxieties about the now desired fetus are intensified and such fears are often spontaneously interpreted in terms of retribution."

3.19.4   *A Prospective Study of Emotional Disorders in Childbearing Women*, R Kumar, K Robson, Brit J Psychiat 144:35-47, 1984

Prior induced abortion was associated with ante-natal depression and anxiety; thoughts about obtaining abortion was associated with both ante-natal and post-natal depression and anxiety.

3.19.5   "Psychiatric Morbidity in a Pregnant Population in Nigeria," OA Abiodun et. al *General Hospital Psychiatry* 15: 125-128, 1993

A previous history of induced abortion was significantly associated with psychiatric morbidity (mostly anxiety and neurotic depression) among 240 married Christian and Muslim women attending an antenatal clinic.

3.19.6   "Psychological and social correlates of the onset of affective disorders among pregnant women," T Kitamura et al, *Psychological Medicine* 23:967-975, 1993

A Japanese study found that among women with previous pregnancy, pregnancy-related affective disorder was recognized among 27% of those expecting their first baby where there had been a previous termination of pregnancy compared to 3% of women who had no previous termination of pregnancy.

3.20   Anniversary Depressive Reactions

3.20.1   "Aftermath of Abortion. Anniversary Depression and Abdominal Pain. J.O," Cavenar Jr A.A. Maltbie, J.L. Sullivan, *Bulletin of the Menninger Clinic* 42(5):433438, 1978

A case study was presented in which a woman had an apparently uneventful abortion, but which resulted in a depressive reaction which arose during the week of her expected delivery, necessitating psychiatric care.

3.20.2   "Adolescent Suicide Attempts Following Elective Abortion," C Tischler, Pediatrics 68(5):670, 1981

Adolescents attempted suicide on the perceived due date for their aborted child.

3.20.3   "Psychoses Following Therapeutic Abortion," J.G. Spaulding, J.O. Cavenar, Am.J.. Psychiatry

135(3):364, March 1978. (A case study of a 24 year old unmarried women who experienced post abortion insomnia, anorexia, agitation and severe depression that necessitated hospitalization 9 months after the time the child would have been conceived.

3.20.4 "Postabortion Depressive Reactions in College Women," N.B. Gould, J.Am. *College Health Association* 28:316320, 1980.

In a study of college women at Harvard University during 1978-79, cases of 3 women who had abortions are described who each experienced depressive reactions at the time of the expected delivery date which adversely affected classroom performance.

3.20.5 "Post-Abortion Perceptions: A Comparison of Self-Identified Distressed and Nondistressed Populations," GK Congleton and LG Calhoun, *The International Journal of Social Psychiatry* 39(4): 255, 1993

Women who reported post-abortion distress were more likely to report depression around the anniversary date of the abortion or the due date for birth compared to women who reported relieving/neutral responses specifically related to the baby, insomnia, inability to concentrate on studies, divisiveness in their relationships with partners, suicidal ideation, bouts of crying, inability to be consoled.

3.20.6 "Anniversary Reactions and Due Date Responses Following Abortion, K," Franco, N. Campbell, M. Taburrino. S. Jurs. J. Pentz, C. Evans, *Psychother Psychosom* 52:151-154, 1989.

In a study of 83 women in a patient-led post abortion support group in Ohio, 30 reported anniversary reactions associated with the abortion or the due date. Mean scores on the Beck Depression Inventory were 6.5 for those reporting anniversary reactions and 5.5 for those not reporting anniversary reactions. Those reporting anniversary reactions frequently reported physical symptoms including abdominal pain, dyspareunia, headaches and chest pain.

3.21 Depressive Reactions from Genetic Abortion

3.21.1 "The psychological sequelae of abortion performed for a genetic indication," B.D. Blumberg, M.S. Globus, K.H. Hanson, *Am.J. Obstet Gynecol* 122(7):799, August 1, 1975.

In a study of 13 families where abortion was undergone due to a genetic defect in the fetus, the incidence of depression among women was as high as 92% among the women and 82% among the men. This was higher than elective abortion. Four families experienced separations during the pregnancy-abortion period.

3.21.2 "Sequelae and Support After Termination of Pregnancy for Fetal Malformation," J. Lloyd and KM Laurence, *British Medical Journal* 290:907-909, March 1985.

Seventy-seven percent of the women experienced an acute grief reaction following termination of pregnancy for fetal malformation. Forty-six percent still remained symptomatic after six months, some requiring psychiatric support. Depression with anxiety, often with considerable repressed anger, was noted. Severity of the reaction ranged from mild tearfulness, sadness, lethargy and insomnia to incapacitating grief with somatic symptoms, and finally to complete withdrawal. There was no opportunity to mourn. Some women had named the baby, usually secretly, which seemed to help the grieving process. Several would have liked some burial or formal recognition of the death. Several had problems severe enough to influence reproductive behavior.

3.22   Short Term Depressive Reactions

3.22.1   "Outcome Following Therapeutic Abortion," E.C. Payne, A.R. Kravitz, M.T. Notman, J.V. Anderson, *Arch Gen Psychiatry* 33:725, June 1976.

A study of 102 women evaluated anxiety depression, anger, guilt and shame in women prior to abortion and at 24 hours, 6 weeks and 6 months following their abortion with respect to a multiple number of variables. Depressive reactions were significantly reduced following abortions although mild to moderate depression was still present in women 6 months after their abortion. Factors that significantly increased the likelihood of post abortion depression were immature object relationships, younger women, Catholic religion, no prior children, previous mental illness, borderline personality, a negative relationship with mother, a bad relationship with children, conflict with lover, ambivalence to abortion.

3.22.2   "Induced abortion operations and their early sequelae," P.I. Frank, C.R. Kay, S.L. Winsgrave, *Journal of the Royal College of General Practitioners* 35:175, 1985.

In this British study those with a history of depression had a rate of post abortion depression which was 2.59 times higher than expected.

3.22.3   "Pregnancy Decision Making as a Significant Life Event: A Commitment Approach," J Lydon et al, *Journal of Personality and Social Psychology* 71(1): 141-151, 1996

Initial commitment to the pregnancy prior to abortion predicted subsequent depression, guilt and hostility postabortion.

3.22.4   "Therapeutic Abortion and a Prior Psychiatric History," J.A. Ewing, B.A. Rouse, *Am J. Psychiatry* 130(1):37, January, 1973.

A North Carolina study of 126 women who had abortions in 1970-71 found that 36% of the women with a history of psychiatric problems reported depression following abortion compared with only 11% of the women who reported no prior psychiatric history. The responses ranged from a few weeks to two years post abortion. Women with a psychiatric history prior to abortion also had higher incidence of crying spells, anxiety, sleeplessness, worry and guilt.

3.22.5   "Depressive Symptoms in Late Adolescent and Young Adult Females: Effects of Pregnancy Resolution," J. Mesaros, D. Larson and J. Lyons, presented to the American Society for

Psychosomatic Obstetrics and Gynecology, New York, New York, March 1990

A case / control of study of depressive symptoms in women 17-25 years of age compared women with prior induced abortion, delivery, spontaneous abortion and never pregnant on the Center for Epidemiologic Studies Depression Scale. Women with prior abortion had the highest frequency of depressive symptoms. Higher scores were found in women where there was a perceived loss of control in the decision to terminate, negative feelings about the termination and little meaningful religious experience.

3.22.6   "Attributions, Expectations and Coping with Abortion," B. Major, P. Mueller, K. Hildebrandt, *J. of Personality and Social Psychology* 48(3):585, 1985.

A study of 247 women who underwent abortions in a free-standing abortion clinic in a large U.S. metropolitan area found that their immediate (30 minutes post abortion) depression level following their abortion was mean of 4.17 (range 0-22) on the Beck Depression Inventory. Three weeks later on a sample of 99 women who later responded the mean response on the Beck Depression Inventory was a mean of 2.93 (range 0-17) on the Beck Depression Inventory.

3.22.7   "Law. Preventive Psychiatry and Therapeutic Abortion," H.I. Levene, F. J. Rigney, *The J. of Nervous and Mental Disease* 151(1):51, 1970.

A California study of 70 women who were granted a therapeutic abortion under California law found that 14% reported an increase in depressive symptomology 3-5 months post abortion.

3.22.8   "Short-term Psychiatric Sequelae to Therapeutic Termination of Pregnancy," B. Lask, *Br. J. Psychiatry* 126:173-177, 1975.

Fifty inpatients from a London hospital who underwent abortion were interviewed 6 months later. Thirty-two per cent had unfavorable outcomes. The outcome was considered unfavorable when the following criteria were fulfilled: (1) the patient regretted termination: (2) the patient had moderate or severe feelings of loss, guilt or self-reproach: (3) there was evidence of mental illness in the same degree as, or more severe than before the abortion. When moderate or severe adverse sequelae were reported, these were usually associated with depressive states. These varied in intensity from mild to sufficiently severe to necessitate hospital admission.

3.22.9   "Women's Self-Reported Responses to Abortion," G.M. Burnell, M.A. Norfleet, *The Journal of Psychology* 12(1):71-76

A study of 158 women who were members of a prepaid health plan in northern California reported in responding to a mailed questionnaire found that 17% reported depression following abortion which was the highest endorsement under a section entitled -worsened adjustment after abortion. The length of time from the time of the abortion and the questionnaire varied. A majority of the women completed the questionnaire within one and a half years after abortion.

3.22.10   "Long-term psychiatric follow-up," C. McCance, P. Olley, V. Edward in *Experience with Abortion*. Ed. G. Horobin, (Cambridge: Cambridge Univ. Press, 1973) 245-300.

This study found that 20% of the original sample of women who underwent induced abortion were depressed 13-24 months thereafter according to the Beck Depression Inventory.

3.22.11 "Psychological Responses of Women After First-Trimester Abortion," B Major et al, *Arch Gen Psychiatry* 57:777, 2000

20% of women had depression 2 years postabortion. Prepregnancy depression was a risk factor for postabortion depression. Negative postabortion emotions increased over time. Younger age and more children preabortion also predicted more negative abortion responses.

3.22.12 "Emotional Distress Patterns Among Women Having First or Repeat Abortions," E.W. Freeman, K. Rickels, G.R. Huggins, *Obstetrics and Gynecology* 55(5):630, May, 1980.

A study of 413 women at the University Hospital in 1977-78 using the SCL-90, a multidimensional self-report inventory measured depression before abortion and 2 weeks following abortion. The adjusted mean value prior to abortion was 1.06. After 2 weeks the adjusted mean value was 0.60 (one abortion) and 0.74 (two abortions). Women who repeated abortions showed significantly higher scores on interpersonal sensitivity, paranoid ideation, phobic anxiety and sleep disturbance compared to women with one abortion.

3.22.13 "Before and after therapeutic abortion," P. Mackenzie, *Canadian Medical Association Journal* 111:667, October 5, 1974.

A 1973 study at Queens University School of Medicine of 150 Canadian women two weeks post abortion had 53% respond to a questionnaire survey. Based on self reports of the women 39% said they were depressed a lot from the pregnancy (21% said they were a little depressed). Two weeks post abortion 4% said they were depressed a lot from the abortion and 28% said they were depressed a little and 39% said they were not at all depressed.

3.22.14 "Induced abortion after feeling fetal movements: Its causes and emotional consequences," C. Brewer, *J. Biosocial Science* 10:203-208.

In a study of 40 women who had abortions between 20-24 weeks gestation. Twenty-five were followed-up 30 months post abortion. Five reported feeling depressed about their abortion. One had taken time off from school or work for this reason. None had sought specialist advice.

3.23 Long Term Depressive Reactions (5 years or more since abortion) - see also Long Term Effects from Abortion

3.23.1 "Psychological profile of dysphoric women post abortion," K.N. Franco, M. Tamburrino, N. Campbell, J. Pentz, S. Jurs, *J. of the American Medical Women's Assoc.* 44(4):113, July/Aug. 1989.

In a survey of 81 women approximately 10 years post abortion who were in a patient led support group for women who described themselves as having poorly assimilated their abortion experience, the mean Beck Depression Inventory Score for all women studied was 5.3 (mild depression). For women with one abortion it was 4.7 (none to minimal depression). For women with multiple abortions it was 9.4 (moderate depression). Other risk factors for post abortion dysphoria were pre morbid psychiatric illness, lack of family support, ambivalence and feeling coerced into having a abortion.

3.23.2   *Post-Abortion Trauma,* Jeanette Vought, (Grand Rapids: Zondervan Publishing House, 1991).

A study of 68 religiously oriented, primarily Protestant women who were studied 10-15 years post-abortion, 76% reported depression as one of the emotional effects of abortion.

3.23.3   "A Survey of Postabortion Reactions," David C. Reardon, (Springfield, IL: The Elliot Institute for Social Science Research, 1987).

In a 1987 Survey of Postabortion reactions among 100 women members of Women Exploited by Abortion an average of 11 years since their abortion, 87% agreed or strongly agreed with the statement, "After my abortion I experienced feelings of depression." Fifty per cent of these women were 20 years of age or younger at the time of their abortion.

3.23.4   *Psycho-Social Stress Following Abortion,* Anne Speckhard, (Kansas City MO: Sheed & Ward, 1987).

In a study of 30 women who reported chronic and long term stress from their abortion 92% expressed feelings of depression following abortion. Fifty per cent of these women had their abortion in the second trimester (46%) or third trimester (4%) of their pregnancy. The majority (64%) had their abortion 5-10 years previously, 20% were less than 5 years and 16% ranged from 11-25 years post abortion.

3.23.5   "Depression associated with abortion and childbirth: A long-term analysis of the NLSY cohort," JR Cougle et al, *Clinical Method & Health Research NetPrints,* April 25, 2001 (Abstract)

This study used the National Longitudinal Survey of Youth which contains a number of psychological variables related to pregnancy outcome. Compared to post-childbirth women, women who had abortions were found to have significantly higher depression scores as measured an average of 10 years after their pregnancy outcome. Post-abortion women were also 41% more likely to score in the "high risk " range for clinical depression compared to non-aborting women. A self-assessment questionnaire administered in 1998 also found that aborting women were 73% more likely to complain of "depression, excessive worry, or nervous trouble of any kind" compared to women with other pregnancy outcomes.

3.23.6   "Psychiatric history and mental status," W.L. Sands in *Diagnosing Mental Illness:Evaluation in Psychiatry and Psychology,* Eds. Freedman and Kaplan, (New York: Athenum, 1973) 31.

"The significance of abortions may not be revealed until later periods of emotional depression. During depressions occurring in the fifth or sixth decades of the patient's life, the psychiatrist frequently hears expressions of remorse and guilt concerning abortions that occurred twenty or more years earlier."

3.24   Psychiatric or Psychological Hospitalization or Consultation

3.24.1   "Postabortion or Postpartum Psychotic Reactions," H David et al, *Family Planning Perspectives* 13(2): 892, 1981

A Danish register linkage study over a three month period found that the rate of psychiatric hospital admissions was 18.4 per 10,000 postabortion women, 12.0 pr 10,000 postpartum women, and 7.5 per 10,000 women of childbearing age generally.

3.24.2   "Risk of Admission to Psychiatric Institutions among Danish Women Who Experienced Induced Abortion: An Analysis Based on A National Record Linkage," Ronald Somers, *Dissertation Abstracts Int'l,* Public Health 2621-B, 1979

The age-adjusted incidence of psychiatric hospitalization was 3.42%, 4.06%, and 6.0% for women with one, two, and three induced abortions respectively compared with 2.56%, 1.97% and 2.15% for women with one, two and three live births respectively. The age-adjusted percentage of psychiatric hospitalization for aborting women was 1.49% for married women, 2.38%for single women, 4.21% for separated women, and 5.16% for divorced women. Aborting women under 30 years of age exhibited higher overall and diagnosis specific psychiatric hospital admission rates than women of this age in general. Teenagers who had abortions had 2.9 times the rate of psychiatric hospital admissions compared to teenage women in general. The highest rate of psychiatric hospital admissions was 9.45% among women age 35-39 with more than one abortion during the study period.

3.24.3   "State-funded abortions vs. deliveries: A comparison of subsequent mental health claims over 6 years," PK Coleman and D Reardon, Poster session presented at the American Psychological Society 12th Annual Convention, Miami, FL, June, 2000

In a study of California women who received state funded medical care and who either had an abortion or gave birth in 1989, postabortion women were more than twice as likely to have from two to nine treatments for mental health as women who carried to term.

3.24.4   "Psychosocial Characteristics of Psychiatric Inpatients with Reproductive Losses," T Thomas et al, *Journal of Health Care for the Poor and Underserved* 7(1):15, 1996

Postabortion women were more likely to require psychiatric hospitalization, have been subjected to sexual abuse, and be diagnosed for psychoactive substance abuse disorder compared to childless women.

3.24.5   "Past Trauma and Present Functioning of Patients Attending a Women's Psychiatric Clinic," EFM Borins and PJ Forsythe, *Am J Psychiatry* 142(4):460, 1985

In a Canadian study of women attending a hospital based women's psychiatric clinic, a past abortion correlated significantly with three or more trauma factors.

3.24.6 *Proceedings of the Conference on Psycho-Social Factors in Transnational Planning*, W Pasini and J Kellerhals, (Washington D.C.: American Institute for Research, 1970) p.44

A three fold increase in previous psychiatric consultations was found in women seeking repeat abortions compared to maternity patients.

3.24.7 *Report of the Committee on the Abortion Law*, RF Badgley et al, (Ottawa:Supply and Services, 1977) pp. 313-321

A Saskatchewan, Canada study found that postabortion women had "mental disorders" 40.8% more often than postpartum women. An Alberta, Canada study found that among women who had abortions, 24% made visits to psychiatrists compared to 3% in the general population.

3.24.8 "Health Services Utilization After Induced Abortion in Ontario: A Comparison Between Community Clinics and Hospitals," T Ostbye et al, *Am J Medical Quality* 16(3):99-106, 2001

A study of Ontario Health Insurance Plan claims in 1995 found that women who were three months postabortion from hospital day surgery had a rate of hospitalization for psychiatric problems of 5.2 per 1000 vs. 1.1 per 1000 for age matched controls without induced abortions. Three month postabortion women who had abortions at a community clinic had a rate of hospitalization for psychiatric problems of 1.9 per 1000 vs. 0.60 per 1000 for age-matched controls who did not have induced abortions. The incidence of postabortion psychiatric hospitalization was significantly higher if there had been preabortion hospitalization for psychiatric problems, preabortion emergency room consultation, or preabortion hospital admissions. Ed. Note: Flaws in the available data and study design limit the value of this study.

Self-Destructive Behavior

3.25 ## Suicide

3.25.1 "Suicides after pregnancy in Finland, 1987-94: register linkage study, M. Gissler et. al.. *Br. Medical Journal* 313: 1431. Dec 7.1996

A Finnish study of women who committed suicide in 1987-94 within one year of a pregnancy found out that the suicide incidence associated with induced abortion was 34.7 per 100,000 postabortion women compared to 13.1 per 100,000 postmiscarriage women and 5.9 per 100/000 postpartum women and a mean annual suicide rate of 11.3 per 100/000 women generally.

3.25.2 "Suicide and/or abortion. 20th Meeting of the Group for Suicide Research and Prevention: The body and suicide," J. Koperschmitt et al, *Psychologie Medicale* 21(4): 446, March, 1989

Abortion can have an important effect on suicidality.

3.25.3   "Suicide After Ectopic Pregnancy," (letter) J. Farhi et al. *New England Journal of Medicine*, March 10,1994, p. 714

A study of Israeli women found that among 160 women treated for ectopic pregnancy 3.75% attempted suicide within one year thereafter and 0.625% committed suicide compared to a matched non-pregnant population rate of 0.04-0.06% and 0.002% respectively.

3.25.4   "Psychopathological effects of voluntary termination of pregnancy on the father called up for military service," DuBouis-Bonneford et al, *Psychologie Medicale* 14(8): 1187-1189, June 1982

Several case studies are presented of 18-22 year old males who came from disadvantaged backgrounds and were recent military recruits. All had extreme depression and/or attempted suicide brought on by the news of their wives or girlfriends having had a voluntary induced abortion. The men believed that becoming a father would make them more mature or respectable and the abortion brought on feelings of self-recrimination and self-punishment.

3.25.5   "Psychiatric Sequelae of Abortion: The Many Faces of Post-Abortion Grief," E. Joanne Angelo, *Linacre Quarterly* 59:69-80, May 1992.

Three cases of completed suicide following abortion are presented. In one case, a 22 year old woman in the military was referred for psychiatric counseling because of an eating disorder. She had made a suicide attempt two days before her scheduled abortion, feeling unable to go through with the abortion or face the rest of her tour of duty as a single parent. Her psychiatrist had advised going through with the abortion. Following the abortion, her use of cocaine and alcohol escalated and her weight continually dropped. She felt a strong desire to be united with her baby. She made several more suicide attempts and despite continuing therapy it did happen.

In another case a 23 year old woman was referred for psychiatric counseling after a suicide attempt involving a planned drunk driving incident. She and had two abortions at ages 17 and 18 while in high school. She was the youngest child of a large family and was afraid to tell her parents for fear they would "drop dead of heart attacks." (The parents were in precarious heath.) She suffered alone with the guilt for 6 years. She had planned to tell an uncle, who was a priest, what had happened, but before she could talk with him he suddenly died of a heart attack. Mourning his death as well as her earlier loses, she had planned her own death both to end her pain and to achieve a reunion with her children and her uncle.

In a third case, an 18 year old male gas station attendant shot himself and died 3 months after his father's unexpected death. Only his closest friend knew that at the time of his suicide he was despondent over his girl friend's abortion. The child had been conceived on the day of his father's death. He had formed a mental image of the child and told his friend he planned to name his son after his father. The loss of the child and what it represented was more than he was able to bear.

3.25.6   "Second-Trimester Abortions in the United States," D. Grimes, *Family Planning Perspectives* 16(6):260, Nov/Dec 1984.

Among the 92 reported deaths of women from second-trimester legal abortion, from 1972-1981, 2 were as a result of suicide.

3.25.7   "Physical and Psychological Injury in Women Following Abortion: Akron Pregnancy Services Survey," L.H. Gsellman, *Association For Interdisciplinary Research Newsletter* 5(4):1-8, Sept/Oct 1993.

(In a survey of 344 post-aborted women receiving services at Akron Pregnancy Services during 1988-1993, 16% reported suicidal impulses, 7% were preoccupied with death and 7% made suicide attempts.

3.25.8   "Adolescent Suicide Attempts Following Elective Abortion," Carl Tischler, *Pediatrics*, 68(5):670 (1981).

Case studies of attempted suicide on the anniversary of what would have been the aborted baby's birth.

3.25.9   *The Psycho-Social Aspects of stress Following Abortion,* Anne C. Speckhard, (Kansas City: Sheed and Ward, 1987)

Thirty women stressed by abortion were interviewed 5-10 years since abortion; 65% had suicide ideation; 31% attempted suicide.

3.25.10   "Therapeutic Abortion and Psychiatric Disturbance Among Women," E.R. Greenglass, *Canadian Psychiatric Association Journal* 21:453-459(1976).

Of 188 women interviewed, five attempted suicide about 2.6 months after abortion; there was evidence of other traumatic difficulties in addition to abortion.

3.25.11   "Post-Abortive Psychoses," Myre Sim and Robert Neisser, in *The Psychological Aspects of Abortion*, ed. D. Mall and WF Watts, (Washington D.C.: University Publications of America, 1979).

Fifty-eight women at an Israeli Government hospital volunteered the information that abortion, induced or spontaneous, had led to their referral to the psychiatric unit; seven had made serious attempts at suicide, three others had threatened suicide.

3.25.12   *Stress. Depression and Suicide: A Study of Adolescents in Minnesota.,* B Garfinkel, H. Hoberman, J. Parsons and J. Walker (Minneapolis: University of Minnesota Extension Service, 1986).

A teenage girl was about 6 times more likely to have attempted suicide if she had an abortion in the last six months compared to teenagers who had not had an abortion in that period (4% vs. 0.7%). Teenage girls attempting suicide in general were more likely to be depressed, to have recently broken up with their boyfriend, and come from chaotic homes. In an interview announcing the study results Dr. Garfinkel stated that impulsiveness, anger and anxiety are the three most important factors in teenage suicide. Too often abortion is taken as either producing an alleviation of stress or being helpful to young people. I think we need to re-examine the issues. *Minnesota Daily,* Oct 29,1986, p. 3/16

3.25.13 "Mental Disorders After Abortion," B. Jansson, *Acta Psychiatrica Scandinavica* 41:87 (1965)

In a Swedish study of 57 women with prior psychiatric problems who subsequently had induced abortions, three committed suicide as determined by long-term follow-up studies 8-13 years after their abortion. In contrast, of 195 women with previous psychiatric problems who carried their children to term, none committed suicide.

3.26   Accidents

3.26.1 "Pregnancy-associated deaths in Finland 1987-1994-definition problems and benefits of record linkage," M Gissler et al, *Acta Obstet Gynecol Scand* 76:651-657, 1997

A Finnish register linkage study identified all deaths that occurred up to 1 year after an ended pregnancy. The mortality rate was 27 per 100,000 births, and 101 per 100.000 abortions. Compared to women of reproductive age with no pregnancy (1.0), the risk of death from an accident following abortion was 2.08 (1.03-4.20, 95% CI) compared to 0.49 (0.18-1.33, 95% CI) for childbearing women.

3.26.2 "Suicide Deaths Associated with Pregnancy Outcome: A Record Linkage Study of 173,279 Low Income American Women," D Reardon et al, *Clinical Medicine & Health Research* clin med/2001 030003 v1 (April 25, 2001)

State funded medical insurance records identifying all paid claims for abortion or delivery in 1989 were linked to the state death certificate registry in a population of low income women in California. Compared to women who delivered (1.0), those who aborted had a significantly higher adjusted risk of dying from accidents (1.82).

3.26.3 "Sexual Experience and Drinking Among Women in a U.S. National Survey," A Klassen, S Wilsnack, *Archives of Sexual Behavior* 15(5): 363-392, 1986; "Women's Drinking and Drinking Problems: Patterns from a 1981 U.S. National Survey," R Wilsnack, S Wilsnack, A Klassen, *Am J Public Health* 74:1231-1238, 1984.

In a random national survey of 917 U.S. women in 1981, 4% of the abstainers and 5% of lighter drinkers reported non-spontaneous abortion compared to 13% for moderate drinkers, 13% for heavier drinkers, and 6% for women who had ever been pregnant. The same survey found that 17% of all women drinkers said they had driven vehicles while drunk or high at least once in the preceding year including 27% of moderate drinkers and 45% of heavier drinkers.

3.26.4 "Alcohol-Related Relative Risk of Fatal Driver Injuries in Relation to Driver Age and Sex," Paul L Zodor, *J Stud Alcohol* 52:302-310, 1991.

A study by the Insurance Institute for Highway Safety based on 1986-87 data found that each 0.02% increase in blood alcohol content nearly doubles the risk of being in a single vehicle fatal crash. The risk of a female 21-24 years of age at a blood alcohol level of 0.05%- 0.09% of dying in a single vehicle accident was reported to be 35 times higher compared to a blood level of 0.00%- 0.01%

3.26.5 "Adolescent Suicide Attempts Following Elective Abortion: A Special Case of Anniversary Reaction," CL Tishler, *Pediatrics* 68 (5):670-671, 1981

A 17 year old upper middle class white girl attempted to kill herself while driving under the influence of alcohol and 29 Bufferin tablets. She smashed her car into a bridge overpass repeatedly, damaging her car beyond repair. She had had an elective abortion approximately seven months prior to the suicide attempt. During the abortion process she calculated the birth date had the fetus been allowed to come to term. The date of the accident was on the perceived birth date of the child.

3.27   Repeat Abortions

3.27.1 "Abortion Surveillance-United States, 1997," *MMWR* Vol 49, No.SS-11, December 8, 2000.

The Centers for Disease Control reported that 48% of U.S. women had repeat abortions in 1997 with 28.4% reporting a second abortion, 12% reporting a third abortion, and 7.6 % reporting a fourth or more abortion.

3.27.2 "Abortion Surveillance-United States. 1992," L.M. Koonin et. al., *MMWR* 45, No. 55-3: 1, May 3,1996

For 1992,1,359/145 legal abortions were reported to CDC, representing a 2.1% decline overall, from the number reported for 1991. 45.8% of women were repeating abortion with 26.9% reporting a second abortion, 10.8% (third), and 6.4% having 4 or more abortions. The abortion ratio was more than nine times greater for unmarried women than for married women. The abortion rate for white women was 15 per 1000 white women compared to 41 per 1000 black women and 32 per 1000 Hispanic women.

3.27.3 "The epidemiology of preterm birth," Judith Lumley, *Bailliere's Clinical Obstetrics and Gynaecology* 7(3): 477, Sept, 1993

A study of more than 300,000 first singleton births in Victoria, Australia from 1986-1990 found that 6.5 per 1000 births were 20-27 gestational weeks where the woman had one prior induced abortion compared to 10.3 per 1000 births (two prior induced abortions) and 23.1 per 1000 births (three or more prior induced abortions). The rate of preterm births at 32-36 gestational weeks was 54.1 per 1000 births where women had one prior induced abortion, 78.7 per 1000 births where women had two prior induced abortions and 120.1 per 1000 births where women had three or more prior induced abortions. For purposes of analysis women who had experienced both induced and spontaneous abortions were excluded.

3.27.4 "Pregnancy Decision Making as a Significant Life Event: A Commitment Approach," J. Lydon, et. al. *J. Personality and Social Psychology* 71(1): 141-151, 1996

Women with prior abortions were found to be more committed to a current pregnancy compared to women with no prior abortion history. Initial commitment predicted subsequent depression, guilt, and hostility among those who aborted.

3.27.5   "Post-Abortion Syndrome as a Variant of Post Traumatic Stress Syndrome," Robert C. Erikson, *Association for Interdisciplinary Research Newsletter,* 3(4) :5-8, Winter, 1991.

Repeat abortion will, to a degree, reflect a re-creation of the social, emotional and relational circumstances present before the initial abortion. Repeat abortions frequently are re-enactments of conflict between drives, and have little to do with ego functions such as learning.

3.27.6   The compulsion to repeat the trauma. Re-enactment, revictimization, and masochism," PA van der Kolk, *Psychiatric Clinics of North America* 12(2): 389-411, June, 1989

Trauma can be repeated in behavioral, emotional, physiologic, and neuroendocrinologic levels. Repetition on these different levels causes a large variety of individual and social suffering. Previously traumatized people tend to return to familiar patterns, even if they cause pain.

3.27.7   "Special Issue on Repeat Abortion,"*Association for Interdisciplinary Research Newsletter* 2(3): 1-8, Summer 1989.

Review of the literature on the incidence and effects of repeat abortions. It including moral and social deterioration, communication breakdown, decline in religious affiliation, emotional or psychological conflicts, replacement pregnancy, self-punishment, abortion as birth control and the evangelization of abortion.

3.27.8   "Repeat Abortion: Blaming the Victims," B. Howe, R. Kaplan, and C. English, *American Journal Public Health,* 69(12):1242-1246, December 1979,

Repeaters were found to be more sexually active than first-timers, thus increasing their risk of unwanted pregnancy even though they used contraception more than initial aborters.

3.27.9   "Women's Health and Abortion. I. Deterioration of Health Among Women Repeating Abortion," *Association for Interdisciplinary Research Newsletter* 5(1):1-8, Winter, 1993.

This article identifies 32 areas of social, medical and psychological health that deteriorate as induced abortion is repeated.

3.27.10   "Repeat Abortion: Is It A Problem?," C. Berger, D. Gold, D. Andres, P. Gillett and R. Kinch, *Family Planning Perspectives,* 16(2):70-75, March/April 1984,

Medical and counseling personnel are troubled by women who come back to their facilities for a repeat abortion. Counseling deficiencies, possible negative media coverage, unclear long-term effects on future child bearing are some of the reasons for concern. This study of Canadian women found that repeaters were more tolerant of abortion than women having a first abortion;

they also had intercourse more frequently than first-time abortion patients [average 11 times per month versus 8 times per month]. Women having repeat abortions were slightly more likely to have been using contraceptives at the time they became pregnant. Repeaters described their relationships as being less satisfactory than first-time patients. More repeaters than first-time patients said they had made the decision by themselves [45 percent vs. 33 percent]. Repeaters reported fewer physical complaints but had more difficulty sleeping.

3.27.11 "Third Time Unlucky: A Study of Women Who Have Had Three or More Legal Abortions," Colin Brewer, *Journal Biosocial Science*, 9:99-105(1977).

Of 50 women having their third or subsequent legal abortion, 23 were pregnant because they claimed their contraceptive method had failed; 24 because of erratic contraceptive use; and three changed their minds after initially welcoming the pregnancy. The study concluded there was a significant relationship between erratic use and a history of consultation for psychiatric reasons, and suggested that unsettled relationships and low educational status also related to erratic use. There was no evidence that abortion was deliberately used as a method of birth control.

3.27.12 "Repeaters-Different or Unlucky?," C. Berger and D. Gold, et al., in P. Sechder, ed.. *Abortion: Readings and Research.* (Toronto: Butterworth Press, 1981).

3.27.13 *Proceeding of the Conference on Psycho-Social Factors in Transnational Family Planning Research,* W. Pasini and J. Kellerhals (Washington: American Institute for Research, 1970), 44-54.

A threefold increase in previous psychiatric consultations was found in women seeking repeat abortions compared with maternity patients.

3.27.14 *Beyond Choice. The Abortion Story No One Is Telling,* Don Baker, (Portland: Multonomah Press, 1985).

A powerful narrative true story of a woman who had three abortions. Demonstrates the moral and social deterioration in her life until she commits her life to Jesus Christ. Excerpts reprinted in the April/May 1987 issue of *The Christian Reader.*

3.27.15 "The Repeat Abortion Patient," Judith Leach, *Family Planning Perspectives*, 9(1):37-39, January/February 1977

Repeat abortion patients are more often dissatisfied with themselves, more often perceive themselves as victims of bad luck, and more frequently express negative feelings toward the current abortion than women who are obtaining abortions for the first time.

3.27.16 "Pilot Surveys of Repeated Abortion," E. Szabady and A. Klinger, *International Mental Health Res. Newsletter* 14:6(1972).

In a study of Hungarian women those women having a repeat abortion were less likely to be in a happy marriage and were more likely to have an abortion independently of their partner.

3.27.17 "Emotional Distress Patterns Among Women Having First or Repeat Abortions," Ellen Freeman, *Obstetrics and Gynecology* 55(5):630-636, May 1980

Repeat abortion patients showed significantly higher distress scores on interpersonal sensitivity, paranoid ideation, phobic anxiety and sleep disturbance, compared with controls. Repeaters also showed a trend in higher scores in somatization, hostility and psychoticism.

3.27.18 "Repeat Abortions-Why More?," Christopher Tietze, *Family Planning Perspectives*, 10(5):286-288, September/October 1978,

Repeaters tended to have more frequent intercourseless satisfying relationships, and more difficulty sleeping. They were less likely to live with their partners. (Women with prior abortion were almost 4 times more likely to have repeat abortion compared to women having an abortion for the first time.

3.27.19 "Women Who Obtain Repeat Abortion: A Study Based Upon Record Linkage," P. Steinhoff, R. Smith, J. Palmore, M. Diamond and C. Chung, *Family Planning Perspectives* 11(1):30-38 Jan/Feb 1979.

Study noted the proportion of induced abortions that are repeat procedures increases over time. Shortcomings in making contraceptives available were cited as the reason. The women's own reporting of repeat abortions was about 20% lower than the actual number determined by record linkage.

3.27.20 "Abortion Recidivism - A Problem in Preventative Medicine," Joseph Rovinsky, *Obstetrics and Gynecology*, 39(5) :649-659, May 1972.

There was a lack of contraceptive motivation in repeaters as an etiologic basis for recurrent unwanted pregnancy; the article cites a case of 17 prior abortions.

3.27.21 "First and Repeat Abortions: A Study of Decision-Making and Delay," M.Bracken and S. Kasi, *Journal Biosocial Science*, 7:473-491 (1975).

Women having a repeat abortion took less time than those having a first abortion; women repeaters were more likely to report medical problems as a reason for contraceptive failure, compared with first-abortion women who were more likely to admit to carelessness. Women having repeat abortions were more likely to mention problems with the contraceptive, while those having first abortions were more likely to have failed to anticipate intercourse. Fewer women repeaters were pregnant by husbands, and unmarried women having repeat abortions had been in relationships of shorter duration than unmarried women having first abortions. Women having first abortions were generally more concerned with moral and ethical issues, worry over the procedure itself and the possibility of complications than were women having repeat abortions, who generally showed more desire to have children.

3.27.22 "Characteristics and Contraceptive of Abortion Patients," S. Henshaw, J. Silverman, *Family*

Planning Perspectives 20(4): 158, July/August, 1988.

A national survey of 9/480 women at U.S. abortion facilities in 1987 by the Alan Guttmacher Institute found that 42.9% of those women surveyed had repeat abortions: 26.9% (second abortion); 10.7% (third abortion); 5.3% (fourth abortion or more).

3.27.23 "Reflections on repeated abortions: The meanings and motivations," Susan Fisher, *Journal of Social Work Practice* 2(2):70-87, May 1986.

The author, a social worker at a London hospital, interviewed more than 1,000 women with crisis pregnancies. Several in-depth case histories are reported. Repeaters were variously described as "chaotic, childlike" (a woman who had 15 abortions in 23 years); "doll-like" (history of numerous suicide attempts); holding "anxiety, rage and confusion" over mother's mental illness; "a delicate child-woman 16 years old with very little human warmth, depressed"; "cold and detached with little feeling"; "a suicidal woman with a history of three abortions, a first suicide attempt at age 15 and the most recent one at age 27, only six weeks ago/drug overdoses, anorexia nervosa and hospitalization for psychiatric treatment." Women had shallow relationships with putative fathers and seemed to select male partners known to be objectionable to the repeaters' parents. Unconscious conflicts and lack of nurturing in family of origin were typical. Relationships with male partners usually terminated following abortion. Repeaters were irregular in keeping appointments and in completing therapy. Some called their unborn child "monster." The author concluded that repeat abortions are both an individual and social problem with physical and emotional suffering as well as a strain on medical and counseling resources.

3.27.24 "A Case Study of Reproductive Experience of Women Who Have Had Three or More Induced Abortions," Elizabeth Lincoln, Ph.D. Dissertation, University of Pittsburgh (1982); *Dissertation Abstracts International* 44(4), October 1983, Order No. DA 8318205.

A study of eight women with three or more abortions found that women had a sex role orientation less modernistic than effective contraceptors, feared health effects, had problematic relationships with partners ,family of origin relationships were characterized by lack of affection and probable subsequent influence on adult relationships, interest in parenting and sexuality. Anger at perceived lack of male interest in contraception combined with poor communication and changing sex role expectations seemed to create conflicts increasing the likelihood of unwanted pregnancy.

3.27.25 "Incidence of Repeat Abortion. Second-Trimester Abortion. Contraceptive Use and Illness within a Teenage Population," Rena Bobrowsky, Ph.D. Dissertation, University of Southern California (1986); *Dissertation Abstracts International* 47(9), March 1987. Copies available from Micrographics Dept, Doheny Library, USC, Los Angeles, CA 90069-0182.

In a study of teenage abortion, 404 women were followed through medical records over a five-year period. Some 38% had a previous abortion and 18% had two abortions within the same year. Repeat aborters were found to have less stable relationships with their partners, more likely to show greater use of contraception post-abortion and have more medical problems that might preclude the safe use of more reliable contraceptives.

3.27.26 "Association of Induced Abortion with Subsequent Pregnancy Loss," A. Levin, S. Schoenbaum, R. Monson, P. Stubbelfield, K. Ryan, *JAMA* 243:2495(1980).

Women who had two or more induced abortions were 2.7 times more likely to have future first-trimester spontaneous abortions (miscarriage) and 3.2 times more likely to have a second-trimester incomplete abortion than were women with no history of induced abortion.

3.27.27 "Repeat Abortions Increased Risk of Miscarriage. Premature Births and Low Birth Weight Babies," *Family Planning Perspectives*, 1(1):39-40, January/February 1979.

Repeated abortion was associated with a 2- to 2.5-fold increase in the rate of low birth weight and short gestation when compared with either one abortion or one live birth.

3.27.28 "Ectopic Pregnancy and Prior Induced Abortion," A. Levin, S. Schoenbaum, P. Stubblefield, S. Zimicki, R. Monson and K. Ryan, *American Journal of Public Health* 72(3):253-256, March 1982.

In a study at Boston Hospital for Women conducted from 1976-1978, the relative risk of ectopic pregnancy was found to be 1.6 for women with one prior abortion and reduced to 1.3 after control of confounding factors. The relative risk for two or more abortions was 4.0 for women with two or more prior induced abortions, which was reduced to 2.6 after control of confounding factors.

3.27.29 "Patterns of Alcohol and Cigarette Use in Pregnancy," J. Kuzma and D. Kissinger, *Neurobehavorial Toxicology and Teratology* 3:211-221(1981)

In a California study of more 12,000 women during 1975-1977, of those having a history of two or more abortions, virtually all (98.5%) consumed alcohol throughout the entire 9 months of a subsequent pregnancy and at higher levels, i.e., up to 3 oz. per day than any of the other categories studied.

3.27.30 "Low Birth Weight in Relation to Multiple Induced Abortions," M.T. Mandelson, C.B. Maden, J.R. Daling, *Am.J. Public Health*, 82 (3):391-394, March, 1993.

In a Washington State Study of 6541 women who delivered a child between 1984-87, 41.6% of the women smoked during this pregnancy if they had a history of 4 or more induced abortions compared with 31.0% smokers (2 prior abortions), 28.1% smokers (1 prior abortion), or 18.0% smokers (no prior abortions).

3.27.31 "The Concept of the Repetition Compulsion," E. Bibring, *Psychoanalytic Quarterly* 12: 486,507 (1943).

"Perhaps the most frequent way of taking the compulsive repetition into the personality is through sexualization when the repetition compulsion becomes linked with masochistic drives."

3.27.32 "Repeat Abortion: Is it a Problem?," C. Berger, D. Gold, D. Andres, P. Gillett and R. Kinch, *Family Planning Perspectives* 16(2):70-75, March/April 1985.

Interviews with medical and counseling personnel at abortion facilities regarding women who return for repeat abortions reveal counseling deficiencies, possible negative media coverage and unclear long-term effects on childbearing as some of the reasons for concern.

3.27.33 "Abortion Work: A Study of the Relationship Between Private Troubles and Public," Kathleen Marie Roe, Ph.D. Dissertation, University of California, Berkeley (1985).

In a study of 90 abortion facility workers in the San Francisco area, over 95% expressed discomfort and surprise at repeaters.

3.27.34 "Contraception and repeat abortion," M. Shepard and M. Bracken, *Journal of Biosocial Science* 11:289-302 (1979).

In a study of women at Yale-New Haven Hospital during 1974-1975, women having repeat abortions were significantly more likely to be divorced than women having first abortions. Women having repeat abortions were more likely to be on public welfare than women having first abortions (38% vs. 25%).

3.27.35 "Dysphoric reactions in women after abortion," K. Franco, M. Tamburrino, N. Campbell, J. Pentz and S. Jurs, *J. of the American Medical Women's Association* 44(4): 113, July/August 1989.

Women reporting multiple abortions had more often considered suicide and scored higher on borderline personality pathology and depression. Some 40% of the 71, women studied reported anniversary reactions. None of the women aborting sought psychotherapy after the procedure.

3.27.36 "The First Abortion And The Last? A Study of the Personality Factors Underlying Failure of Contraception," P. Niemela, P. Lehtinen, L. Rauramo, R. Hermansson, R. Karjalienen, H. Maki and C-A Stora, *International Journal of Gynaecol. Obstet.* 19:93- 200(1981).

A Finnish study compared women seeking their second abortion to women who had successfully contracepted after their first abortion Repeaters rated lower in control of impulsivity, emotional balance/realism, self-esteem and stability of life as well as reflecting a lesser capacity for integrated personal relationships. Repeating women more often had a history of broken legalized or non-legalized partner relationships. Partners of repeaters took less responsibility for contraception even though the women had left them greater responsibility in this respect. Solidarity with partners was weaker in the repeaters even though the women felt greater admiration for their partners. Repeating women were less mature and more impulsive, indicating a "split" mechanism and immaturity of ego development which verged on a borderline level disturbance.

3.27.37 "Single and repeated elective abortions in Japan: a psychosocial study," T Kitamura et al, *J Psychosom Obstet Gynecol* 19:126-134, 1998.

A Japanese study found that women with two or more abortions had a longer dating period, were likely to have a non-arranged marriage, smoked more cigarettes, had an early maternal loss experience or a lower level of maternal care during childhood compared to women with women with a first abortion.

3.27.38 "Mourning and Guilt Among Greek Women Having Repeated Abortions," D. Naziri, A. Tzararas, *Omega* 26(2): 137-144,1992-93

In a clinical study of the bereavement process of Greek women following one or more induced abortions, it was concluded that strong identifications with both father and mother images were present in the women. It was concluded that abortion might be a replacement/displacement of a reparatory character in relation to the "family romance" of each woman. In several cases of repeated abortion, mourning and guilt not only refer to a murdered and lost person of the fetus, but also principally to the death and loss of an object of ambiguous desire.

3.27.39 "The Repeat Abortion Patient," Judith Leach, *Family Planning Perspectives* 9(1):37, January/February 1977.

In a study of repeat abortion patients in the Atlanta area, 21% of the repeat aborters vs. 8% of the first-time aborters reported they had no religious affiliation. The disparity was especially striking in the private clinic population, among whom eight times as many repeat abortion patients as first-time aborters said they had no religious affiliation (20% vs. 2.5%).

3.27.40 "Risk of Admission to Psychiatric Institutions Among Danish Women Who Experienced Induced Abortion: An Analysis Based Upon Record Linkage," Ronald Somers, Ph.D. Dissertation, University of California, Los Angeles (1979), *Dissertation Abstracts International*, Order No. 7926066.

A study of the Danish Central Psychiatric Register of all women who had been admitted between April 1,1973 and December 31/1975 found that psychiatric admissions increased with the self-reported number of past abortions (no abortions, 1.90%; one abortion, 3.4%; two abortions, 4.0%; three abortions, 6.0%). No increase was observed as number of live births increased; women aged 35-39 with two or more abortions had higher rates of psychiatric admission than younger women with two or more abortions.

3.27.41 "Increased Reporting of Menstrual Symptoms Among Women Who Used Induced Abortion," L.H. Roht, M.A. Fanner, H. Aoyama and E. Fonner, *Am. Journal of Obstetrics and Gynecology* 127:356-362, February 15,1977.

A study of 3,222 female residents in Southern Japan in 1971, based upon a mailed questionnaire, found that women perceived menses to occur more frequently and be of shorter duration as the number of reported prior abortions increased. "Nervousness" increased as number of prior abortions increased: 150/1,000 women (no prior abortion); 228/1,000 (one prior abortion); 256/1/000 (two or more prior abortions).

3.27.42 "Induced Terminations of Pregnancy: Reporting States," 1988, K. Kochanek, *Monthly Vital Statistics Report* 39(12): 1-32 (Suppl.), April 30,1991, Table 9, p. 20

In 1988 among the 14 reporting states, 297,251 induced abortions were performed. Some 25.5%

had a second abortion, 9.0% had a third abortion and 8.7% had a fourth abortion or more. Overall, 44.1% were repeating abortion, 39.6% of white women were repeating abortion vs. 53.0% of black women.

3.27.43 "The Social and Economic Correlates of Pregnancy Resolution Among Adolescents in New York by Race and Ethnicity: A Multivariate Analysis," Theodore Joyce, *Am. J. Public Health* 78(6):626-63, (1988).

Teenagers who experienced one prior abortion were approximately four times more likely to terminate a current pregnancy by abortion compared to teenagers with no prior abortion history. Medicaid tended to increase the likelihood of carrying pregnancies to term. Married adolescents were more likely to carry a pregnancy to term than unmarried adolescents.

3.28 Eating Disorders

3.28.1 "Self-Induced Abortion in a Bulimic Woman," C.M. Bulik et. al., *Int'l J. Eating Disorders* 15(3): 297-299,1994.

A case of a woman was presented who deliberately induced abortion via self-imposed starvation and vigorous exercise. She had a history of severe obsessive-compulsive and narcissistic personality disorders as well as a lifelong pattern of denial of affect and illness.

3.28.2 "The Impulsivist: a multi-impulsive personality disorder," J.H. Lacey et. al., *Br. J. Addiction* 81: 641-649,1986.

There are strong associations between eating disorders, substance abuse, impulse control, self-harm and personality disorders.

3.28.3 *Post-Abortion Trauma: 9 Steps to Recovery,* Jeanette Vought, (Grand Rapids: Zondervan, 1991) 110.

In a 1990 study of 68 religiously oriented (primarily Evangelical and Lutheran) 10-15 years post-abortion, found 8.8% of the women identified themselves as having suffered from eating disorders (bulimia and anorexia). Of these women, 66.7% had increased problems with their eating disorder after their abortion. And additional 51.5% indicated they had problems with overeating and 23.5% expressed problems of under eating. Overeating behavior increased 54.3% following their abortion and under eating behavior increased 50.1% after their abortion.)

3.28.4 "Pregnancy : Outcome and Impact on Symptomatology in a Cohort of Eating-Disordered Women," MA Blais et al, *Int J Eat Disord* 27:140-149, 2000

There was an elevated incidence of eating disorders among women with therapeutic abortions which was not found among women with live births or spontaneous abortions.

78

3.28.5 "Recurrent Abortions in a Bulimic: Implications Regarding Pathogenesis," R.S. El-Mallakh, A.Tasman, *Intl. J. Eating Disorders* 10(2):215-219,1991.

A woman with severe bulimia used repeated pregnancies and abortions to achieve the same calming function as repeated binge eating and vomiting. It was suggested that her behavior was compatible with the view that bulimics use their own bodies as transitional objects and that the cycle of incorporation and expulsion is central to affect regulation. The woman was suicidal and preoccupied with death.

3.28.6 *The Psycho-Social Aspects of Stress Following Abortion,* Anne C. Speckhard, (Sheed and Ward: Kansas City, 1987)

In a study of 30 women who were stressed by abortion, 23 percent reported extreme weight gain, generally defined by the subjects as a 20-pound weight gain or more. Extreme weight gain was usually attributed to increased eating to calm oneself. Extreme weight loss was reported by 30 percent of the sample; 23 percent classified themselves as experiencing a period of anorexia nervosa. This was self defined, although many subjects reporting anorexia included evidence such as loss of 25 percent of body weight, cessation of menses, hospitalization and/or clinical diagnosis of anorexia nervosa.

3.28.7 *Aborted Women: Silent No More,* David C. Reardon, (Chicago: Loyola Press, 1987) 24.

In a study of 252 women who were members of Women Exploited by Abortion, two women were reported to suffer from anorexia nervosa which they attributed to their abortions. At least one woman suffered from excessive weight gain after her abortion, as she tried to bury her guilt in food.

3.28.8 "Ritual Mourning in Anorexia Nervosa," R.K. McAll and F.M. McAll, *The Lancet,* August 16,1980, p. 368.

Of 18 patients with anorexia nervosa treated in the hospital without improvement, 15 experienced total relief of symptoms following a process of ritual mourning for deceased family members who had not previously been mourned. Two patients were male. In 17 of the cases, family histories revealed a total of 25 violent deaths or deaths by suicide, five terminations of pregnancy for non-medical reasons and eight miscarriages. In one case a 17-year-old girl had anorexia nervosa since age 14 and had been hospitalized three times. At the time of referral she was unable to get out of bed. Her mother had an earlier pregnancy aborted. Without the knowledge of the patient, who was considered too ill to be involved/the parents went through a form of service in a church for the aborted child. When the patient was later told about this she admitted an awareness of the existence of her unborn "sister" but said she had not mentioned this for fear of being locked up in a mental hospital. She was immediately able to get up and in a very short time was successfully attending a college. In another case, a man of 41, had first been diagnosed as having anorexia at age 22. At the time of the examination he was not only anorectic but also severely depressed. On close questioning he admitted to having precipitated the abortion of his wife's first child. Within a week of his admission, and after following through with a process of mourning for and committal of the child, he was no longer depressed and was eating normally. The authors suggest that "hidden guilt, either in the patient or in a close member of the family, or lack of adequate recognition for a lost member of the family may be a causative factor. Providing a means of repentance, mourning for and committal of the dead can lead to dramatic relief of symptoms in the affected person, in addition to the emotional release experienced by other involved members of the family."

3.28.9 "Value of Family Background and Clinical Features as Predictors of Long Term Outcome in Anorexia Nervosa," H. Morgan and G.F.M. Russell, *Psychological Medicine* 5:355-37, (1975).

A disturbed relationship between the patient and other members of the family, and premorbid personality difficulties are predictors of unfavorable outcome.

3.28.10 "Diseases of the Nervous System," Asbury, McKhana, McDonald, Vol. 1(Philadelphia: WB Saunders, 1986)

Anorexia nervosa is a disorder usually affecting affluent young women 14-17 years of age but occasionally found even earlier or even up to age 40-50. The person is preoccupied with body weight, under eats even to possible starvation or self-destruction, and becomes depressed, very impatient and irritable. Anorexia nervosa is frequently associated with distressed and disturbed family relationships, suggesting a psychogenic aspect. Some have suggested that anorexia nervosa represents an aspect of affective disorder. Extreme perfectionism and self-criticism are often common traits. Mortality rates range from 4-16 percent depending on the study.

3.28.11 "A Study of 56 Families with Anorexia Nervosa," R.S. Kalucy, *British Journal of Medical Psychology* 50:381-395(1977).

A central feature was the threat to family values and stability which such events posed. Deaths and illnesses often involved waiting and then mechanisms of identification seemed important. For example/a daughter's illness was preceded by identification with the loss of another sister from leukemia; in another a father's wasting from achalasis.

3.28.12 "Avoidance of Anxiety and Eating Disorders," J. Keck and M. Fiebert, *Psychological Reports* 58: 432-434 (1986)

Female patients with eating disorders appeared to use an obsession with food and weight as a form of escape.

Substance Abuse

3.29 General Background Studies (Substance Abuse)

3.29.1 "Substance abuse and post-traumatic stress disorder comorbidity," P.J. Brown, J. Wolfe, *Drug and Alcohol Dependence* 35: 51-59,1994

Reviews the existing literature on the subject. In the relatively few studies which have assessed post-traumatic stress disorder, there is a common-co-occurring diagnosis among substance abusers.

3.29.2   "Fragmantation of the Personality Associated with Post-Abortion Trauma," Joel O Brende, *Association for Interdisciplinary Research in Values and Social Change Newsletter* 8(3):1-8, Jul/August 1995.

Victims of post-traumatic self-fragmentation often use alcohol, tranquilizers, and other substances.

3.29.3   "Sharp rise reported in fetal alcohol syndrome," *Minneapolis Star Tribune*, April 7,1995, p. 7A

According to a study by the Centers for Disease Control, the rate of babies born with health problems caused by fetal alcohol syndrome increased from 1 per 10,000 births in 1979 to 6.7 per 10,000 births in 1993. Despite growing awareness that avoiding liquor prevents the syndrome, about one-fifth of women continued to drink even after they learned they were pregnant.

3.29.4   "The Spectrum of Fetal Abuse," J.T. Condon, *J. Nervous and Mental Disease* 174(9): 509- 516, Sept, 1986

The fetus is a (potential) recipient par excellence for projection and displacement. Strategies aimed at reducing fetal abuse could more profitably focus on the determinants of the dysfunctional maternal-fetal relationship rather than "education" although clearly necessary but which may be insufficient for a major impact.

3.29.5   "A Study of Alcoholism in Women," James H. Wall, *American Journal of Psychiatry* 93:943,952(1937).

In women excessive drinking is more highly individual and is more intimately associated with a definite life situation. Both sexes have in common a narcissistic type of personality with increasing inability to adjust to reality and adult responsibility.

3.29.6   "Women and Alcohol: A Review," Sheila B. Blume, *Journal of the American Medical Association* 256(11): 1469, September 19,1986.

Review of the literature.

3.29.7   "Some Backgrounds and Types of Alcoholism Among Women," T. Fort and A.L. Porterfield, *Journal Health and Social Behavior* 2:282-292(1961).

Thirty-four women members of Alcoholics Anonymous were interviewed; 47% evidenced a sudden onset of alcoholism immediately following a specific stressful event.

3.29.8   "Life Issues as Social Determinants for the Meaning of Being a Woman," *Alcoholic-A Theory of Loss,* Gloria Ann Gelfand, Ph.D thesis, Columbia University Teachers College, 1985.

3.29.9   "Suicide and Alcoholism-Interpersonal Loss Confirmed as a Predictor, G," E. Murphy, J. Armstrong, S. Hermele, J. Fischer and W. Clendenin, *Archives of General Psychiatry* 36:65-69, January 1979.

3.29.10 "Drinking During Pregnancy and Spontaneous Abortion," J. Kline, P. Shrout, Z. Stein, *The Lancet,* July 26,1980, pp. 176-180.

Even moderate consumption of alcohol during pregnancy is a risk factor for, and may be a cause of spontaneous abortion. More than one-quarter of pregnant women drinking twice a week or more are likely to abort, compared with 14 percent of women who drink less often. Heavy drinking has been associated with fetal alcohol syndrome, minor and major malformations, stillbirths, prematurity, low birth weight, placental weight, and birth length.

3.29.11 "Alcohol. Smoking, and Incidence of Spontaneous Abortions in the First and Second Trimester," S. Harlap and P.H. Shiono, *The Lancet,* July 26,1980, pp. 173-176.

Increased risk of second-trimester miscarriage was noted in drinkers. Drinking and smoking were found to be independent risk factors for spontaneous abortion. The effect of drinking was greater than that of smoking.

3.29.12 "Alcohol Abuse During Pregnancy: An Epidemiologic Study," R. J. Sokol, S. Miller and G. Reed, *Alcoholism: Clinical and Experimental Research* 4(2): 135-145, April 1980.

A study of 12,127 pregnancies at a single institution found complications by maternal alcohol abuse of 1.7 percent. Patients tended to be older multigravidas who were not currently married. Their obstetric histories were marked by an excessive incidence of previous spontaneous abortions, low birth weights and fetal anomalies. They were more likely to smoke and abuse drugs. The risk of intrauterine growth retardation was estimated to be increased 2.4-fold in association with alcohol abuse alone, 1.8-fold with smoking alone, and 3.9-fold with combined smoking/alcohol use.

3.29.13 "The Effects of Moderate Alcohol Consumption During Pregnancy on Fetal Growth and Morphogensis," Hanson, et al.. *Journal of Pediatrics* 92(3), 457-460 (March 1978).

Data from this study of 163 selected offspring of mothers at a Seattle hospital suggested that the risk of having a newborn child with Fetal Alcohol Syndrome (FAS) increases proportionately with the average daily alcohol intake. If average maternal ingestion is less than one ounce of absolute alcohol per day/the apparent risk for abnormalities appears to be low. In the range of one to two ounces of absolute alcohol per day, the risk may approach 10 percent. Among women who drank an average of two or more ounces of ethanol daily, 19 percent had infants who were considered abnormal.

3.29.14 "Women's Drinking and Drinking Problems: Patterns from a 1981 National Survey," Richard Wilsnack, S. Wilsnack and A. Klassen, *American Journal of Public Health* 74(11):1231-1238, November 1984

Adverse drinking consequences and episodes of extreme drinking were most common among women aged 21-34. Women with extremely high consumption levels were more likely to have histories of obstetrical and gynecological problems. (Some 17% of all women drinkers, 27% of moderate, 45% heavier drove a car while feeling drunk or high at least once during the past year.

3.29.15 "Alcohol-Related Relative Risk of Fatal Driver Injuries in Relation to Driver Age and Sex," P.L. Zador, *Journal of Studies on Alcohol*, 52(4): 302 ,1991.

A study based on driver fatalities in single-vehicle crashes, it was estimated at each 0.02 percentage increase in the blood alcohol content (BAC) of a driver with a non-zero BAC nearly double the risk of being in a fatal crash. At a BAC in the 0.05-0.09% range the likelihood of a crash was at least 9 times greater than at zero BAC for all age groups. Females had a higher relative risk than males. See also "Trends in Alcohol-Related Traffic Fatalities, by Sex-United States." Centers For Disease Control, *JAMA* 268(3): 313, July 15,1992. Citing various studies.

3.29.16 "Effects of Maternal Marijuana and Cocaine Use on Fetal Growth, B," Zuckerman, D. Frank, R. Hingson, H. Amaro, *New England J. Med.* 320:762-768, March 23,1989.

Cocaine or marijuana use increases risk of shorter gestation, low birth weight and spontaneous abortion. Some 80% of marijuana users and 80% of cocaine users also smoked. Alcohol use also was higher in drug users than non-users. Cocaine users had 22% incidence of sexually transmitted disease vs. 12-13% for other groups.

3.29.17 "Surgeon General's Advisory on Alcohol and Pregnancy," *FDA Bulletin* 11(2) (1981)

In a recent report to the president and Congress, it was stated that alcohol consumption during pregnancy can harm the fetus especially in the early months. Decreased birth weights have been noted in some women who average only one ounce of absolute alcohol per day during pregnancy. Sizable and significant increases of spontaneous abortions at reported alcohol consumption as low as one ounce of absolute alcohol twice per week. A woman who consumes alcohol at amounts consistent with a diagnosis of alcoholism risks bearing a child with fetal alcohol syndrome. (Fetal alcohol syndrome is frequently associated with mental retardation, central nervous system disorders, growth deficiencies, facial abnormalities, and other malformations.)

3.30 Substance Abuse and Induced Abortion

3.30.1 "Fetal Alcohol Syndrome (FAS) Primary Prevention Through FAS Diagnosis: II. A Comprehesive Profile of Birth Mothers of Children with FAS," SJ Astley et al, *Alcohol & Alcoholism* 35(5): 509-519, 2000.

In a study of birth mothers of children with fetal alcohol syndrome, 31.3 % reported having used abortion as birth control.

3.30.2   "Substance Abuse in Pregnant Women: Recent Experience at the Perinatal Center for Chemical Dependence of Northwestern Memorial Hospital," L.G. Keith et al, *Obstet. Gynecol.* 73: 715,1989

In a study of pregnant women who used drugs, cocaine users averaged 1.8 abortions, opiate users averaged 1.0 abortions, cocaine plus opiate users averaged 1.9 abortions, and non-drugs using controls averaged 0.6 abortions.

3.30.3   "Drug Use as a Risk Factor for Premarital Teen Pregnancy and Abortion in a National Sample of Young White Women," B. Mensch, D.B. Kandel, *Demography* 29(3): 409, August, 1992.

In the National Longitudinal Survey of Youth, illicit drug use among adolescents increased the likelihood of an abortion fivefold.

3.30.4   "Prevalence of Illicit Drugs Detected in the Urine of Women of Childbearing Age in Alabama Public Health Clinics," *Public Health Reports* 109(4): 530, July/Aug. 1994

In a 1991 Alabama study of women attending maternity, family planning and obstetrical clinics throughout the state, the prevalence of positive findings for any drug, marijuana or cocaine significantly increased with an increasing number of abortions.

3.30.5   "The Incidence and Effects of Alcohol and Drug Abuse in Women Following Induced Abortion," Thomas W. Strahan, *Association for Interdisciplinary Research Newsletter* 3(2): 1-8 Summer, 1990

Summary of the literature

3.30.6   "Alcoholism in Women: Social and Psychological Concomitants," E.S. Lisansky, Quarterly Journal of Studies in Alcohol 18:588,609(1957). (Prior abortion listed as one of the reasons for drinking.

3.30.7   "Stressful Life Events and Alcohol Problems Among Women Seen at a Detoxification Center," E.R. Morrissey and M.A. Schuckit, *Journal of Studies on Alcohol* 39(9): 1559-1576, 1978

Eighty-nine percent of 262 women had experienced a prior gynecological event; 18% had prior abortions. Problem drinkers and secondary alcoholics were likely to have experienced alcohol-related problems subsequent to abortion. Problem drinkers and secondary alcoholics had a wide variety of health and social problems.

3.30.8   *The Psycho-Social Aspects of Stress Following Abortion,* Anne Catherine Speckhard, (Sheed and Ward: Kansas City, 1987)

Sixty percent of 30 women experiencing psychosocial stress following abortion reported increased alcohol use. A majority reported their first heavy use of drugs or alcohol in conjunction with stress related to abortion.

3.30.9 "Post-Abortion Trauma, 9 Steps To Recovery," Jeanette Vought (Grand Rapids: Zondervan, 1991) p. 111-112.

In a 1990 study of 68 religiously oriented women (primarily Evangelical and Lutheran) 10-15 years post-abortion, 37% of the women reported they frequently used alcohol and 21% frequently used drugs. Of the women who used alcohol, 48% began drinking after their abortion experience. Of the women who used drugs, 42.9% started using them after their abortion experience.

3.30.10 "Physical and psychological Injury in Women Following Abortion: Akron Pregnancy Services Survey," L.H. Gsellman, *Association for Interdisciplinary Research Newsletter* 5(4):1-8, Sept/Oct 1993.

In a survey of 344 postabortion women receiving a variety of services Akron Pregnancy Services, Akron, Ohio during 1988-1993 ,17% reported alcohol/drug abuse as a psychological problem following abortion. In a sub-sample of African-American women, 6% reported alcohol/drug abuse as a psychological problem following abortion.

3.30.11 "Patterns of Alcohol and Cigarette Use in Pregnancy," J. Kuzma and D. Kissinger, *Neurobehavioral Toxicology and Teratology* 3:211-221(1981).

In a California study of more than 12,000 women during 1975-1977, of those having a history of two or more abortions, virtually all (98.5%) consumed alcohol throughout the entire 9 months of a subsequent pregnancy and at higher levels than any of the other categories studied (up to 3 oz. per day) Overall, 51% of the women drank and 35% smoked during the pregnancy.

3.30.12 "Sexual Experience and Drinking Among Women in a U.S. National Survey," A. Klassen and S. Wilsnack, *Archives of Sexual Behavior* 15(5): 363-392 (1986)

In a 1981 random survey of 917 women in the U.S., 4% of the abstainers had a prior reported non-spontaneous abortion compared to 5% for light drinkers (under 0.22 oz. absolute alcohol per day), 13% for moderate drinkers (0.22-0.99 oz. absolute alcohol per day) , and 13% for heavy drinkers (at least 1 oz. absolute alcohol per day) compared to 6% for all ever pregnant women. Moderate and heavy drinkers combined exceeded lighter drinkers in abortion experience to a statistically significant degree.

3.30.13 "Characteristics of pregnant women who engage in binge alcohol consumption," J Gladstone et al, *Can Med Assoc J* 156 (6): 789-808, 1997

Women who were binge drinkers during their pregnancy had a significantly higher rate of previous therapeutic abortions.

3.30.14 "Overdose and termination of pregnancy: an important association?," H. Houston, L. Jacobson,

Br. J. General Practice 46: 737-738, Dec. 1996

A significant association was found between a recorded and treated drug overdose either before or after an induced abortion with a majority of such events occurring within two years of each other.

3.30.15 *Aborted Women: Silent No More,* David C. Reardon (Chicago: Loyola Univ. Press, 1987).

According to anecdotal reports substance abuse occurred in women following induced abortion to overcome nightmares or insomnia, as an attempt to reduce grief reactions, and to repress the abortion experience itself.

3.30.16 "Therapeutic Abortion on Psychiatric Grounds," S.A. Drower and E.S. Nash, *South Africa Medical Journal* 54(2): 604-608 Oct 7/1978.

Increased use of alcohol, tobacco, drugs and tranquilizers was found in women who aborted compared to women who were refused abortion and had a variety of pregnancy outcomes where each group had presented for abortion for psychiatric reasons at a Capetown, South Africa hospital.

3.30.17 *Women,* Drinking and Pregnancy, Moria Plant, (London: Tavistock Publications, 1985)

In a Scottish study of 1,008 women, those with a history of induced abortion had significantly higher self-reported levels of alcohol consumption in pregnancy than those with a history of stillbirth, spontaneous abortion, or having had a mentally or physically handicapped child.

3.30.18 "Drug Use Among Adolescent Mothers: Profile of Risk," H. Amaro, B. Zuckerman and H. Cabral, *Pediatrics* 84:144-150, July 1989.

In a study of inner-city adolescent mothers, those with a history of induced abortion were twice as likely to be involved in alcohol, marijuana or cocaine compared with non-using controls.

3.30.19 "Drug Use and Other Determinants of Premarital Pregnancy and Its Outcome: A Dynamic Analysis of Competing Life Events," K Yamaguchi and DB Kandel, *Journal of Marriage and the Family* 49:257, 1987

A study of young women in the state of New York found that the current use of illicit drugs (other than marijuana) was 6.1 times higher if there was a history of a prior abortion. In contrast, women with postmarital births were much less likely (0.14) to report current use of illicit drugs.

3.30.20 "Abortion and Subsequent Substance Abuse," DC Reardon, PG Ney, *Am J Drug Alcohol Abuse* 26(1): 61-75, 2000

Women who aborted a first pregnancy were five times more likely to report subsequent substance abuse compared to women who carried to term.

3.30.21 "Characteristics of pregnant women exposed to cocaine in Toronto between 1985 and 1990," K

Graham and G Koren, *Can Med Assoc J* 144(5): 563, 1991

In a Toronto study of pregnant women, cocaine users had a higher mean average of elective abortions compared to non-users of drugs.

3.30.22 "Health issues associated with increasing use of "crack" cocaine among female sex workers in London," H Ward et al, *Sex Transm Infect* 76(4): 292-293, 2000

34% of female sex workers in London reported using " crack" cocaine in 1995-1996. Crack use was associated with abortion and with hepatitis C infection.

3.30.23 "Cocaine Use During Pregnancy: Prevalence and Correlates," D.A. Frank, B. Zuckerman, H. Amaro, K. Aboagye, *Pediatrics* 82(6):888-895, December 1988.

In a study of drug abuse among Boston inner-city women during pregnancy/those using cocaine were twice as likely to have a history of two elective abortions (19% vs. 9%) and three times more likely to have had three or more elective abortions (9% vs. 3%) than non-cocaine using controls. Cocaine users were more likely to drink alcohol, use cigarettes, marijuana, opiates and other illicit drugs compared to cocaine non-users.

3.30.24 "Direct and Indirect Interactions of Cocaine with Childbirth Outcomes," L Singer et al, *Arch Pediatr Adolesc* Med 148: 959-964, 1994

A retrospective review of hospital charts over a one year period compared women who tested positive for cocaine during pregnancy compared with matched controls who did not use cocaine found that cocaine use was the best predictor of increased incidence of abortions.

3.30.25 "Perinatal cocaine and methamphetamine exposure: Maternal and neonatal correlates," A.S. Oro and S.D. Dixon, *Journal of Pediatrics* 111:571-578(1987).

In a San Diego study of drug use, women who used cocaine and/or methamphetamine averaged 1.7 abortions compared with 1.2 abortions for non-drug using controls. Women who used heroin or methadone were more likely to have had abortions (2.4 vs. 1.2) than non-drug using controls. Infants exposed to both heroin and either cocaine or methamphetamine had mothers with the highest number of pregnancies (5) and abortions (2.7). These infants had the highest percentage of no prenatal care, prematurity/poorer growth, small birth weight and fetal distress.

3.30.26 "Psychosocial Characteristics of Psychiatric Inpatients with Reproductive Losses," T Thomas et al, *Journal of Health Care for the Poor and Underserved* 7(1): 15, 1996

Women hospitalized for major psychiatric disorders with a history of abortion were significantly more likely to have received the diagnosis of psychoactive substance abuse (DSM-IIIR criteria) and significantly more likely to report substance abuse, alcohol abuse and cocaine abuse compared to women with no live birth.

3.30.27 "Abortion in Adolescence," Nancy B. Campbell/ K. Franco and S. Jurs, *Adolescence* 23(92):813-

823, Winter 1988.

A study at the Medical College of Ohio compared differences in 35 women who had their abortions as teenagers with 36 women who had their abortions after the age of 20. Antisocial and paranoid disorders as well as drug abuse and psychotic delusions were found to be significantly higher in the group who aborted as teenagers. Adolescents were more likely to retreat into sexual activity or drug and alcohol abuse.

3.31   Smoking

3.31.1   "Morbidity and Mortality in Children Associated With the Use of Tobacco Products by Other People," J.R. DiFranza, R.A. Lew, *Pediatrics* 97(4): 560 April, 1996

Based on meta-analysis it was concluded that the use of tobacco products by adults has an enormous adverse impact on the health of children.

3.31.2   "The Relationship Between Idiopathic Mental Retardation and Maternal Smoking During Pregnancy," C.D. Drews et. al. *Pediatrics* 97(4): 547, April, 1996

A study by researchers at Emory University suggested that maternal smoking may be a preventable cause of mental retardation in children.

3.31.3   "Characteristics of Women by Smoking Status in the San Francisco Bay Area," E.A. Holly et al.. *Cancer Epidemiology, Biomarkers & Prevention*: 1: 491-497, Sept/Oct 1992

Women smokers were more likely than non-smokers to consume larger quantities of coffee, soft drinks, liquor and beer; more likely to have had first sexual intercourse before age 16; had a greater number of lifetime sexual partners; were more likely to have been pregnant and report a history of chlamydia, gonorrhea and/or pelvic inflammatory disease.

3.31.4   "Pregnancy Decision Making as a Significant Life Event: A Commitment Approach," J Lydon et al, *J. of Personality & Social Psychology* 71(1): 141-151, July, 1996.

57 women from either Los Angeles or Montreal were interviewed during a clinic visit for a pregnancy test, and subsequently received positive test results. They were interviewed a second time two days later. A third interview took place a month after the women had undergone an induced abortion or carried to term Those women continuing the pregnancy reported smoking fewer cigarettes at the third interview compared to the first interview, while those who had abortions did not report a change in smoking behavior. see Changes in Smoking and Drinking During Pregnancy, CA Hilton, JT Condon, Aust NZ Obstet Gynaecol 29:18, 1989 (An Australian study found that the primary reason influencing smoking and drinking behavior during pregnancy was that doing so might harm the baby.).

3.31.5   "Psychological responses following medical abortion (using mifepristone and gemepost) and surgical aspiration," R Henshaw et al, *Acta Obstet Gynecol Scand* 73:812, 1994.

A study of Scottish women who had an induced abortion by use of either mifepristone and gemepost or vacuum aspiration found that at 16 days postabortion, anxiety scores correlated with the number of cigarettes smoked, with the most anxious women having the heaviest smoking habits.

3.31.6   "Increased Smoking Rates in Women Following Induced Abortion," Thomas W. Strahan, *Association for Interdisciplinary Research Newsletter* 2(2):5-8, Spring, 1989

Review of the literature.

3.31.7   "Pregnancy and Patterns of Tobacco Use: Shifts and Directions," in Forbes, Frecker, Nostbakken, ed. *Proceeding of the Fifth World Conference on Smoking and Health*, Vol. 1 (Winnipeg, Canada: Ottawa Council on Smoking and Health, 1983) 117-120.

Data on tobacco use before, during and after pregnancy showed that 80 percent of the women surveyed were aware of smoking's adverse effects. The proportion of smokers declined from 49 percent before pregnancy to 35 percent during pregnancy. The major reasons cited for not smoking were less desire to smoke and concern for the infant. After pregnancy/however, smoking increased again to before pregnancy frequency.

3.31.8   "An Overview: Maternal Nicotine and Caffeine Consumption and Offspring Outcome," J.C. Martin, *Neurobehavioral Toxicology and Teratology* 4(4): 421-27, July-August 1982.

Smoking during pregnancy generally results in a 150-200 mg. reduction in weight, a 20 percent increase in neonatal death for those smoking a pack per day/and a 35 percent greater chance of neonatal death for those smoking a pack per day. There is also a possible increase in congenital anomalies, decrease in growth rate, and a compromise in cognitive function in early and middle childhood. Only 12-13 percent of smoking women curtail their habit during pregnancy, and it has been estimated that 4,600 of the 87,000 infant deaths in the U.S. during the prenatal period would have been prevented if their mothers had not smoked.

3.31.9   "Smoking and Women. Tragedy of the Majority," J. F. Fielding, *New England Journal of Medicine,* 317(21), November 19/1987, pp. 1343-1345.

Since the release of the first Surgeon General's report on smoking and health in 1964, the prevalence of female smokers had declined at a considerably slower rate than that of male smokers. The decline in adult male smokers has been 21.4 percent, as compared with only 5.8 percent in women. Currently, 25.7 percent of adult women smoke as compared with 31.5 percent of men. Smoking reduces fertility, increases the rate of spontaneous abortion of chromosomally normal fetuses/and increases the incidence of abruptio placenta, placenta previa, bleeding during pregnancy and premature rupture of the membranes. Because of these effects, smoking results in many thousands of preventable fetal and neonatal deaths. Pregnant women must understand that giving their unborn child the best chance of being normal at birth and surviving the perinatal period requires that they stop smoking. Organizations that have been actively working for women's rights might consider devoting some attention to helping women wean themselves from a habit that is usually unwanted and known to be self-destructive.

3.31.10 "Managing the Uncomplicated Pregnancy," J.M. Bengston, R. Petrie and J.C. Shank, *Patient Care,* December 15,1987, pp. 56-93.

Very detailed listing of items to consider during pregnancy. It states that risks to patient and baby associated with smoking include miscarriage, premature birth, stillbirth, abruptio placenta and placenta previa, low birth weight, sudden infant death syndrome, neurobehavioral deficits, and susceptibility to respiratory infections during infancy.

3.31.11 "Mixed Messages for Women: A Social History of Cigarette Smoking," Virginia L. Emster, *New York State Journal of Medicine,* 85(7): 335-34, July, 1985; also "Getting Women Hooked: Defending the Indefensible, Women and Children Last?" J.L. Stenfeld, *N.Y. State J. Med.* 83(13): 1257, Dec, 1983; "Precious Baby." Mary Ann Comer, *N.Y. State J.Med.* 83(13): 1292, Dec, 1983.

This valuable collection of articles written by the health profession should be read in connection with articles in the same journal in July 1985. The articles attack the feminist movement and urge the medical profession to become more active in the smoking and health field. For example, the article "Precious Baby" states, "Ms. Magazine [May 1983 issue] was devoted entirely to the topic of women's health without a clear emphasis on the leading cause of preventable disease and death in women-cigarettes. In its 13 year existence Ms. has never published an article on smoking but has carried hundreds of pages of cigarette advertising." Apparently many women in the feminist movement smoke themselves. See *New York State Journal of Medicine*, December 1983, p. 1258.

3.31.12 "Women's Smoking Trends and Awareness of Health Risk," R. Tagliacozzo and S. Vaughn, *Preventive Medicine* 9:384-387(1980).

Several studies have reported results indicating that in treatment programs designed to stop smoking, women are less successful than men in achieving and maintaining abstinence. Cites several studies.

3.31.13 *United States Public Health Service. Adult Use of Tobacco,* (Atlanta: U.S. Department of Health, Education and Welfare, Center for Disease Control, Bureau of Health Education, 1975).

Women are more likely to report that they use cigarettes to deal with emotional upset than men. Women are more likely than men to affirm, "When I feel blue or want to take my mind off troubles, I smoke cigarettes," and "I light up when I feel angry about something."

3.31.14 "Personality Variables Associated With Cigarette Smoking," Richard W. Coan, *Journal of Personality and Social Psychology* 26(1): 86-104(1973).

Valuable study on the differences between smokers and non-smokers. Male smokers had the greatest extroversion while female non-smokers had the greatest introversion. Smokers tended to experience more distress or disturbance than non-smokers. There is a tendency for men to be more liberal than women, and for smokers to be more liberal than non-smokers. Nonsmokers tend to attach greater importance to deliberate and planned action, while smokers favored spontaneity. Smokers tended toward uncontrolled complexity rather than organized simplicity in their preferences and thought processes. Smokers tended to manifest aesthetic rather than practical interests. Smokers tended to show more tolerance if not actual hunger for varied ideas/ emotional and perceptual effects, complexity and perhaps even confusion. Non-smokers had a greater need for control, order and simplicity. Women tend to be more psychologically sensitive than men-they are aware of a greater range of effects in their private experience. Smokers have a higher level of anxiety than non-smokers. Smokers manifest more psychomatic symptoms, more pretension, more guilt proneness, more ergic tension, a higher Taylor anxiety score, more unrealistic fantasy content, less self-control over internal processes, more nervous tension. Evidently smokers dwelled more on the past than non-smokers but future time perspective was highest in the male smokers and lowest in the female smokers. Future time perspective represents percentage measures based upon the subject's assignment of his recent topics of conversation to the categories of past, present and future.

3.31.15 "Smoking in Pregnancy: a study of psychosocial and reproductive risk factors," AW Morales et al, *J Psychosom Obstet Gynaecol* 18(4): 247, 1997

A British study found that women with a higher incidence of smoking in pregnancy were more likely to have previous miscarriages and terminations.

3.31.16 "The pregnant smoker: a preliminary investigation of the social and psychological influences," C Haslam et al, *Journal of Public Health Medicine* 19(2): 187-192, 1997

Pregnant smokers, when asked, 'What in particular, causes you to have an urge to smoke?'; two-thirds gave an emotional state (stress, boredom, feeling upset) for their answer.

3.31.17 "Characteristics of young female smokers in a Swedish primary health care area," J Liljestrand et al, *Scand J Primary Health Care* 11:157, 1993

A 1990 Swedish study found that women smokers were significantly more likely to have prior legal abortions (19%) compared to non-smokers (9%). There were no differences between smokers and non-smokers where there were prior miscarriages or live born children.

3.31.18 "Induced abortion is not a cause of subsequent pre-term delivery in teenage pregnancies," TT Lao and LF Ho, *Human Reproduction* 13(3): 758, 1998.

In a Hong Kong study, 39% of teenage mothers with a history of induced abortion who delivered were smokers compared to 14.4% of teenage mothers who delivered but had no induced abortion history.

3.31.19 "Relation between smoking in reproductive age women and disorders in reproduction," D Hrub'a and P Kachl'ik, *Ceska Gynekol* 62(4): 191-196, 1997.

A study of women teachers in the Czech Republic found that smokers significantly more often had abortions of unwanted pregnancies compared to non-smokers.

3.31.20 "Outcome of First Delivery After 2nd Trimester Two-Stage Induced Abortion. A Controlled Historical Cohort Study," O. Meirik and K.G. Nygren, *Acta Obstetricia et Gynecological Scandinavica* 63(1): 45-50(1984).

A positive correlation between maternal smoking and history of abortion was found in an historical cohort study of the outcome of the first birth after a legal second trimester two-stage abortion induced with saline or prostaglandin. It was concluded that low birth weight of infants born to aborters may be related as much to maternal smoking as to the previously induced abortion.

3.31.21 "Pregnancy Complications Following Legally Induced Abortion: An Analysis of the Population with Special Reference to Prematurity," E.B. Obel, *Danish Medical Bulletin* 26:192-199(1979).

A study of 7,327 pregnant women at two Copenhagen hospitals found 63 percent smokers where there was one or more prior induced abortions, 51 percent smokers where there was a history of one or more spontaneous abortions, 49 percent smokers where there was a previous live birth, and 55 percent smokers where there was no previous history of pregnancy. After 28 weeks gestation 43.1% still smoked during pregnancy if the last pregnancy was terminated by abortion compared to only 32.1 % if live birth or 30.2% for no previous pregnancy.

3.31.22 "Characteristics of Pregnant Women Reporting Previous Induced Abortions," S Harlap and A. Davies, *Bulletin World Health Organization*, 52:149(1975).

Smokers have twice the rate of reporting previous induced abortion than non-smokers i.e. 12 percent vs. 6 percent based upon standardized rates among Arab and Israeli women.

3.31.23 "Early Complications of Induced Abortion in Primigravidae," K. Dalaker, K. Sundfor, and J. Skuland *Annales Chirurgiae et Gynaecologiae* 70(6): 331-336(1981).

A statistically significant difference was found between the smoking habits of women under 19 years and those over 19. The incidence of pelvic inflammatory disease after the abortion was highest in the group of patients who, in addition to having a high frequency of smokers/ were characterized by a low age of menarche and a low rate of married or cohabit status. (Abstracted in Smoking and Health Bulletin, U.S. Department of Health and Human Services, Public Health Services [1982}, p. 396)

3.31.24 "Ectopic Pregnancy and Myoma Uteri: Tetragenic Effects and Maternal Characteristics," E. Matsunaga and E. Shiota, *Teratology* 21:61-69 (1980).

Ectopic pregnancy was found to be associated with lower parity, previous ectopic pregnancy and maternal smoking and drinking. The frequency of fetal malformations was 11.6 percent among 43 recovered from ectopic pregnancies, compared with 6.2 percent among 97 from myomatous pregnancies, and 3.3 percent among 3/1474 from normally implanted pregnancies not complicated by myomas. Incidence of smoking was 9.4 percent in the myomatous pregnancy group, 29.2 percent in the ectopic pregnancy group, and 15.1 percent in the prior induced abortion group. (Japanese study at National Institute of Genetics)

3.31.25 "Association of Induced Abortion with Subsequent Pregnancy Loss," A. Levin, S.C. Schoenbaum, R. Monson, P.G. Stubblefield and K. Ryan, *Journal of the American Medical Association* 243:2495-2499, June 27, 1980.

(Women patients of Boston Hospital had smoking rates of 31.7 percent with no prior induced abortion, 40.3 percent with one prior abortion and 51.7 percent with two or more prior abortions.

3.31.26 "Low Birth Weight In Relation To Multiple Induced Abortions," M.T. Mandelson, C.B. Maden, J.R. Daling, *AmJ. Public Health,* 82(3):391-394, March, 1992.

In a Washington State study of 6541 white women who delivered a child between 1984-87, 41.6% of the women smoked during this pregnancy if they had a history of 4 or more induced abortions compared with 31.0% smokers (2 prior abortions), 28.1% smokers (1 prior abortion) or 18.0% smokers (no prior abortions).

3.31.27 "A study on the effects of induced abortion on subsequent pregnancy outcome," C. Madore, W.E. Hawes, F. Many, A.C. Hexter, *Am. J. Obstet. Gynecol.* 139: 516, 1981.

A California case-control study in 1976-78 of women with a history of one or more previous induced abortions compared to control subjects without a history of abortion found that 11.8% of women with an abortion history smoked 1 pack of cigarettes per day compared to 8.1% of controls which was statistically significant.

3.31.28 "A Prospective Study of Smoking and Pregnancy," S. Kullander and B. Kallen, *Acta Obstet. Gynec. Scand.* 50:83-94(1971).

A study of 6,363 Swedish women during 1963-64 found that 56.1% of the women smoked who had induced abortions compared with 43.3% smokers among women having given birth. Information on whether the pregnancy was wanted was obtained on 4,843 women. Among those reporting wanted pregnancies 41.5% were smokers vs. 52.4% among women who reported unwanted pregnancies (later carried to term). Some 18.9% of the women with wanted pregnancies smoked 10 or more cigarettes per day vs. 27.1% of women reporting unwanted pregnancies.

3.31.29 "Outcome of First Delivery After Second Trimester Two Staged Induced Abortion: A Controlled Historical Cohort Study," O. Meirik, K.G. Nygren, *Acta Obstet. Gynecol. Scand.* 63(1):45-50 (1984)

In a later study of 4,719 Swedish women during 1970-1978, 58.1% of those women with a history of abortion smoked (37.4% smoked 10 or more cigarettes per day) compared with 40.4% smokers among parity-matched controls (21.1% of parity-matched controls smoked 10 or more cigarettes per day) and all Swedish women generally in 1975 (37.8% smoked and 18.9% of all Swedish women smoked 10 or more cigarettes per day).

3.31.30   "Smoking During Pregnancy and Child Maltreatment: Is There An Association?," J. Chessare, J. Pascoe and E. Baugh, *Int'l J. Biosocial Research* 8(1): 37-42, (1986).

Women who smoked during pregnancy were three times more likely to be reported for maltreatment in the first 18 months after birth compared with non-smoking mothers. (22.6% vs. 7.6%)

3.32   Long-Terms Effects of Abortion

3.32.1   "Induced Elective Abortion and Perinatal Grief," Gail B. Williams, *Dissertation Abstracts Int'l.* 53(3): 1296B, Sept. 1992.

A study of 83 white women with one first trimester abortion, no documented psychiatric history and no self-reported prenatal losses in the last 5 years an average of 11 years postabortion. The Grief Experience Inventory was used as a test instrument and found a range of scores from 27-82. 50 represents at least minimal grief on 12 bereavement/research scales. Various scales measured included anger/hostility, social isolation, loss of control, death anxiety, loss of vigor, physical symptoms, dependency, somatization, sleep disturbance, loss of appetite, optimism/despair, denial. It was concluded that some women experienced persistence of various aspects of grief for long periods of time following induced abortion.

3.32.2   *The Psycho-Social Aspects of Stress Following Abortion,* Anne C. Speckhard, (Kansas City: Sheed and Ward, 1987)

In a study of 30 women stressed by abortion after 5-10 years following their abortion, women reported feelings of sadness, regret, remorse or a sense of loss [100 percent]; feelings of depression [92 percent]; feelings of anger [92 percent]; feelings of guilt [92 percent]; fear that others would learn of the pregnancy and abortion experience [89 percent]; many expressed surprise at the intensity of the emotional reaction to the abortion [85 percent]; Other adverse reactions included feelings of lowered self-worth [81 percent]; feelings of victimization [81 percent]; preoccupation with the characteristics of the aborted child [81 percent]; feelings of depressed effect or suppressed ability to experience pain [73 percent]; and feelings of discomfort around infants and small children [73 percent]. In this study the most common behavioral reactions included frequent crying [81 percent]; inability to communicate with others concerning the pregnancy and abortion experience [77 percent]; flashbacks of the abortion experience [73 percent]; sexual inhibition [69 percent]; suicide ideation [65 percent] and increased alcohol use [61 percent].

3.32.3   "Aborted Women: Silent No More," David C. Reardon, (Chicago: Loyola Press, 1987)

In a detailed study of 252 women with prior abortions who are members of Women Exploited by

94

Abortion approximately 10 years after their abortion, 95% were now dissatisfied with the abortion choice and 94% attributed negative psychological effects to their abortion.

3.32.4 "Mental Disorders After Abortion," B. Jansson, *Acta Psychiatrica Scandinavica* 41:87 (1965).

In a Swedish study of 57 women with prior psychiatric problems who subsequently had induced abortions, three committed suicide as determined by long-term follow-up studies 8-13 years after their abortion. In contrast, of 195 women with previous psychiatric problems who carried children to term, none committed suicide.

3.32.5 "Risk of Admission to Psychiatric Institutions Among Danish Women Who Experience induced Abortion," Ronald L. Somers, Ph.D. Thesis/ UCLA (1979)

Among women with 2 or more abortions the rate of psychiatric admissions among women 35-39 (approx. 9%) was about 4 times higher than women 25-29 years of age (approx. 2.3%) and 8-18 times higher than women 20-24 years of age (0.5-1.1%) during 1973-1975.

3.32.6 "Psychological Aspects of Abortion," Edna Ortof in *Psychological Aspects of Pregnancy, Birthing and Bonding,* ed. Barbara L. Blum (New York: Human Sciences Press, 1980)

Several examples of post-abortion dreams are provided. One woman had the following dream 11, years after a self-induced abortion:

"I was in my old home town with two girlfriends and about to go horseback riding... (but) we couldn't get a horse. Then some lady came over and handed me a bundle wrapped in a sheet and blankets/ like a baby. I was delighted to hold it... when I opened the bundle ... there was a kid there and it looked like it was shrinking. Like it was wasting away and I wanted the mother to come and take it away before it would die in my arms... The more I looked, the more anxious I got." The therapist reported this woman had an enormous sense of unfinished business about the pregnancy and abortion. She still had periodic intercourse without use of contraceptives with the prospective father hoping to "undo" that event. At times her guilt was overwhelming and her sense of loss increased with the passing years.

3.32.7 *A Survey of Post-Abortion Reactions,* David C. Reardon, (Springfield, Illinois: Elliot Institute, 1987)

A 1987 survey of 100 women an average of 11 years post-abortion who were contacted through state Women Exploited by Abortion chapters found that only 54% felt they had fully reconciled their abortion experience; 62% experienced the majority of their negative experience one year or more post-abortion; 97% regretted having the abortion; 62% said they felt more callused and hardened; 70% felt a need to stifle feelings; 45% said they had feelings of relief after abortion; 42% became sexually promiscuous; 50% reported aversion to sexual intercourse or sexual unresponsiveness; 54% thought the abortion choice was inconsistent with their own ideals; 64% ended the relationship with their sexual partner following the abortion (41% within one month, 9% more within 6 months and 14% more within one year.

3.32.8   *The Long-Term Psychological Effects of Abortion,* Catherine A Barnard, (Portsmouth, NH: Institute for Pregnancy Loss, 1990) Summarized in *Association for Interdisciplinary Research in Values and Social Change Newsletter* 3(4):1 (1991)

A random sample of 984 women who had abortions during 1984-84 at a clinic in Baltimore, Maryland were selected for study. However, only 160 women could be contacted 3-5 years later, Of the 160 contacted only 80 actually completed the research packets. Research instruments used were the DSM-IIIR, Impact of Events Scale, and the Millon Clinical Mulitaxial Inventory. The prevalence of Post Traumatic Disorder was 18.8%. High stress levels ranging from 39-45% were prevalent in such areas as sleep disorers, hypervigalence, or flashbacks. The variables that predicted high stress reactions were: a negative relationship with mother, a past history of emotional problems in the family of origin, a conflictual relationship with the father of the child, and poor aftercare at the clinic. The number of reported prior abortions did not predict the incidence of PTSD. 30% of the women had abortions between 14-18 years of age and few were religious at the time of their abortion.

3.32.9   "Methodological considerations in empirical research on abortion," RL Anderson et al in *Post-Abortion Syndrome. Its Wide Ramifications,* ed. Peter Doherty (1995) 103

A study at Pine Rest Christian Hospital in Grand Rapids, Michigan which provided psychiatric outpatient services, compared women who presented with a history of elective abortion and sought psychiatric outpatient services in response to a negative adjustment to abortion (the abortion distressed group), to a control group which also had a history of elective abortion but who presented for outpatient psychiatric services for reasons which were not abortion related. (the abortion non-distressed group). The average length of time from the abortion to the time of the study was 9 years. Seventy-three percent (73%) of the abortion distressed group met the criteria for Post Traumatic Stress Disorder (DSM-IIIR) which was significantly higher than the abortion non-distressed group. Women in the abortion distressed group more often reported they believed abortion to be morally wrong compared to the abortion non-distressed group. There were no significant differences among groups in psychopathology as measured by MMPI-2, on overall social support, or religiosity. Abortion distressed women experienced fewer recent adverse life events compared to abortion non-distressed women.

3.32.10 *Canonical variates of postabortion syndrome,* Helen P Vaughan, (Portsmouth, NH: Institute for Pregnancy Loss, 1990)

Questionnaires were distributed nationwide to 62 crisis pregnancy centers to women who had reported symptoms of postabortion syndrome and 232 questionnaires were returned. The mean length of time from their abortion was 11 years. It was found that postabortion syndrome was comprised of anger, guilt, grief, depression, and stress reactions. Two different dimensions of negative postabortion adjustment were noted. One dimension included high levels of anger and guilt, with a significant absence of any grief feelings. The second dimension showed high guilt and stress with a significant absence of anger. The various personality characteristics and circumstances of women in each dimension were discussed.

3.32.11 " Psychological Profile of dysphoric women postabortion," KN Franco et al, *Journal of the American Medical Women's Association* 44(4): 113, 1989

Eighty-one women in a patient-led postabortion support group years who described themselves as having poorly assimilated their abortion experience 1-15 years postabortion were studied. 78% were single at the time of their abortion and only 19% married the father of the child. The Bech Depression Inventory for women with one abortion was 4.7(none to minimal depression) and for women with multiple abortions was 9.4(moderate depression). The Millon Clinical Mulitaxial Inventory (MCMI) suggested personal pathology in the form of anxiety (48%), somatoform disorders (58%), and dysthymia (36%). Those with multiple abortions scored on the borderline personality subscales. Some 48% of the group underwent psychotherapy after their abortion; 50% of women with multiple abortions made a suicide attempt sometime after their abortions; anniversary reactions were clearly reported by 42% of the sample. For additional studies on this sample of postabortion women see "Anniversary Reactions and Due Date Responses Following Abortion," K Franco et al, *Psychother Psychosom* 52:151, 1989; "Abortion in Adolescence," NB Campbell et al, *Adolescence*, 23(92), 1988

3.32.12 *Post-Abortion Trauma,* 9 steps to Recovery, Jeanette Vought, (Grand Rapids: Zondervan, 1991).

In a study of women in a religiously-based postabortion recovery group 10-15 years post-abortion, 90% reported guilt and shame related to their abortion, 74% feelings of isolation, 60% expressed anger toward others, 24% were more fearful of sexual intercourse after their abortion, 31% tried to avoid pregnant women, 53% said they desired to get pregnant again to compensate for their loss; 76% suffered from depression, 78% struggled with low self-esteem and 49% said they felt alienated from God. Following their abortion, women reported insomnia (25%), negative and hurtful relationships with men (38%, abortion had a negative effect on parenting (32.4%), frequent alcohol use (17.8%), frequent drug use (9.2%) as well as other negative personal or relational problems.

3.32.13 "Physical and Psychological Injury Following Abortion: Akron Pregnancy Services Survey," L.H. Gsellman, *Association For Interdisciplinary Research Newsletter* 5(4):1-8, Sept/Oct 1993.

In a questionnaire study of 344 post-abortal women receiving a variety of services at a pregnancy service center an average of 6 years following their abortion, 66% expressed guilt, 54% expressed regret or remorse, 46% had an inability to forgive self, 57% reported crying or depression, 38% reported lower self-esteem and 36% reported anger or rage, 16% reported suicidal impulses and 7% made suicide attempts. 18.4% of the abortions were at 13 weeks gestation or more; 22% reported two abortions and 4.3% reported three or more abortions.

3.32.14 "Prolonged Grieving After Abortion. A Descriptive Study," D Brown et al, *The Journal of Clinical Ethics* 4(2):118, 1993.

Upon request, women from a large protestant congregation in Florida wrote descriptive letters on the negative effects of abortion. 45 letters contained sufficient information to compile statistical information, 81% were first trimester abortions and 71% occurred after Roe v Wade was decided. 42% reported negative emotional sequelae that lasted over 10 years. Frequently mentioned long term experiences included guilt feelings (73.3%), fantasizing about the aborted fetus(57.8%), masking their experience with the appearance of well-being (35.5%), suicide ideation (15.5%), recurrent nightmares(15.5%), marital discord (15.5%), phobic responses to infants (13.3%), as well as fear of men (8.9%) and disinterest in sex (6.7%).

3.33 Replacement Pregnancies/Rapid Repeat Pregnancies After Abortion

3.33.1 "Adolescent Mourning Reactions to Infant and Fetal Loss," NH Horowitz, *Social Casework* 59:551, 1978.

Replacement pregnancies may follow adolescent abortion.

3.33.2 "Post-Abortion Perceptions: A Comparison of Self-Identified Distressed and Non-Distressed Populations," GK Congleton and GC Calhoun, *The Int'l Journal of Social Psychiatry* 39(4): 255, 1993.

Women experiencing postabortion stress were more likely to report a desire to replace the fetus, report depression around the anniversary date or due date, and immediately experience feelings of loss compared to women reporting relieving/neutral postabortion experiences.

3.33.3 "Post-Abortion Trauma; 9 Steps to Recovery," Jeanette Vought (Grand Rapids: Zondervan, 1991)

53% of women in a religiously-based postabortion recovery group stated they desired to get pregnant again to compensate for the loss.

3.33.4 "Physical and Psychological Injury in Women Following Abortion: Akron Pregnancy Services Survey," L Gsellman, *Association for Interdisciplinary Research in Values and Social Change Newsletter* 5(4): 108, Sept/Oct, 1993

In a questionnaire survey of post-abortion women who were obtaining a variety of services at a pregnancy services center between 1988-93, 23% stated they desired to get pregnant again as a psychological reaction to abortion.

3.33.5 "Selection bias in a study on how women experienced induced abortion," H Soderberg et al, *Eur J Obstet & Gynecol* 77:67, 1998.

Swedish researchers at Lund University calculated that of approximately 33,000 induced abortions in Sweden each year, that about 6000 of these women will become pregnant again within 12 months, with half of them carrying to term, and the other half undergoing another induced abortion. (Non-participants in the follow-up study seemed to have a sense of guilt that they did not wish to discuss. These non-participants were significantly more likely to conceive again within 12 months and carry to term compared to study participants.)

3.33.6 "Conception rates after abortion with methotrexate and misoprostol," MD Creinin, *Int'l J Gynaecol Obstet* 65: 183-188, 1999.

25% of women who had abortions using methotrexate and misoprostol became pregnant again within the next 12 months. The vast majority of these pregnancies resulted in another induced abortion.

3.33.7 "Contraception and Repeat Abortion: An Epidemiological Investigation," MJ Shephard and MB Bracken, *J Biosocial Science* 11:289, 1979.

In a Connecticut study of abortion and contraceptive practice, it was found that 42% of women repeating abortion had had an abortion within the previous year.

3.33.8 "Repeat Pregnancies Among Metropolitan Area Teenagers, 1971-1979," MA Koenig and M Zelnik, *Family Planning Perspectives* 14(6):341, Nov/Dec 1982.

Among metropolitan teenagers age 15-19 whose first premarital pregnancy ended in abortion, 27% had a second premarital pregnancy within 12 months, 49.8% within 18 months and 74.9% within 24 months postabortion.

3.33.9 "Rapid Repeat Pregnancy and Experiences of Interpersonal Violence Among Low-Income Adolescents," M Jacoby et al, *Am J Prev Med* 16(4):318-321, 1999.

A Michigan study of low income women aged 13-21 found that within 12 months of a prior pregnancy outcome (delivery, spontaneous abortion, elective abortion), 43.6% of the women were again pregnant within 12 months, and by 18 months 63.2% had experienced at least one additional pregnancy. Women whose pregnancies ended in spontaneous or elective abortion were more likely to experience rapid repeat pregnancy than women who carried to term.

3.34   Sterilization

3.34.1 "Women regretting their sterilization," H.M. Vemer, P. Colla, D. Schoot, W. Willemsen, P.B. Bierkens and R. Rolland, *Fertility and Sterility* 46(4): 724 (1986).

In a Dutch study, 118 sterilized women who came to the hospital between 1978-84 for a reversal were compared to a set of matched control women, each of whom was sterilized on or about the same date and at the same hospital as the woman requesting reversal. A change in marital status was more frequent in patients requesting reversal compared with controls. Some 20% of the sterilization in the regretting group took place at the time of an obstetrical procedure (mostly induced abortion) compared with only 2% of the controls.

3.34.2 "A comparison of definable traits in women requesting reversal of sterilization and women satisfied with sterilization," A. Leader, N. Galan, R. George, PJ. Taylor, *Am. J. Obstetrics and Gynecology* 145:198 (1983)

In a study at the University of Calgary, a group of 159 women who requested reversal of sterilization was compared to 160 women who were satisfied with their sterilization. Dissatisfied women were more likely to have had an abortion and were more likely to have had their sterilization at the time of the abortion (10.1 vs. 3.2%) compared to the satisfied women.

3.34.3　"Therapeutic Abortion. Fertility Plans and Psychological Sequelae," E. Greenglass, *American Journal of Orthopsychiatry* 47(1): 119, January 1977.

One hundred eighty-eight Canadian women were interviewed about 36 weeks following their abortion in 1972-73. At the time of the abortion, 27 women were sterilized (14.4%).)

3.34.4　"Safety of Post-Abortion Sterilization Compared with Interval Sterilization," M. Cheng, J. Cheong, S. Chew, H. Choo, M. Belsey and K. Edstrom, *The Lancet*, September 29,1979, p. 682

In a study by the World Health Organization of women who initially desired sterilization after abortion, 33% changed their minds or were unable to keep their appointments for sterilization six weeks after the abortion.

3.34.5　"Psychological profile of dysphoric women post-abortion," K. Franco, M. Tamburrino, N. Campbell, J. Pentz and S. Jurs, *J. of the American Medical Women's Assoc.* 44 (4): 113-115, July/August 1989.

Some 21% of the women in a post-abortion support had been medically sterilized after their abortion. Physicians should be aware that a small number of women may request hysterectomies and tubal ligations as self-punishment post abortion.

3.34.6　"Taking Liberties with Women: Abortion. Sterilization and Contraception," W. Savage, *International Journal of Health Services* 12(2): 293-307 (1982).

Reproductive freedom is being denied to women when sterilization is used without adequate counseling on the risks or reversibility or when it is made a precondition for performing an abortion. The article cites several studies on women who regretted their sterilization following abortion.

Impact of Abortion On Others

3.35　Men And Abortion

3.35.1　"Psychopathological effects of voluntary termination of pregnancy on the father called up for military service," DuBouis-Bonneford et al, *Psychologie Medicale* 14(8): 1187-1189, June 1982

Several case studies are presented of 18-22 year old males who came from disadvantaged backgrounds and were recent military recruits. All had extreme depression and/or attempted suicide brought on by the news of their wives or girlfriends having had a voluntary induced abortion. The men believed that becoming a father would make them more mature or respectable and the abortion brought on feelings of self-recrimination and self-punishment.

3.35.2 "Emotional distress among couples involved in first-trimester induced abortions," P Lauzon et al, *Canadian Family Physician* 46:2033-2040, Oct 2000

A study of short term distress reactions following abortion found that many men were highly distressed with both men and women having similar reactions.

3.35.3 "Early Adult Psychological Consequences for Males of Adolescent Pregnancy and Its Resolution," M. Buchanan, C. Robbins, *J. Youth and Adolescence* 19(4): 413, 1990.

In a Texas study of 2522 young men who were first surveyed as 7th grade students in 1971, 15% had been involved in a non-marital pregnancy by age 21. 56% of black men had girlfriends who had the child but did not marry or cohabitate, while 28% married and had the child while 16% were ended by abortion. White adolescent males tended to end non-marital adolescent pregnancies by abortion (58%) and 34% chose to marry or cohabitate. Although numbers were small, 55% of Hispanic men married or cohabitated as a result of an adolescent pregnancy. Men whose girlfriends had abortions were more distressed than the men whose girlfriends continued the pregnancy to term.

3.35.4 "Portraits of Post-Abortive Fathers Devastated by the Abortion Experience," Thomas Strahan, *Association for Interdisciplinary Research in Values and Social Change* 7(3): 1-8, Nov/Dec 1994.

Grief patterns, repressed feelings and emotions, loss of manhood or fatherhood, substance abuse, guilt, suicidal behavior and loss of relationships are described by men following abortion of the child they fathered.

3.35.5 "Abortion Attitudes and Experiences in a Group of Male Prisoners," Lindy A. Pierce, *Association for Interdisciplinary Research in Values and Social Change* 6(2): 1-8, Jan/Feb, 1994

This study is based on interviews during 1987-1988 of men in a Kentucky prison. The men were predominantly pro-life. 62% opposed abortion without stating any exceptions; 14% opposed abortion except for health, rape, or incest; and 24% said they would permit abortion more generally but still had reservations.

3.35.6 "Adolescent Males' Abortion Attitudes: Data from a National Survey, W," Marsiglio, C.L. Shehan, *Family Planning Perspectives* 25(4): 162, July/Aug, 1993

A national survey of 1880 males aged 15-19 found that a majority of males disagreed with abortion if the woman couldn't afford to care for the child, if the man would not support the child, if the woman wanted the abortion for any reason, and if the woman wanted an abortion but the man did not.

3.35.7 "Restoring Fatherhood Lost," Warren Williams; "Remembering Thomas: Case Study," Phil McCombs; "Forgotten Fathers and Their Unforgettable Children," David Reardon; "Men and Abortion, Grief and Healing," W.F. Brauning, *Post-Abortion Review* 4(4): 1-8, Fall, 1996.

Valuable collection of brief articles.

3.35.8 *Post-Abortion Trauma: 9 Steps To Recovery,* Jeanette Vought, (Grand Rapids: Zondervan, 1991) 131-143.

Describes anecdotal reports of men in postabortion counseling who feel extreme anger and helplessness in not having a voice in the abortion decision. The anger may turn inward and lead to depression which further damages relationships and creates isolation.

3.35.9 "Husband mourns outcome of wife's painful decision," R. Christopher Moore, *American Medical News,* October 24, 1991, p.24.

The husband was a medical doctor, his wife a lawyer. The wife decided on an abortion over the husband's objections. He said, "Even though I was the father and wanted to care for my child, I couldn't unless my wife wanted to have it. She controlled new life, our child's life and my life. I controlled nothing."

3.35.10 "Men and Abortion," Wayne Brauning, address to Healing Visions VI Conference, June 1992, National Office Post-Abortion Reconciliation and Healing, P.O. Box 07477, Milwaukee, WI, 53207.

In counseling men whose partners aborted, rage, powerlessness and isolation have been predominant.

3.35.11 "Many in Survey Who Had Abortion Cite Guilt Feelings," G. Skelton, *Los Angeles Times,* March 19, 1989, p.28.

In a random telephone survey conducted in March, 1989 by the Los Angeles Times, 7 % of the 1050 men interviewed acknowledged as having been the father of an aborted child. Guilt was felt by almost two-thirds and regret by more than one-third.

3.35.12 "Fathers and Fetuses," George W. Harris, *Ethics* 96:594-603, April 1986.

Conspicuously absent from most discussions of the abortion issue are considerations of third-party interests, especially those of the father. A survey of the literature reveals an implicit assumption by most writers that the issue is to be viewed as a two-party conflict-the rights of the fetus versus the rights of the mother-and that an adequate analysis of the balance of these rights is sufficient to determine the conditions under which abortion is morally permissible.

3.35.13 "Men's reactions to their partner's elective abortions," A.A. Rothstein, *American Journal of Obstetrics and Gynecology* 128:831-837, August 15, 1977.

In a study of 60 men who accompanied their wives or girl friends for elective abortion, less than half knew the type of abortion their partners were having. When asked what they knew, just over one third who claimed understanding were able to give fully accurate explanations of the procedure.

3.35.14 "Adolescent Males. Fatherhood and Abortion," A.A. Rothstein, *Journal of Youth and Adolescence* 7(2):203-204 (1978).

In a study of 35 adolescent males, most prominent were regressive wishes for nurturance, competition with one's own father, and efforts to meet paternal ego ideals of maturity and responsibility. Cases examined in detail revealed rage, fear of abandonment and total despair.

3.35.15 "Doesn't a Man Have Any Say? Fathers Go to Court to Stop Abortions," *Newsweek,* May 23, 1988 p. 74.

Thwarted fathers in unhappy relationships are more likely to go to court to attempt to stop abortions.

3.35.16 "How Abortion Affects Fathers," Regis Wailing, *Liguorian,* Liguori Publications, Box 701, Liguori, MO 63057, January 1988, pp. 26-31.

The article describes a university psychology class viewing a film on pre-natal development when suddenly a young male student rushed from the room and leaned against the wall outside, sobbing, and said, "I didn't know it was a baby. I never would have paid for it if I had known it was a baby.' Another man was described as a former seminarian who left the seminary in the late 1960's and had a hard time adjusting. When his girl friend became pregnant, he pleaded in vain with her not to have an abortion. He has had a major alcohol problem ever since.

3.35.17 "Pregnancy Termination for Genetic Indications: The Impact on Families," R. Furlong and R. Black, *Social Work in Health Care* 10(1): 17-34, Fall 1984.

Fathers were particularly adversely impacted by genetic abortion and many would not even talk about it.

3.35.18 "Abortion and Men." Linda Bird Francke, *Esquire,* September 1978, pp. 58-60.

The article cites several ways in which repressed emotions in men following induced abortion will reveal themselves in various ways: one man feared that a living son would be sacrificed for the aborted one; another felt sadness when he heard a certain song; another experienced periodic impotence and depression. The author concludes, "Abortion is a far greater dilemma for men than researchers, counselors, and women have even begun to realize ... and [men] sometimes have more trouble dealing with abortion than women."

3.35.19 "Abortion as Fatherhood Lost: Problems and Reforms," Arthur Shostak, *The Family Coordinator* 28:569-574(1979).

In a study of the impact of abortion on males many relationships between unmarried partners appeared unable to survive the strains inherent in the abortion experience. A sizable minority reported the persistence of day or night dreams about the chiild-that-never-was, and some represented these moments as times of guilt, sadness and remorse.

3.35.20 "Whose Freedom of Choice? Sometimes it takes two to untangle," Judith Paterson, *The Progressive* 46(l):42-45, April 1982.

Article includes case histories of men adversely impacted by abortion and also has an extensive discussion by professional psychologists and psychiatrists who have counseled men on the after-effects of abortion. The article quotes Andre Watson, health educator for the Men's Center of Planned Parenthood in Washington, who like many others in his field thinks conflict over abortion often affects a relationship and sometimes destroys it. "For better or for worse, an abortion brings out the stark, naked truth of a relationship." Psychologist Arnold Medvene was quoted as saying, "Abortion is undeniably a death experience, a loss experience with immense reverberations for everybody. If all of that gets blocked, it is bound to have a dramatic and destructive impact on the relationship." Dr. Neil Bernstein, a clinical psychologist, emphasizes the effect of "denial and distancing." Psychiatrist Richard Epstein says that abortion evokes powerful and complex feelings in men as well as women, and that the individuals react in accord with the psychological level at which they experience the abortion. The article notes that many women handle the implications of abortion alone, while men repress them to a dangerous degree.

One man worried about the negative spiritual consequences and thought women have trivialized the issue by emphasizing the right to control their own bodies. Another was amazed at the intensity of his objections to the destruction of his offspring and surprised at the rift between his political posture and his paternal feelings. A black man expressed a sense of heritage and importance of perpetuating himself.

3.35.21 "Abortion: How Men Feel About One of Biggest Issues in a Woman's Life," James L. Collier, *Glamour Magazine*, February 1980, pp. 164-165, 243-244.

The article quotes Uta Landy of the National Abortion Federation: "They [men] behave much differently from the women who call in too. They'll never admit they're directly involved. It's always "this girl, ' never 'my girl friend.' And they're mainly concerned about safety. Frequently, women ignore what you tell them about the guidelines, they're so anxious to get the abortion over with, but men will pay strict attention. Many take down what you tell them word for word." The National Abortion Federation was quoted as saying that 40% of the calls on their hotline are from males. Clinical psychologists who studied male reactions to abortion concluded men had even stronger guilt feelings than women. Men wanted to be present or even go through the abortion themselves.

3.35.22 "Abortion: Are Men There When Women Need Them Most?," Carol Lynn Mithers, *Mademoiselle*, April 1981, p. 231.

The author notes that about 3 million people had abortions last year. Only half of them were women. A program director for family planning clinics observed, "Abortion is a difficult experience for everyone concerned. That includes men. A man may escape the physical trauma, but it's unlikely he'll come through unscathed." A woman, in describing a boyfriend's reaction to abortion, said it "freaked him out."

A macho 29-year-old male said, "Yeah, I still think about it. Not often but sometimes My brother and his wife are having a baby in the next few months and that brings it to mind-they're having a kid. I'm not."

A 34-year-old man: "I wasn't broken up by the experience. I was saddened though. Even if you have no set moral or philosophical problems with abortion, it's still taking something away from both of you." A 28-year-old said, "I thought. What a shame! This is the combination of her and me and would be such a beautiful child."

Another 28-year-old expressed a lack of empathy and said, "I thought I knew all about abortion and I thought it was a real routine procedure but it didn't hit me till afterward that it's also very emotionally distressing. I'm more sympathetic about that now. Maybe I would have been before if I'd known what to expect."

A casual relationship broke up following abortion. A 28-year-old male said, "I was 22, she was 17. We had only been casual lovers. When she discovered she was pregnant I first tried to deny it. I feared I might be trapped into marriage. She said she wanted the child but I insisted abortion was the best idea. I didn't even like her very much."

A 28-year-old man: "We were students; our biggest problem was where to go for dinner. Afterward, there was a loss of freedom. We were more sober. After the abortion there was no way that relationship was going to work. That's what makes me so sad, because in many ways it was the nicest one I'll ever have."

A 29-year-old businessman whose girlfriend began seeing another man after her abortion: "The whole experience was like being hit by an emotional battering ram. It broke her down where she was in a real weak and vulnerable condition. I wasn't there for her."

3.35.23 "How abortion affects men," John Stanhope, *Faith Today*, May/June 1988, pp. 26-27.

The article quotes abortionist Henry Morgentaler as saying abortion is a silent agony for many men. There is still little information on the subject. From what is available, there seems to be some indication that men go through the same grief, remorse and sadness that characterize post-abortion syndrome in women.

3.35.24 *The Anatomy of Bereavement*, Beverly Raphael, (New York: Basic Books, 1983) 240.

Some fathers will feel angry and cheated by the women's decision to terminate their child, whether or not they would be prepared to care for it as a father. Many men involved in the termination of a pregnancy they have fathered will experience grief too and may need recognition of mourning for the lost child.

3.35.25 "Psychiatric Sequelae of Abortion: The Many Faces of Post-Abortion Grief, E," Joanne Angelo, *Linacre Quarterly* 59:69-80, May, 1992.

In a clinical case, an 18 year old male gas station attendant shot himself and died 3 months after his father's unexpected death. Only his closest friend knew that at the time of his suicide he was despondent over his girl friend's abortion. The child had been conceived on the day of his father's death. He had formed a mental image of the child and told his friend he planned to name his son after his father. The loss of the child and what it represented was more than he was able to bear.

3.35.26 "The Effects of Abortion on a Marriages," Janet Mattinson, Abortion: Medical Progress and Social Implications, *Ciba Foundation Symposium* 115, 1985, pp. 165-177.

Marriage problems involving adverse reactions of men to induced abortion are reported in a British study of several case histories at Tavistock Clinic. Inability to conceive, withdrawal, inability to function to seek employment, sexual and interpersonal conflicts, extramarital affairs, loss of trust, seeking abortion as a form of punishment for a spouse and a heightened sense of inferiority were identified.

3.35.27 "A Program of Group Counseling for Men Who Accompany Women Seeking Legal Abortions," Robert A. Gordon and Cheryl Kilpatrick, *Community Mental Health Journal* 13(4):291-295 (1977).

In a program of group counseling for men developed at a Wisconsin abortion clinic, men expressed anxiety, helplessness, guilt, self-blame and regret. Men used denial, intellectualization, rationalization and withdrawal in an attempt to cope with stress. Men often attempted to be invulnerable, a "real man" by denying any expression of feelings. Many men said they did not express their feelings to their partners and instead felt the need to be a source of support by presenting a strong front. Themes of discussion included (a) issues of right and wrong, particularly in connection with religious beliefs; (b) viewing fetal material as non-human; (c) disinterest in bringing a child into such a "troubled" world.

3.35.28 *Men and Abortion. Lessons. Losses and Love,* Arthur Shostak and Gary McLouth, (New York: Praeger, 1984).

In follow-up of 75 post-abortion men 25% had broken up with their partner although only 3% had stated on the day of the abortion that abortion was contributing to the breakup. Unexpected guilt and remorse, relief from tension, anger at the woman, were cited as some of the reasons for breaking up. Sex relations and contraceptive questions caused new stress immediately after the abortion. This study involved people in committed relationships (only 4% were casual).

3.35.29 "Psychological Factors That Predict Reaction to Abortion," D.T. Moseley, *Journal of Clinical Psychology* 37(2):276-279, April 1981.

A woman's relationship with her partner was determined as a crucial factor in her post-abortion adjustment. Liberated women tended to devalue the significance of the partner in conception.

3.35.30 "Fatherhood and Abortion: Psychological and Psychopathological Reactions," P Benvenuti, P. Borri, P. Buzzoni, L. Clerici and M.R. Monti, *Rivista di Patologica Nervosa e Mentale* 104:255-268(1983).

Despite the scant psychological and medical interest in the reactions of men to abortion, there is considerable emotional involvement in lost parenthood both for the man and the woman. The involvement by men may manifest itself in persecutory or depressive anxiety and psychosomatic symptoms. Rarely, psychopathological symptoms such as depression and behavioral disorders may appear. The appearance of these reactions is linked to problems and conflicts aroused by prospective fatherhood leading to a comparison between fulfilled fatherhood and fatherhood lost.

3.35.31 "Adolescent Males: Fatherhood and Abortion," A.A. Rothstein, *Journal of Youth and Adolescence* 7(2):203-204 (1978).

A study of 35 adolescent males whose sexual partners were undergoing abortion at Bronx Municipal Hospital found that males had regressive wishes for nurturance, competition with one's own father, and efforts to meet parental ego ideals of maturity and responsibility. In the cases examined in detail rage, fear of abandonment and total despair were observed. Little is known about the reaction or developmental difficulties of adolescent males as a result of their implication in abortion. This is one of the few studies on the subject.

3.36   Abortion's Impact on Siblings

3.36.1 "Children's Disturbed Reactions to their Mother's Miscarriage," A.C. Cain et al *Psychosomatic Medicine* 26:58-66(1964).

Important background article on the subject.

3.36.2 "Effects of Sibling Death on the Surviving Child: A Family Perspective," R. Krell and L. Rabkin, *Family Process* 18:471-477, December 1979.

Describes such family maneuvers as conspiracy of guilt, survivor reactions, substitution for the lost child, the haunted child (silence), the resurrected child (substitution). Therapy with survivor families is described as a difficult task involving the working through of short-circuited and unresolved grief reactions, unraveling of multiple distortions of identity and clarifying of mystifying communication.

3.36.3 "A Consideration of Abortion Survivors." Philip G. Hey, *Child Psychiatry and Human Development* 13(3): 168-178, Spring 1983.

It is hypothesized that approximately 50% of the children in the Western world are or soon will be abortion survivors, i.e., they are children who have had siblings terminated by induced abortion.

3.36.4   "The Surviving Sibling: Another Victim of Abortion," *National Right to Life News* [Washington D.C.], September 25, 1986.

The article quotes Dr. Edward Sheridan of Georgetown University Hospital who observed that children may become aware of an induced abortion through overheard conversations or by being directly told by their parents. Frequently, even a very young child will "sense", the mother's pregnancy and then become confused when the anticipated brother or sister does not materialize. If no explanation is given, this confusion may lead the child to somehow feel responsible for the loss. If the child becomes aware that the mother actively chose to "get rid" of the sibling, the survivor may begin to fear her. The mother becomes the agent of death instead of life.

3.36.5   "The Survivor Syndrome: Siblings and Abortion," *National Right to Life News* [Washington D.C.], January 15, 1987, p. 19.

The article quotes Dr. E. Joanne Angelo, a practicing psychiatrist and assistant clinical professor at Tufts University School of Medicine, who observed that siblings of aborted children may be children who are having trouble going to school and being separated from their parents. The children are "replacement children", born after their parents suffered the loss of another child through sudden infant death syndrome, miscarriage or abortion. The children picked up their fears from their parents, not from outside the home. If abortion was the catalyst for the "replacement child, " the child may also suffer from the mother's often unresolved, and perhaps unacknowledged, grief over the loss of the unborn child.

3.36.6   "The Aborted Sibling Factor: A Case Study," A.H. Weiner and E.C. Weiner, *Clinical Social Casework Journal,* Human Services Press (1984), pp. 209-215.

Case study of 5-year-old girl whose mother had multiple abortions. The girl was very frightened of her mother, dreamed of being killed and tore her doll's head and arms off.

3.36.7   "Child's Reaction to Mother's Abortion: Case Report," J.O. Cavenar, J.G. Spaulding and J.L. Sullivan, *Military Medicine* 144(6):412-413 (1979).

A five-year-old boy was referred for psychiatric evaluation because of aggressive behavior toward his sister, poor peer relationships and multiple tics. He learned of his mother's abortion when he was only slightly over 2 years old. He thought he had undergone mutilative surgery as punishment for his aggressive and hostile impulses and via identification with his mother viewed himself as mutilated and castrated.

3.36.8   "Ritual Mourning for Unresolved Grief After Abortion," K. McAll and W. Wilson, *Southern Medical Journal* 80(7):817-821, July 1987.

Includes several case studies drawn from the experience of the authors with the effects of induced abortion or miscarriage on over 400 people with whom they have counseled. A report is given of a 7-year-old girl initially diagnosed as epileptic. She had unpredictable episodes of shouting at her parents, stamping her feet and falling unconscious. She often hurt herself when she fell. Drugs were of no help to her. When in counseling with her parents she added the name of a sibling who she said was her best friend. When her parents attempted to correct her she called her mother a murderer who had thrown her sister away. The mother then admitted to a pregnancy where the doctor gave her a rough examination and she lost the baby. Following prayer and mourning for the lost child the family was helped to recover.

3.36.9 "Infant Abortion and Child Abuse," Philip G. Ney in *The Psychological Aspects of Infant Abortion and Child Abuse,* eds. D. Mall and W.F. Watts, (Washington D.C.: University Publications of America, 1979) 33.

Describes a case of severe child neglect where the mother was depressed as a result of an earlier coerced abortion and the father had rejected the child and had left the family.

3.36.10 "Ritual Mourning in Anorexia Nervosa," RK McAll and FM McAll, *The Lancet,* August 16, 1980, p. 368.

The authors report on 18 patients who were treated in a hospital without initial improvement. Fifteen experienced a total relief of symptoms after ritual mourning. Two patients were male. In 17 of the cases, family histories revealed a total of two violent deaths or deaths by suicide, five terminations of pregnancy for non-medical reasons and eight miscarriages. In one case a 17-year-old girl who had anorexia nervosa since 14 and had been hospitalized three times. Her mother had an earlier pregnancy aborted. She admitted the existence of her unborn "sister" but had not mentioned it for fear of being locked up in a mental hospital.

3.36.11 "Parental high concern and adolescent-onset anorexia nervosa," . A case-control study to investigate direction of causality, P Stonebridge, SG Gowers, *Br J Psychiatry* 176:132-137, 2000

Mothers of adolescent girls who had anorexia nervosa were found to have a history of second trimester abortion as well as other identified pregnancy losses.

3.36.12 "Pregnancy Termination for Genetic Indications: The Impact on Families," R. Furlong and R. Black, *Social Work in Health Care* 10(1): 17-34, Fall 1984.

A study was made of 22 children whose mothers had undergone induced abortion because of a serious fetal defect. Nineteen of the 22 exhibited some adverse reaction according to observations of the parents. The children included several adult children and reactions ranged from mild to severe. Of four young children who supposedly knew nothing about the abortion, three exhibited some adverse reaction including sleep walking, regression in motor behavior and searching for the baby by touching the mothers stomach. Sadness, guilt and separation anxiety were noted. A 7-year-old girl who was given a full explanation exhibited a severe reaction of horror, had trouble sleeping, refused close physical contact with the mother, had a morbid interest in the abortion procedure raising questions about her attitude about future childbearing.

3.36.13 "Ritual Mourning for Unresolved Grief After Abortion," K. McAll and W. Wilson, *Southern Medical Journal* 80(7):817-821, July 1987.

A professional man had conducted a long search for therapists on behalf of his 26-year-old daughter who was sexually promiscuous with men about 30 years older. She was the cause of much gossip, impeded the attainment of his goals and the cause of violent arguments in the family. The woman's mother had undergone an abortion several years before the marriage to the father and the mother's life prior to her marriage had many parallels to her daughter's. After the mother mourned for the aborted child and expressed her love for it, the problems of the daughter ceased.

3.36.14 "Psychiatric Sequelae of Therapeutic Abortions," Jesse O. Cavenar, A.A. Maltbie and J.L. Sullivan, *North Carolina Medical Journal* 39:101-104, February 1978.

A 28-year-old professional man who had entered psychoanalysis for anxiety, career indecisiveness, and inability to become emotionally involved with a woman. He visited his mother to ask about various memories he had recovered in analysis. His mother confessed to an abortion when she was 17 and pressured her son to marry and provide her with grandchildren apparently as an attempt to atone for or undo her own abortion. The authors concluded that abortion may have a profound emotional effect on other family members and permanently alter intrafamilial relationships.

3.36.15 "Great Joy for All-Praise Reports," newsletter of Pastor and Mrs. Timothy D. Hansen, *Igreja Evangelica da Renovaqao*, Brazil, December 1, 1987.

A woman was married for a number of years but was apparently unable to bear children. Upon prayer with the woman it was discerned that the woman's mother had been involved in deep sin. When mentioned to the woman she began to weep and weep and said, "Yes, my mother is a prostitute and has had 29 abortions." After prayer for the woman she forgave her mother. The missionaries reported, "That was five months ago. We have just learned [the woman] is five months pregnant." Ed. Note: This is the highest number of abortions known to us.

3.37 Impact of Abortion on Marriage and Family

3.37.1 "The Effects of Abortion on Marriage and Other Committed Relationships," Teri Reisser, *Association for Interdisciplinary Research in Values and Social Change* 6(4): 1-8, May/June 1994

Anecdotal reports include breakup of relationships, communication problems, threats to family loyalty, increased isolation, loss of self-concept, sexual dysfunction, and interference with relationships to existing or future children as problems related to induced abortion.

3.37.2 "Post-Traumatic Stress Disorders in Women Following Abortion: Some Considerations and

Implications for Marital/Couple Therapy," Dennis A. Bagarozzi, *Int'l Journal of Family and Marriage* (Dehli, India) Vol. I, No. 2: 51-68, 1993

A clinical study of 18 women referred for sexual/marital therapy found that the women suffered from post-traumatic stress disorder although women denied that the abortion was a traumatic experience. Impacted grief, guilt, and unresolved mourning were primary issues. See also "Identification, Assessment and Treatment of Women Suffering from Post-Traumatic Stress After Abortion." Dennis A. Bagarozzi, *Journal of Family Psychotherapy* 5(3): 25,1994.

3.37.3   "Post-Abortion Survivors Syndrome," (letter), Philip G. Ney, *Canadian Journal of Psychiatry* 38 (8): 577-578, Oct., 1993.

Post-Abortion survivors syndrome is found in children and adults. It consists of symptoms stemming from deep conflicts because they may have been aborted. All have existential guilt, a sense of worthlessness, and a feeling of impending disaster. Eight types of abortion survivors syndromes are described.

3.37.4   *Invisible Loyalties,* I. Boszormeny and G. Spark (New York: Harper and Row, 1973) 149.

Until the post-Victorian age the issues of family loyalty were largely unformulated because they were taken for granted. Our age, on the other hand, denies these issues with the help of myths of individual material success and the endless struggle against the threat of authority.

From earliest times great playwrights and novelists have always pictured man as part of a relational motivation system. Autonomy purchased through outwardly complete separation and denial of relatedness tends to be offset inwardly by the accumulation of guilt and responsibility.

3.37.5   "Childbirth is A Family Experience," John G. Howells in *Modern Perspectives in Psycho-Obstetrics* (1980) 127-149

The family is a complete organism, a unity in its own right, as well as an individual. The individual is an organized system; so too is the family. The family has a structure, paths of communication, characteristics, elements as any organized system. Like an individual, it has a psyche-the family group psyche. Any event in every part of this organized system impinges on every part of the rest of the system. Every experience within the organized system belongs to the system. Thus, childbirth and its attendant pregnancy is an experience that belongs to the family as a whole.

3.37.6   "Social Stresses on the Family," Reuben Hill, *Social Casework* 39:139-150(1958).

Stressor events must be seen as a variable rather than as a constant in family crisis research. Family crises can be classified as dismemberment, accession or demoralization. Various stages of adjustment include [1] attempts to deny the problem; [2] attempts to eliminate the problem; (3) disorganization; (4) attempts to reorganize in spite of the problem; [5] efforts to escape the problem; [6] reorganization of the family without the missing member; (7) reorganization of the entire family. These stages parallel closely the stages of adjustment and recovery to bereavement.

The sexual area is one of the most sensitive areas of family life. In crises involving interpersonal recriminations, where the crisis is regarded as the fault of any one member, the position of that member is greatly devalued. Intrafamily events such as illegitimacy, nonsupport, mental breakdown, infidelity, suicide and alcoholism are usually more disorganizing to the family because they arise from troubles that reflect poorly on the family's internal adequacy.

3.37.7   "Family Boundary Ambiguity: A New Variable in Family Stress Theory," Pauline Boss and Jan Greenberg, *Family Process* 23:535-546(1984).

Boundary ambiguity is defined as the family not knowing who is in and who is out of the system. The family may perceive a physically absent member as psychologically present or a physically present member as psychologically absent. The culture can support the denial of a physical loss and thereby make it more difficult for the family to grieve and close out the missing member. An example is given in regard to stillbirth where the belief system only accorded viable babies mourning rites.

3.37.8   "The Fund of Sociability," Robert S. Weiss, *Trans-Action,* July/August 1969, pp 36-43.

Relationships with other people are essential and their loss can be traumatic. Relational functions necessary for well-being are intimacy, social integration, opportunity for nurturant behavior, reassurance of worth, assistance or guidance.

3.37.9   "The Effects of Abortion on a Marriage," Janet Mattinson, in *Abortion: Medical Progress and Social Implications,* Pitman (London: Ciba Foundation Symposium, 1985)165-177.

Patients seeking help for troubled marriages may have a past abortion experience for which they have been unable to mourn at the time of the abortion and they may show a delayed grief reaction. It may be mild or persistent or may occur in more extreme form many years later. Sometimes husbands are more affected than wives. Examples of counseling issues included inability to function, sexual and interpersonal conflict, compulsive sexual affairs outside marriage, development of inferiority feelings, inability to conceive.

3.37.10   "Predictive Factors in emotional Response to Abortion: Kind's Termination Study-IV," E.M. Belsey, H. Green, S. Lal, S. Lewis and R.W. Beard, *Social Science and Medicine* (2) 71-82(1977)

In a British study of marital adjustment 3 months post abortion, 42% of the women said they were less close to their sexual partners vs. 22% who said they were more close. Unsatisfactory or mediocre marital adjustment before the abortion increased the likelihood of marital or sexual adjustment problems following the abortion.

3.37.11   "Induced abortion and psychosexuality," F Bianchi-Demicheli et al, *J Psychosom Obstet Gynecol* 21(4): 213-217, 2000

Reviews the limited published literature on the subject. Sexual dysfunction was reported in up to

30% of women after abortion.

3.37.12 "Sexuality, partner relations and contraceptive practices after termination of pregnancy," F Bianchi-Demicheli et al, *J Psychosom Obstet Gynecol* 22(2): 83-90, 2001

A Swiss study interviewed women before abortion and 6 months postabortion. 18% reported a decrease in sexual desire, and 17% reported orgasmic disorders.

3.37.13 "Sexual Dysfunction Related to Induced Abortion," Thomas Strahan, *Association for Interdisciplinary Research in Values and Social Change Research Bulletin* 11 (4): 1-8, Sept/ Oct, 1997

Various studies and anecdotal reports reveal that both men and women may have sexual impotency, aversion to sex, loss of intimacy, unexpected guilt, and extra-martial affairs as a result of induced abortion.

3.37.14 "The Hostility of Parents to Children: Some Notes on Infertility. Child Abuse and Abortion," Victor Calef, *International Journal of Psychoanalytic Psychotherapy* l(l):76, February 1972.

A case report by psychiatrist Victor Calef of marital difficulty following induced abortion included anxiety, sexual dissatisfaction, husband's lack of interest in wife and in sex. The wife said she had no guilt over the abortion. The psychiatrist concluded that the guilt over the abortion was displaced onto the doctor who performed the abortion, while guilt over the pregnancy was displaced onto the husband. It was concluded that the woman experiences the request and permission for abortion as a rejection of her sexuality.

3.37.15 "Abortion As A Stigma: In the Eyes of the Beholder," Gerdi Weidner and William Griffitt, *Journal of Research in Personality* 18:359-371(1984).

A recent study among university students in an introductory psychology course at a large midwestern U.S. university revealed that involvement in an abortion has a stigmatizing effect for both men and women. Abortion involvement produced a negative perception in members of the opposite sex who considered them less desirable partners to date or marry. Males involved in abortion received strong ratings of rejection only from female subjects , and females involved in abortion were rejected only by male subjects.

3.37.16 "Low Birth Weight in Relation to Multiple Induced Abortions," M.T. Mandelson, C.B. Madden, J.R. Daling, *Am.J. Public Health,* 82(3): 391, March, 1992.

In a Washington State Study of 6541 white women who gave birth to their first child between 1984-87, 33.5% of the women reported 4 or more abortions were unmarried compared to 27.5% of women (2 abortions), 24.0% of women (1 abortion) and 20.5% of women (no abortions).

3.37.17 "The Rights and Responsibilities of Men in Abortion Situations," Shirley Rosenwasser, L.S. Wright and R.B. Barber, *Journal of Sex Research* 23:97-105, February 1987.

Abortion adversely impacts upon the parental attitude towards the legal obligation of a parent to provide for the care and support of a child. In a study conducted at a state supported university in Texas, male and female students were asked whether or not a woman should be able to legally sue the father for child support if he was willing to pay for an abortion and the woman decided to keep the child. Some 59% of the men and 40% of the women thought the woman should not be able to sue for child support under those circumstances.

3.37.18 *Men and Abortion. Lessons. Losses and Love,* Arthur Shostak and Gary McLouth, (New York: Praeger, 1984).

In a study of 1,000 men who accompanied women to abortion clinics in the U.S., 48% of the males did not think a man should be required to pay child support as at present-if the woman refused his request that she have an abortion.

3.37.19 "Emotional Distress Patterns Among Women Having First or Repeat Abortions," Ellen Freeman, K. Rickels, G. Huggins, C. Garcia and I. Palin, *Obstetrics and Gynecology* 55(5):630-636, May 1980.

Lack of communication by partners following induced abortion is reported. In a study on emotional distress patterns among women following induced abortion it was observed that "repeat aborters continued to have significantly higher emotional distress scores in dimensions relating to interpersonal relationships." In other words, they had trouble getting along with others.

3.37.20 "Psychological Problems of Abortion for the Unwed Teenage Girl," Cynthia D. Martin, *Genetic Psychology Monographs*, 88:23-110(1973)

In a San Diego study of unmarried adolescents who obtained abortions for mental health reasons two out of three had poor relationships with both parents prior to the abortion which tended to further deteriorate following the abortion.

3.37.21 "Repeat Abortion: Is it A Problem?," C. Berger, D. Gold, D. Andres, P. Gillett and R. Kinch, *Family Planning Perspectives* 16(2):70-75, March/April 1984.

In a study comparing first-time aborters with repeaters, 45% of the repeaters said they made the decision by themselves compared with 33% of the first-time aborters.

3.37.22 "Pilot Surveys of Repeated Abortion," E. Szabady and A. Klinger, *International Mental Health Res.* Letter 14:6(1972).

In a Hungarian study, those women having a repeat abortion were less likely to be in a happy marriage and were more likely to have an abortion independent of their partner.

3.37.23 "First and Repeat Abortions: A Study of Decision-Making and Delay," M Bracken and S. Kasl, *Journal of Biosocial Science* 7:473-491(1975).

A 1975 report of social relationships of women following induced abortion concluded that women having repeat abortions are in less stable social situations compared with women who seek abortion for the first time. Their relationships were of shorter duration than unmarried women having first abortions.

3.37.24 "Maternal Perinatal Risk Factors and Child Abuse," M. Benedict, R. White, and P. Comely, *Child Abuse and Neglect*, 9:217-224(1985).

A study of 532 Baltimore mothers (two thirds black) found that mothers who maltreated their children were significantly more likely to have had a prior stillbirth or reported abortion (18.2% vs. 12.4%). With two prior stillbirths or abortions or combination thereof, the abuse rate was nearly doubled (4.3% vs. 2.4%). It was concluded that reproductive history may provide important clues in eliciting more precisely what family dynamics may be related to subsequent maltreatment.

3.37.25 "Motivation of Surrogate Mothers: Initial Findings," Philip Parker, *American Journal of Psychiatry* 140(1): 117-118, January 1983.

In a Michigan study of 125 women who applied to be commercial surrogates, 35% either had a voluntary prior abortion (26%) or had relinquished a child for adoption (9%). Women felt, often unconsciously, that surrogate motherhood would help them master unresolved feelings through previous voluntary loss. Women stated, "It would be their baby, not mine"; "I'd be nest watching"; and,"I'll attach myself in a different way-hoping its healthy."

3.37.26 *Living Through Personal Crisis,* Ann Kaiser Steams (New York: Ballantine Books, 1984).

Describes a delayed reaction in a woman who became pregnant and underwent an abortion. Her relationship with the man who got her pregnant had ended without his being able to share in her troubled feelings over the abortion. Later, when she fell in love again, she found herself mistrusting her new lover and men in general. She also had a renewed sadness over the prior abortion. (Illustrates how abortion circumstances may impair new attachments.)

3.37.27 *Taking Chances: Abortion and the Decision Not to Contracept,* K. Luker (Berkeley: University of California Press, 1975).

A study based upon interviews with 50 predominantly unmarried women who had repeat abortions found that many had become pregnant to either test their partners' commitment to the relationship, or to hurry it along to a marriage. When their partners did not commit, the women resorted to abortion.

3.37.28 "Psychiatric Sequelae of Therapeutic Abortions," Jesse O. Cavenar, A.A. Maltbie and J.L. Sullivan, *North Carolina Medical Journal* 39:101-104, February 1978.

(Grief in a grandmother over a lost grandchild is reported; a 28-year-old professional man who had entered psychoanalysis for anxiety,career indecisiveness and inability to become involved emotionally with a woman visited his mother to ask about various memories he had recovered in analysis. His mother confessed to [having] an abortion when she was 17 and pressured her son to marry and provide her with grandchildren apparently as an attempt to atone for or undo her own abortion. The authors conclude abortion may have a profound emotional effect on other family members and permanently alter intrafamilial relationships.

3.37.29 "Therapeutic Abortion. Clinical Aspects," Edward Senay, *Archives of General Psychiatry* 23:408-415, November 1970.

Patients who mention problems following induced abortion almost invariably want help for long-term marital problems. Rarely do they talk about the abortion spontaneously.

3.37.30 *Rachel Weeping: The Case Against Abortion,* James Burtchaell (San Francisco: Harper and Row, 1982,1984) 13

There seems to be some hostility at work which alienates women choosing abortion from even the helpful enjoyment of whatever intimate trust they had previously (and possibly unrealistically) thought they shared with their kinfolk and mates. A decision is produced-apparently the result of freshly independent and straightforward deliberation-yet shadowed by much unspoken and undigested thought. Then it is rushed to completion without the sharing of minds and hearts one would hope for even in matters of far less importance.

3.37.31 "The Family at Bay," Donald DeMarco, *Human Life Review* 8(4):44-54, Fall 1982.

The family as the fundamental unit of society is the reality. But legislators and judges, knowingly or unknowingly, can and do ignore this reality. A great deal of judicial thinking in recent years has been grounded in the premise that the individual is the fundamental social unit. A prime example of a woman's newly created "right" to individual privacy in the matter of abortion... Once the mother was legally relieved of the duty to care for her unborn child and was given the liberty of destruction, the stage was set for the severing of every other family relationship.

3.37.32 "The Abortion Experience in Private Practice," David H. Sherman et al in *Women and Loss: Psychobiological Perspectives,* ed. William F. Finn et al., *The Foundation of Thanatology Series, Volume 3,* (New York: Praeger Publ., 1985) 98-107.

In a study of 100 women at a private clinic at Mount Sinai School of Medicine, 75% of the women were married or had long-term ongoing relationships. All had knowledge about contraception and had easy access to medical care; 66% had at least a college degree; 71% were employed full-time; 57% had incomes over $20,000 per year; 81% had one abortion, 14% two) and 5% (three); one-third had a pregnancy before abortion, one-third had a child since aborting, and for one-third the abortion was their sole obstetrical history. Some 46% agreed that the abortion was a major crisis in their lives. Most women experienced loss and grief rather than joy and freedom. Relationships were suddenly and unexpectedly shaken. Some 48% believed their relationship with their male partner was significantly altered (approximately equally split positive and negative); 33% felt their sexual life was negatively affected to some degree; 52% were reluctant to tell people they had an abortion. Sadness, a sense of loss or emptiness, guilt, anger, anxiety and/or confusion was recalled by many. None ever expressed joy. Residual emotions diminished with time. Women with Catholic backgrounds and those with previous abortions more frequently expressed abortion as a form of infanticide.

3.37.33 "Personal Communication," (letter from Sarah J.O. Ricketts to Thomas W. Strahan), April 3,1989.

In working with post-abortion support groups involving women who are seeking counseling and healing, usually one third to one half of the women are siblings of those who had been aborted as well as having had abortions themselves. They frequently report a generational abortion pattern in the family, including grandmother, aunts, uncles, brothers, sisters. These women appear to have a more impenetrable denial (numbness) of emotions of grief following their own abortions.

3.37.34 "Ethical Issues in Clinical Obstetrics and Gynecology," Benjamin Freedman, *Current Problems in Obstetrics, Gynecology and Fertility,* 8(3): 1-47, March 1985.

Obstetrics and gynecology is among several medical specialties... that are especially likely to perceive the family unit, rather than a single patient, as the proper focus of primary health care.

3.37.35 "The Post-Abortion Experience-Abortion's Secondary Victims," *National Right to Life News,* January 15,1987.

Includes articles on *The Survivor Syndrome: Siblings and Abortion, Men and Abortion,* and *A Grandmother Grieves for Her Lost Grandchild.*

3.37.36 "The Aborted Sibling Factor: A Case Study," A. Weiner and E. Weiner, *Clinical Social Work Journal,* 1984, pp. 209-215.

A 5-year-old girl tore her doll apart and drew a picture of a child falling down the stairs following her mother's induced abortion.

3.37.37 "Child's Reaction to Mother's Abortion: A Case Report," Jesse O. Cavenar, J.E. Spaulding and J.L. Sullivan, *Military Medicine* 144(6): 412A13 (1979).

3.37.38 "A Consideration of Abortion Survivors," Philip Ney, *Child Psychiatry and Human Development* 13(3): 168-169, Spring 1983.

Argues that since approximately 50% of Western children are abortion survivors, there is a need to analyze their individual and collective responses.

3.37.39 "Ritual Mourning in Anorexia Nervosa," R.K. McAll and F.M. McAll, *The Lancet,* August 16,1980, p. 368.

Concludes that hidden guilt, either in the patient or in a close member of the family, or lack of adequate recognition or mourning for a lost family member may be a causative factor in anorexia nervosa-the article includes two abortion related examples involving family members.

3.37.40 "Seesaw Response of a Young Unmarried Couple to Therapeutic Abortion. I," Wallerstein and M. Bar-Din, *Archives of General Psychiatry* 27:251-254 (1972)

3.37.41 "Men's Reactions to Their Partner's Elective Abortion," A.A. Rothstein, *American Journal of Obstetrics and Gynecology* 128:831-837 (1977)

3.37.42 "Out of Wedlock Abortion and Delivery: The Importance of the Male Partner," James M. Robbins, *Social Problems* 31(3):334-350 February 1984

Women who aborted tended to be less strongly tied to their partners following abortion.

3.37.43 *Parental Loss of a Child,* ed. Therese A. Rando, esp. chapter on "Induced Abortion." Betty Harris, (Champaign, Ill: Research Press Co., 1986)

3.37.44 "The Effects of Abortion on a Marriage," Janet Mattinson, 1985; *Abortion: Medical Progress and Social Implications,* Pitman, (London: Ciba Foundation Symposium 115), pp. 165-177.

Patients apparently unable to mourn the loss of a child at the time of the abortion may show a delayed grief reaction. Therapeutic work needs to concern itself with the earlier loss. Sometimes husbands are more affected than wives. Husbands and fathers are much neglected in the British follow-up studies of abortion, except [rarely] through the subjective reports of the women.

3.37.45 *Men and Abortion. Lessons. Losses and Love,* Arthur B. Shostak, (New York: Praeger Publishers 1984) xiv.

Men are seriously affected by their abortion experiences, and their memories are extremely sharp and cogent when recalling these experiences.

3.37.46 "The Psychological Sequelae of Abortion Performed for a Genetic Indication, B," Blumberg, M. Golbus and K. Hanson, *American Journal of Obstetrics and Gynecology* 122(7):799-808, August 1,1975.

Stresses attendant to selective abortion produce undesirable marital consequences. Two families out of 13 experienced separation during the pregnancy, even prior to the performance of amniocentesis; in each case the separation was related to problems engendered by their genetic circumstances. Separation occurred in two families after the selective abortion; although the separations were for less than six weeks, they produced repercussions which threatened marital stability for many months or years afterward.

3.37.47 "Repeat Abortion: Is It a Problem?," C. Berger, D. Gold, D. Andress, P. Gillett and R. Kinch, *Family Planning Perspectives* 16(2):70-75, March/April 1984.

Repeaters described their relationships as being less satisfactory than first-time abortion patients; more repeaters than first-timers said they had made the decision by themselves [45% vs. 33%].

Abortion tends to be communication restricting rather than communication enhancing.

3.37.48 "Abortion: Predicting the Complexity of the Decision-Making Process. M," Friedlander, T. Kaul and C. Stimel, *Women and Health* 9(1):43-53, Spring 1984.

Observes that "women experience difficulties in decision-making which exceed immediate concern and may include moral dilemmas, problems in relationships, role conflicts and career decisions, among others."

3.37.49 "First and Repeat Abortions: A Study of Decision-Making and Delay. M," Bracken and S. Kasi, *Journal Biosocial Science* 7:473-491 (1975).

Fewer women repeaters were pregnant by husbands, and unmarried women having repeat abortions had been in relationships of shorter duration than unmarried women having first abortions.

3.37.50 *Rachael Weeping: The Case Against Abortion,* James Burtchaell, (San Francisco: Harper and Row, 1982,1984) 8.

One has the impression that the pregnancy crisis and abortion disclosed rather than caused the falling away of friends and mates. In case after case there seem to have been no previous bonds generous and giving enough - despite the frequency with which they were anointed as "caring" and "loving -to sustain much claim on either good sense or energetic support. In many instances, the women simply woke up to find that they had been on their own all along, despite the couplings. When the emergency erupts, bonds that have long been frayed and rotted simply snap. Comments on case histories of abortion circumstances described in *The Ambivalence of Abortion,* Linda Bird Francke (1978).

3.37.51 "Therapeutic Abortion. Clinical Aspects," Edward Senay, *Archives of General Psychiatry* 23: 408-415, November 1970.

Alter some months most patients appear either to have resolved the abortion crisis completely or to have successfully repressed it, for they report not having thought about the experience in some time. Patients who mention problems almost invariably want help for long-term marital problems. Rarely do they talk about the abortion spontaneously.

3.37.52 "Abortion in Relationship Context," Vincent M. Rue, *International Review of Natural Family Planning,* 9:95-121, Summer 1985

Like the Trojan horse, abortion is only beginning to be seen for what it truly is and does. There is evidence to suggest that induced abortion promoted "mystification and masking" within the family, which is dysfunctional for the individual. In relationships abortion provides "pseudo-homeostasis," that is, a stability through non-adjustment which promotes even more serious relational disequilibrium. For men it increases masculine insecurity and provides alienation, role conflict, and for some, limited relief. For women it provides relief, but also induces a heavy burden of guilt, secrecy and intra-psychic conflict. Clinically, if an unwanted pregnancy is a mistake or problem, then abortion becomes a denial of the problem. Psychologically, then, abortion reinforces defective problem-solving behavior. The article concludes that abortion exists for women, yet it is against women, men and children. Like an anesthetic, abortion comfortably numbs all from experiencing the burden of pregnancy. Abortion has become a social eraser of choice, individually, quickly/and secretly eliminating all traces of the pregnancy problem. And yet, traces always remain. Within the depths of male-female relations, the indelible marks of violation reappear.

3.37.53 "A Report on 1.000 Men and the Impact of Abortion on Their Family Life," Arthur Shostak, presented at the 1984 meeting of the American Sociological Society ,San Antonio, Texas, August 29,1984.

The author interviewed 1,000 men in the waiting room of abortion clinics and gave a report on his findings. He describes his own waiting room experience as a "bruising experience." Males spoke with relief of the rapidity and resoluteness of the decision-making process, the insignificance of the cost challenge and their firm conviction that power here belonged exclusively to their sex partner. They were not entirely without discontent. Specifically, a minority worried about the moral character of abortion. Many were bitter about the treatment they received from the abortion clinic, and quite a few had objections to their status in current abortion law. Sixty-eight per cent felt males involved in abortions did not have an easy time of it; 47% worried that such individuals generally had disturbing thoughts about it afterwards [39% were uncertain about this prospect]; 52% had "occasional" and 29% "frequent" thoughts of the fetus prior to the abortion. Thirty-nine per cent thought a fetus was a person; 26% felt abortion was the killing of a child; 17% thought the act they were involved in was immoral; 10% recalled urging adoption as an option; 17% recommended childbirth followed by single parenthood which they would support financially and emotionally; 45% recalled urging abortion.

3.37.54 "Families. Sex and the Liberal Agenda," Allan C. Carlson, *The Public Interest,* Winter 1980 p. 77

In place of the nuclear family, dominant voices in sociology and family counseling journals are now describing the emergence of new normative concepts. There should be no bias towards marriage and children. Everything is open. All habitual and cultural attitudes may be questioned. All values are on trial. Uninhibited Sexuality-Sexual gratification represents one of life's ultimate values. Access to regular sexual satisfaction should be viewed as a basic human right. The Problem of Children-Sexuality should be totally separated from procreation. Parenting should be undertaken only after a careful weighing of social, cultural and economic costs. ... Unwanted pregnancies should be aborted.

Violence

3.38 "Wantedness" as a Factor in Child Abuse

3.38.1 "Child Abuse: A Study of the Child's Perspective," Philip G. Ney *Child Abuse and Neglect* 10:511-518(1986).

In a study of 57 children admitted to the Child and Family Psychiatric Unit at Christchurch Hospital, New Zealand, a three-way study of abuse experience via mother, child and staff was undertaken. When wantedness by mothers was compared to abuse, there was no significant correlation between mothers not wanting their child and either the extent or severity of any kind of abuse. Some 85% of these children were wanted after they were born. Mother's ambivalence about their pregnancies appears to have been greatest during the early stages.

3.38.2 "The Hostility of Parents to Children: Some Notes on Infertility, Child Abuse and Abortion," Victor Calef, *International Journal of Psychoanalytic Psychotherapy* 1(1) :76, February 1972

A case of extensive therapy of a woman patient is described by a psychiatrist. The woman physically abused her children and also aborted an apparently "unwanted" pregnancy. The pregnancy was not, in fact, unwanted but due to pathological behavior had to be "destroyed." Unresolved conflicts in the woman's family of origin were uncovered, i.e., resentment against her father for failing to protect the woman from her cruel mother.

3.38.3 *Child Abuse: An Interactional Event,* A. Kadushin and J.A. Martin, (New York: Columbia University Press, 1981) 236

A study of non-sexual physical abuse by parents in Wisconsin found that less than 5% of the mothers had considered either abortion or adoption as a means of "unburdening" themselves of the child. Three out of four parents had a positive reaction to the child at birth.

3.38.4 "Antecedents of Child Abuse," W.A. Altemeier, S. O'Connor, P. Vietze, H. Sandler and K. Sherrod, *Journal of Pediatrics* 100(5):823 (1982)

In a Vanderbilt University study of 1,400 low-income mothers, it was found that mothers who had physically injured their children did not differ significantly from the non-abusing mothers in money available to raise a child, in considering abortion or adoption, readiness for motherhood or current feelings about the baby; abusing mothers had more aggressive tendencies, were more likely to think they had unfair treatment as a child and were more likely to have lost a child to foster care or avoidable death.

3.38.5 "Social aspects of the battered baby syndrome," M.S. Smith, R. Hanson and S. Noble, *Br. J. Psychiatry* 125:568(1974).

A British study of 134 battered children under five years of age compared to children under five years who were emergency hospital admissions with no battering found that abortion had been considered by only 12% of the mothers of battered children vs. 2% of controls, which was not considered statistically significant. Family size and family income was similar between the two groups but battered children were more likely to be illegitimate and mothers of battered children tended to be more isolated than controls.

3.39   Child Abuse and Its Relationship to Abortion

One of the arguments advanced for the legalization of abortion was that it would reduce child abuse. However, there is evidence that it may increase abuse and neglect of children as the following articles indicate.

3.39.1   "Smoking during pregnancy and child maltreatment," J. Chessare J. Pascoe, and E. Baugh, *International Journal for Bio-Social Research* 8:1-6(1986).

Women who continue to smoke during pregnancy had three times higher child abuse reporting rates in the 18 months following delivery than women who did not smoke during pregnancy. Ed. Note: women with a history of abortion are more likely to smoke during subsequent pregnancies compared to women with no history of abortion.

3.39.2   "Maternal Perinatal Risk Factors and Child Abuse," M. Benedict, R. White and P. Comely, *Child Abuse and Neglect* 9:217-224(1985).

A Johns Hopkins study of 532 Baltimore mothers in maltreating families (two-thirds black) found that mothers tended to be younger, have shorter birth intervals, less prenatal care and were significantly more likely to have had a prior stillbirth or reported abortion or a prior child death. Some 18% of abusing families had one or more prior stillbirth or abortion vs. 12% of non-abusing families. Where there were two stillbirths or abortions or a combination thereof, the rate was nearly doubled (4.3% vs. 2.4%). The authors called these findings "provocative" and concluded that reproductive history and the circumstances surrounding past pregnancies may provide important clues of what family dynamics may be related to subsequent maltreatment.

3.39.3   "Smoking in pregnancy:a study of psychosocial and reproductive risk factors," AW Morales et al, *J Psychosom Obstet Gynaecol* 18(4):247, 1997

A British study found that women who were more likely to smoke during pregnancy were more likely to have had previous miscarriages and terminations, more likely to report marital difficulties, and more likely to physically discipline their one year old infants. see also "Smoking during pregnancy and child maltreatment," J Chessare et al, *Int'l Journal for Biosocial Research* 8:1, 1986 (Women who continued to smoke during pregnancy had three times higher child abuse reporting rates compared to women who did not smoke during pregnancy.)

3.39.4   "Association of Drug Abuse and Child Abuse," PK Jaudes and E Ekwo, *Child Abuse & Neglect* 19(9): 1065-1075, 1995

A study at a Chicago urban medical center of children exposed to drugs in utero found that the risk of subsequent abuse or neglect was 80% higher among children whose mothers had previously planned abortion after controlling for confounding variables.

3.39.5 "Drug Use Among Adolescent Mothers: Profile of Risk," Amaro, Cabral, Zuckerman, *Pediatrics,* 84(1):144, July 1989.

In Boston inner city study of adolescent mothers in 1984-86, mothers with a prior elective abortion were twice as likely to use alcohol, marijuana, cocaine or opiates than non-drug users (33% v. 16%). Drug users were nearly three times more likely to report being threatened, abused or involved in fights during pregnancy than non-users (24% v. 9%).

3.39.6 "Post-Abortion Trauma. 9 Steps to Recovery," Jeanette Vought, (Grand Rapids: Zondervan, 1991).

In a study of 68 women in a post-abortion support group 10-15 years post-abortion, 32% reported lacking patience with their children, 29% reported sometimes being verbally or emotionally abusive with them, 20% acknowledged frequent anger toward their children, 15% admitted feelings of unexpected rage toward their children and 13% felt they over disciplined their children--29% also reported being over-protective of their children and 14.7% reported having difficulty bonding to their children.

3.39.7 "Two Hidden Predisposing Factors in Child Abuse," Emanuel Lewis, *Child Abuse and Neglect* 3:327-330(1979).

With all bereavement which occurs during or shortly before or after pregnancy, mourning tends to be inhibited. Quick replacement pregnancies impede the mourning of stillbirth; stillbirth can often lead to marital difficulty and if there is a family difficulty in containing violence, the child may be battered; child abuse is a pathological mourning reaction.

3.39.8 "Relationship Between Abortion and Child Abuse, Philip," Ney, *Canadian Journal of Psychiatry* 24:610-620(1979).

Death to Canadian children from social causes rapidly increased after early abortion became available on demand in 1969; British Columbia and Ontario, with the highest rates of abortion, are also the provinces with the highest rates of child abuse. Newfoundland, Prince Edward Island and New Brunswick, with low rates of abortion, have low rates of child abuse. Rates of increase of child abuse parallels increases in abortion. Rather than preventing child abuse, abortion on request may be a cause of the increase in battered and murdered children because, (1) Having an abortion may decrease an individual's instinctual restraint against the occasional rage felt toward those dependent on her care. (2) Allowing infants to die by permissive abortion might diminish the social taboo against aggressing the defenseless. (3) Abortion may devalue children, thus increases guilt and self-hatred, the parent may displace it onto a child. (5) A woman's choice for abortion increases the hostile frustration of some men, intensifying the battle of the sexes for which children are scapegoated. (6) Abortion of the first child may truncate the developing mother-infant bond, thereby diminishing future mothering capability. (7) A previous abortion may result in depression which interferes with the mother's capacity to bond to her newborn.

3.39.9 "Induced Abortion as a Precipitating Factor in Child Abuse or Neglect: Case Studies," *Association for Interdisciplinary Research Newsletter* 4(1), Spring, 1991, p.7

Severe anger and hostility shortly before undergoing an induced abortion spilled over to precipitate an act of reported physical abuse on a 9 year old child by the mother.

3.39.10 *A Survey of Post-Abortion Reactions,* David C. Reardon, (Springfield, Illinois: The Elliot Institute, 1987).

In a 1987 survey of 100 women who were contacted through state Women Exploited by Abortion chapters/ 22% reported being sexually abused as a child and 22% reported being physically abused as a child.

3.39.11 "The Spectrum of Fetal Abuse in Pregnant Women," John T. Condon *Journal of Nervous and Mental Disease* 174(9):509-516, September 1986.

"The fetus is a (potential) recipient par excellence for projection and displacement. The symbiotic relationship between the mother and unborn child... can provide a setting in which ambivalence or hostility can be acted out as assault or maltreatment."

3.40   Child Neglect or Failure to Bond

3.40.1 "The correlates of antenatal attachment in pregnant women," JT Condon et al, *Br J Med Psychol* 70(Pt. 4): 359-372, Dec, 1997.

Women having low maternal-foetal attachment were characterized by high levels of depression and anxiety, low levels of support outside the partner relationship, and high levels of control, domination, and criticism within the partner relationship.

3.40.2 "Infant Abortion and Child Abuse: Cause and Effect," Philip G. Ney, in *The Psychological Consequences of Abortion* Ed. D. Mall and W.F. Watts, (Washington D.C.: University Publications of America, 1979)

Neglect of a subsequent child was related to the depression in a mother from a previous abortion.

3.40.3 "Relationship Between Induced Abortion and Child Abuse and Neglect: Four Studies," Philip G. Ney, T. Fung, A.R. Wickett, *Pre- and Perinatal Psychology Journal* 8(1):43-63, Fall, 1993.

A mother with a history of psychiatric problems and a prior abortion subsequently married and gave birth to a child. Although she was excited at the pregnancy "as soon as they handed me the baby, I handed him back. It was a weird sensation." Later when she returned home she began screaming and hitting her baby, tossing him violently on the bed and desperately trying to stop his crying, "I used to get pissed off when he cried. I never felt close, not as much as I thought I would." She concluded, "If I had had the first child, I would not have been frightened and wouldn't have this problem."

3.40.4　"Some maladaptive syndromes of pregnancy and the puerperium," Richard L. Cohen, *Obstetrics and Gynecology* 27(4):562-570 (1966).

A history of abortions, periods of sterility, traumatic deliveries, or loss of children...may interfere with the mother's emotional growth. Quoting J. Rose, "The Prevention of Mothering Breakdown Associated with Physical Abnormalities of the Infant" in *Prevention of Mental Disorders in Children*, G. Caplan ed. (New York: Basic Books, 1961.)

3.40.5　*Canonical Variates of Post-Abortion Syndrome*, Helen P Vaughan, (Portsmouth, NH: Institute for Pregnancy Loss, 1990) 51

10% of stressed women felt that their abortion had a negative effect on subsequent bonding to and parenting children.

3.40.6　"The disturbance of the mother-child relationship by unsuccessful attempts at abortion," G. Caplan, *Mental Hygiene* 38:67-80(1954).

An unsuccessful attempt at abortion was found to be a direct cause of a disturbed mother-child relationship. Sixteen cases were studied.

3.40.7　"Motivation of Surrogate Mothers: Initial Findings," Philip Parker, *American Journal of Psychiatry* 140(1):117-118, January 1983.

In a study of 125 women who applied to be commercial surrogates, 35% either had a voluntary prior abortion (26%) or had relinquished a child for adoption (9%). Women felt, often unconsciously, that surrogate motherhood would help them master unresolved feelings of previous voluntary loss. Women stated, "It would be their baby, not mine," "I'm only an incubator," "I'd be nest watching" and, "I'll attach myself in a different way- hoping it's healthy." For an example of comment on commercial surrogacy, see "Death without dignity for commercial surrogacy: The case of Baby M. G. Annas," *Hastings Center Report* 18(2):21-24 (1988).

3.40.8　"Antecedents of Child Abuse and Neglect in Premature Infants," R. Hunter, N. Kilstrom, E. Kraybill and F. Loda, *Pediatrics* 61(8):629-635, April 1978.

In a study of 282 infants admitted to the newborn intensive care unit of a hospital, 255 were eventually discharged home to their parents. Ten of the 255 were subsequently reported for physical abuse (2) or neglect (8) during the first year of life. Reported families were noted to be severely isolated without adequate social support, frequent marital maladjustment, financial problems, poor use of medical services, inadequate child care arrangements, inadequate child spacing, lower birth weight, congenital defects in abused child at birth, expressed disappointment over the sex of the baby and 40% claimed to have seriously considered abortion, compared to only 7% of those who were not reported. Forty-one infants of the 255 discharged to their homes were considered high risk for abuse or neglect, yet few of these infants were reported for maltreatment. Parents of reported infants were most likely to be rated by the interviewer as impulsive, apathetic-futile, childish-dependent, or retarded or illiterate.

3.40.9 "Breaking the Cycle in Abusive Families," R. Hunter and N. Kilstrom, *American Journal of Psychiatry* 136(10):1320 (1979)

Repeat families representing 9 out of 10 families who had been reported primarily for neglect and who had been part of an earlier study/were compared with 40 nonrepeating families where there had been child abuse in the family of origin but not with current offspring. Repeating parents had less working through of childhood misfortunes. Non-repeaters were more active in churches or other social groups and were more hopeful. Ed. Note - Factors such as isolation, hopelessness, lack of social support and despair seemed to indicate a spiritual need in the abusing or neglecting families.

3.41 Family Violence and Abortion

3.41.1 "Past Trauma and Present Functioning of Patients Attending a Women's Psychiatric Clinic," E.F.M. Borins, P.J. Forsythe, *Am. J. Psychiatry* 142(4): 460, April, 1985

Physical or sexual abuse was significantly related to abortion, and abortion and trauma were significantly correlated in a sample of 100 women attending a psychiatric clinic.

3.41.2 "Women Psychiatric Outpatients Reporting Continuing Post-Abortion Distress: A Preliminary Inquiry," D. Hanley, H. Piersma, D. King, D. Larson. D. Foy, Presented at the Eight Annual Meeting of the International Society for Traumatic Stress Studies: Los Angeles, Oct. 23,1992.

In a study of women at an outpatient mental health facility approximately two-thirds of post abortion women reported having been physically and/or sexually abused as children, adolescents, or adults before and/or after their abortions.

3.41.3 "Child sexual abuse, HIV sexual risk, and gender relations of African-American women," GM Wingood, RJ DiClemente, *Am J Prev. Med* 13(5): 380-384, 1997

Women who reported a history of childhood sexual abuse were 50% more likely to have had an abortion.

3.41.4 "Psychosocial and behavioral factors associated with physical and sexual abuse among HIV infected women," LA Bedimo et al, Int Conf AIDS, 1998; 12:219 (abstract no. 14185)

Among women attending a HIV outpatient program in New Orleans, Louisiana, 45% reported ever experiencing sexual abuse, 82% acquired HIV through heterosexual contact. Among those sexually abused, 27% first experienced it before the age of 17. Factors associated with a history of sexual abuse included having a history of abortion (33% vs. 9%).

3.41.5 "The Prevalence of Domestic Violence Among Women Seeking Abortion," SL Glander et al, *Obstetrics and Gynecology* 91:1002, 1996

A study of urban women seeking abortions at a single abortion facility found that 39.5% reported prior abuse.

3.41.6 "Stressful Life Events and Alcohol Problems among Women Seen at a Detoxification Center," E.R. Morrissey and M.A. Schuckit, *J. Studies on Alcohol* 39(9):1559 (1978).

A 1976 Seattle, Washington study of women at a detoxification center found that problem drinkers and secondary alcoholics were found to be significantly more likely to have experienced alcoholic related problems subsequent to an abortion. Sixty-four percent of the secondary alcoholics and 32% of the problem drinkers reported physical fights while drinking.

3.41.7 *Psycho-Social Stress Following Abortion,* Anne Speckhard (Kansas City, MO: Sheed&Ward, 1987).

In a study of 30 women reporting stress following abortion 92% reported feelings of anger, rage or hostility toward others following the abortion. Feelings of anger were alternately directed at self, one's partner, medical professionals or significant others who were viewed as having taken a coercive role in the abortion decision.

3.41.8 "Women Who Seek Therapeutic Abortion: A Comparison with women Who Complete Their Pregnancies," C. Ford, P. Castelnuovo-Tedesco, K. Long, *American Journal of Psychiatry* 129(5):58/ November, 1972.

In a study of women seeking abortion for mental health reasons compared with a control group of pregnant women not seeking abortion, the abortion group was found to be more likely to have received psychiatric treatment (42.5% v. 21.1%) and much more likely to exhibit masochistic behavior patterns (35% v. 6%). Many women in the abortion group had been involved in relationships with men which they described as abusive and assaultive. Other women had engaged in self-destructive behavior such as cutting themselves with knives or scissors. Other women were involved in self-defeating behavior such as supporting irresponsible husbands or were married to alcoholics and/or philanderers.

3.42 Abortion as a Risk Factor for Violence During Pregnancy

3.42.1 "Violence During Pregnancy and Substance Abuse," Amaro, Fried, Cabral, Zuckerman, *Am. J. Public Health* 80(5): 575, May, 1990.

A prospective study of 1243 pregnant women who were predominately poor, urban minority women at Boston City Hospital during 1984-87 found that 7% reported physical or sexual violence during pregnancy. A prior elective abortion increased the relative risk of violence during pregnancy. (RR 1.68) Victims of violence were more likely to have had a history of depression, suicide, current unhappy feelings about the pregnancy, lack of support during pregnancy and were more likely to be heavy users of alcohol or illicit drugs.

3.42.2 "Domestic violence during pregnancy. The prevalence of physical injuries, substance abuse, abortions and miscarriages," LW Hedin, PO Janson , *Acta Obstet Gynecol Scand* 79(8):625-630, 2000.

Among 207 women from three different antenatal clinics in Goteborg, Sweden, 30 were abused during the current pregnancy. A higher proportion of abused women had undergone one or more abortions compared to the non-abused group.

3.42.3 "Pregnancy outcomes and health care use: Effects of abuse," J Webster et al, *Am J Obstet Gynecol* 174:769, 1996

An Australian hospital evaluated past and present abuse during pregnancy and found that abused women were significantly more likely to have had a higher incidence of miscarriage, two or more induced abortions, or neonatal death compared to non-abused women.

3.42.4 *Beyond Choice,* Don Baker, (Portland, Oregon: Multonomah Press, 1985).

A father still grieving the loss of his first child by abortion (coerced by his wife's parents) was upset about a subsequent pregnancy which occurred shortly after the abortion. Once in a fit of anger during an argument over finances, he struck his pregnant wife in the stomach. Five days after the birth of the baby, he left for work and never returned. A brief note said, "I'm sorry Deb. We couldn't have the baby we wanted and now we have got one I can't stand. It's too much for me to handle, Tim." His wife, Debbie, never saw Tim again.

3.42.5 "Physical Abuse in Pregnancy," Hillard, *Obstetrics and Gynecology* 66:185 (1985).

In a study of 742 pregnant women seen at the University of Virginia Obstetric clinics in 1982-83,10.9% indicated they had experienced physical abuse at some time in the past; 4.1% reported abuse during their current pregnancy. Those in currently abusive relationships were more likely to have considered abortion (34%) compared to controls (21%).

3.42.6 "Protecting the Children of Battered Women," Richard M. Tolman, *Journal of Interpersonal Violence* 3(4):476-483, December 1988.

A recent example of induced abortion as a result of coercion and violence of the father against the mother and unborn child is reported. The husband beat the wife extensively over the course of a 13-year marriage. He beat her during pregnancies, punching her in the face and stomach, and kicking her between the legs. Following the birth of their first two children, he had forced her to have two abortions she did not want. The wife became pregnant a third time when the husband forced her to have sex with him which resulted in the birth of their third child after the wife refused to have an abortion. The husband reportedly called the third child a "raw piece of meat." The case was referred to by social workers as "not atypical."

3.42.7   "Sixty Battered Women," Elaine Hilberman and Kit Munson, *Victimology* 2:460-470(1977-1978).

An unborn child may be used as a focal point for family violence. In a study of sixty battered women referred by the medical staff of a rural health clinic, the women involved reported changes in the pattern of family violence during pregnancy. There was increasing abuse for some with the pregnant abdomen replacing face and breasts as the target for battering with abortions and premature births as the result. Others reported less abuse with pregnancy and one woman deliberately stayed pregnant to avoid violence.

3.43   Homicide of Women During and Following Pregnancy

3.43.1   "Pregnancy-associated deaths in Finland 1987-1994- definition problems and benefits of record linkage," M Gissler et al, *Acta Obstet Gynecol Scand* 76:651-657, 1997.

A Finnish register linkage study identified all deaths that occurred up to 1 year after an ended pregnancy. The mortality rate was 27 per 100,000 births and 101 per 100,000 abortions. Compared to women of reproductive age with no pregnancy (1.0), the relative risk of death from homicide following abortion was 4.33 (1.03-18.2, 95% CI) compared to a relative risk of 0.31 (0.02-4.42, 95% CI) following childbirth.

3.43.2   "Enhanced Surveillance for Pregnancy-Associated Mortality-Maryland, 1993-1998," IL Horton and D Cheng, *JAMA* 285(11): 1455-1459, 2001.

247 pregnancy-associated deaths were identified from any cause during pregnancy or within 1 year of delivery during 1993-1998. 182 deaths (73.7%) of the pregnancy-associated deaths followed a live birth and 53 deaths occurred among pregnant women who were undelivered; 84 deaths occurred within 42 days of delivery, and 103 deaths occurred 43-365 days following delivery or termination of pregnancy; 50 deaths from homicide were identified among pregnant women or women who had been recently pregnant. An editorial noted that the enhanced surveillance revealed that when an expanded definition of maternal mortality is used, threats from a woman's social environment, like homicide, may be found to be more deadly than those from a biological environment.

3.43.3   "Hidden from View: violent deaths among pregnant women in the District of Columbia, 1988 - 1996," CJ Krulewitch et al, *J Midwifery Women's Health* 46(1): 4-10, 2001

651 autopsy charts were examined from 1988-1996 in the DC office of the Chief Medical Examiner. Among these, 30 (4.6%) documented evidence of pregnancy and 95.4% were not pregnant. Among the 30 deaths where pregnancy was documented, 13 (43.3%) were victims of

homicide. Among non-pregnant women, homicide was the leading manner of death (32.3%); 75% of those who were pregnant died from gunshot trauma; 3 out of 4 women with evidence of pregnancy who were victims of homicide were in their first 20 weeks of pregnancy. Many of the accused perpetrators in the study had the same address as the victim which suggests the possibility of domestic violence.

3.43.4   "Violence during Pregnancy and Substance Use," H Amaro et al, *Am J Public Health* 80(5): 575, 1990

A prior elective abortion increased the risk of violence during pregnancy by 68%,   compared to no abortion history among a sample of poor, urban, mostly minority women.

3.43.5   "Pregnancy outcomes and health care use: Effects of abuse," J Webster et al, *Am J Obstet Gynecol* 174:769, 1996

An Australian hospital evaluated past and present abuse during pregnancy and found that abused women were significantly more likely to have had a higher incidence of miscarriage, two or more induced abortions, or neonatal death compared to non-abused women.

3.43.6   "Domestic violence during pregnancy," LW Hedin and PO Janson, *Acta Obstet Gynecol Scand* 79:625-630, 2000

A Swedish study compared physically abused women with non-abused women during pregnancy. In the group of abused women a higher proportion had undergone one or more abortions than in the non-abused group. Smoking and alcohol use were strongly associated with physical and sexual abuse.

3.43.7   "Mediation of Abusive Childhood Experiences: Dissociation and Negative Life Outcomes," E Becker-Lausen , *Am J Orthopsychiatry* 65(4): 560, 1995

Dissociation was significantly related to reports of females of previously becoming pregnant and having an abortion in high school. Individuals who detach from reality by dissociation may disregard clues that may otherwise warn them of danger and become " sitting ducks" for later abuse.

Sexual Assault Pregnancy and Abortion

3.44   Rape

3.44.1   *Victims and Victors. Speaking Out About Their Pregnancy,* Abortion and Children Resulting from Sexual Assault, ed. David C Reardon, Julie Makimaa, and Amy Sobie (Springfield, IL: Acorn Books, 2000)

Analysis of pregnancy arising from rape or incest including anecdotal stories of women.

3.44.2   "Report of Sandra Mahkorn, MD," *Issues in Law and Medicine* 14(4):433-441, Spring, 1999.

Discusses the myths and realities of pregnancy following sexual assault. If a woman becomes pregnant following sexual assault, it is often difficult to determine if the pregnancy was the result of the assault, or another voluntary sexual encounter. DNA testing is available. Unfortunately, victims are often not aware of this option prior to a decision to abort.

3.44.3   "Rape-related pregnancy estimates and descriptive characteristics from a national sample of women," MM Holmes et al, *Am J Obstet Gynecol* 175(2): 320-324, 1996

A national probability sample of U.S. women found that rape-related pregnancy was 5% among victims of reproductive age (12-45) ; 32.4% did not discover they were pregnant until the second trimester ; 32.2% opted to keep the infant, 50% had an abortion, 5.9% placed the infant for adoption, and 11.8% had a spontaneous abortion.

3.44.4   "Issues in statutory rape law enforcement: the views of district attorneys in Kansas," HL Miller et al, *Family Planning Perspectives* 30(4): 177-181.

The 1996 federal welfare reform law calls for reduction of adolescent pregnancy rates through aggressive enforcement of statutory rape laws at the local and state level. A survey of Kansas district- attorneys found that 74% favored aggressive enforcement, but only 37% believed the public would support aggressive enforcement.

3.44.5   "Prevalence of sexual assault: A survey of 2404 puerperal women," A.J. Satin et al ,*Am J. Obstet. Gynecol.* 167: 973-975, 1992

A study of indigent women at Parkland Memorial Hospital in Dallas who delivered infants in 1991 found that five percent of puerperal women reported a history of sexual assault. These women have more frequent pregnancy complications but achieve normal pregnancy outcomes.

3.44.6   *Lime 5. Exploited by Choice,* Mark Crutcher, (Denton, Texas: Life Dynamics, Inc, 1996).

This book contains a valuable chapter on rape and sexual assault on women by those who are involved in the abortion industry.

3.44.7   "Sexual Abuse as a Factor in Adolescent Pregnancy and Child Maltreatment," D. Boyer, D. Fine, *Family Planning Perspectives* 24(1): 4, Jan/Feb 1992

Among 535 young women, 80% of whom were age 15-19, and who had become pregnant as adolescents, two-thirds had been sexually abused. Some 55% had been molested, 42% had been victims of attempted rape and 44% had been raped. Among those who had been raped 11% became pregnant. The average age at first rape was 13.1 (SD=3.1); the age of the perpetrator was 22.6 (SD=8.4)

3.44.8   "Pregnancy and Sexual Assault," Sandra K. Mahkom, in *The Psychological Aspects of Abortion* ed. D. Mall and W.F. Watts, (Washington D.C.: University Publications of America, 1979), 53-72.

In a fraction of a percent of rape cases, pregnancy does occur and it is a matter to be seriously and sympathetically addressed. In a study of 37 women who became pregnant following rape, 28 chose to continue their pregnancy, 5 chose abortion and 4 could not be determined. Seventeen women were extensively counseled. With supportive counseling two out of three women changed from initially negative attitudes to a positive viewpoint. None changed to a more negative viewpoint throughout the course of their pregnancy. It was found that the pregnant woman becomes progressively aware of the individuality and innocence of the fetus or unborn child. See also "Sexual Assault and Pregnancy," S. Mahkorn and W. Dolan in *New Perspectives on Human Abortion*, ed. T. Hilgers, D. Horan and D. Mall (Washington D.C.: University Publications of America, 1981), 182-198.

3.44.9   *His Eye is on the Sparrow,* Ethel Waters and Charles Samuels (Garden City [N.Y.]: Doubleday & Co., 1951).

Ethel Waters, the famous Black actress, authored the above titled book. (She is quoted as follows: "Some people disclaim their natural habitat. I always named my origin. It didn't hold me back and neither did my color. I was born in poverty. My father raped my mother when she was twelve years old. I was born out of wedlock.")

3.44.10 "Facing the Hard Cases," Mary Meehan, *Human Life Review* 9(3): 19-36, Summer 1983.

The revulsion people feel for the crime of rape carries over to the rape victim and any child who may have resulted from the unwelcome union. The child is never thought of as an entity deserving of consideration-only a blot to be removed."

3.44.11 "Aborted Women: Silent No More," David C. Reardon, (Chicago: Loyola Press, 1987).

Testimony of Debbie "Nelson" who was raped and had an abortion: "I still feel that I probably couldn't have loved that child conceived of rape, but there are so many people who could have loved that baby dearly. The man who raped me took a few moments of my life, but I took that innocent baby's entire life. That is not justice as I see it." Testimony of Jackie Bakker: "When I learned I was pregnant (from rape), my boyfriend and all my friends-including my girlfriend (who was also raped but not pregnant) deserted me. They all acted like I was the plague."

3.44.12 "Rape and Abortion: Don't Forget Robin," Mary Meehan, *Human Life Review* 16(1):55-62, Winter, 1990

Cites a number of instances of pregnancy following rape with a favorable outcome. Racism is a possible implicating factor in support of abortion following rape.

3.44.13 "Rape: An Organized Approach to Evaluation and Treatment," Hunt, *American Family Physician* 15(1): 154-158(1977).

Abortion was suggested if pregnancy results from rape.

3.44.14 "The Rape Victim: Psychodynamic Considerations," . Notman and Nadelson, *Am. J. Psychiatry* 133(4):408-412 (1976).

Good overview of the impact of rape on a woman.

3.45 Incest

3.45.1 *Victims and Victors. Speaking Out About Their Pregnancy,* Abortion, and Children Resulting from Sexual Assault, ed. David C Reardon, Julie Makimaa, and Amy Sobie (Springfield, IL: Acorn Books, 2000)

Analysis of pregnancy arising from rape or incest including anecdotal stories of women.

3.45.2 "Report of Sandra Mahkorn, MD," *Issues in Law and Medicine* 14(4):433-441, Spring, 1999.

Discusses the myths and realities of pregnancy from incest.

3.45.3 *The Secret Trauma,* Diana E.H. Russell, (New York: Basic Books, 1986)

There are a few studies on the prevalence of incestuous abuse of women. In a 1978 San Francisco study of 930 adult female residents, 16% reported at least one experience of incestuous abuse before age 18. Only 4 of these cases (2%) were ever reported to the police. 4.5% of the 930 women reported having been sexually abused by a father; 4.9% by an uncle, 2% by a brother and 1.2% by a grandfather. Female abusers constituted only 5% of the total number of abusers. Sexual abuse by stepfathers was far more prevalent than sexual abuse by biological fathers. 17% of the women raised by a stepfather were sexually abused by him before age 14 compared to only 2% of the women who were raised by biological fathers.

3.45.4 *Incest,* Herbert Maisch, tr. Colin Beame, (New York: Stein and Day Publications, 1972).

In a German study of 13 cases in which incest resulted in pregnancy, three of the male partners suggested abortion and three others actually tried to abort their own daughters or step-daughters (two were successful). Ed. Note: The state would have an interest in childbirth in case of incest to prevent the possible cover-up of a crime.

3.45.5 "Inconsistencies in genetic counseling and screening for consanguineous couples and their offspring: the need for practice guidelines," RL Bennett et al, *Genet Med* 1(6):286-292, Sept/Oct 1999

A survey of board certified genetic counselors found wide variation in the risk figures quoted to consanguineous couples and their offspring with birth defects and mental retardation (1% to 75% for incest between first-degree relatives, and 0.25% to 20% for first cousin unions). The need for genetic practice guidelines was expressed.

3.45.6   *Aborted Women: Silent No More,* David C. Reardon, (Chicago: Loyola Press, 1987).

Traumatic testimony of Edith Young, who became pregnant by her stepfather following rape/incest. Her mother and stepfather procured an abortion for her without telling her what was to happen. Twenty-six years later she still had emotional and physical scars from her incest and abortion experience. She said, "The abortion has not been in my best interest.. " it only saved their reputations, solved their problems", and "allowed their lives to go merrily on."

3.45.7   "Physical and Psychological Injury In Women Following Abortion: Akron Pregnancy Services Survey," L.E.H. Gsellman, *Association For Interdisciplinary Research Newsletter* 5(4):1-8, Sept./Oct. 1993.

A pregnancy services center in Akron, Ohio reported, in one case, that a father's incest had been covered by abortion five times. In another, abortion and two miscarriages covered three pregnancies caused by incest. Both young women had been immediately forced back into their abusive homes because abortion hid the deeds of the perpetuator.

3.45.8   "Adolescent Abortion Option," G. Zakus and S. Wilday, *Social Work in Health Care* 12(4):77-91, Summer 1987.

Women with a history of sexual abuse, including incest, molestation, rape may respond with great anxiety to abortion plans, encompassing even the initial pelvic exam. Oh a conscious or unconscious level these women may associate gynecological and abortion procedures with previous aggressive violations. One such case involved a teenager with an incestuous relationship with her father, who required hospitalization and use of a general anesthetic to do a suction procedure.

3.45.9   "The Consequences of Incest: Giving and Taking Life," G. Maloff in *Psychological Aspects of Abortion,* ed. D. Mall and W.F. Watts (Washington D.C.: University Publications of America, 1979) 73-110.

Extensive overview article.

3.45.10   "Reflections on Repeated Abortions: The Meanings and Motivations," S. Fisher, *J. of Social Work Practice* 2(2):70-87, May 1986.

The case of Ellen, a 19-year-old unmarried woman, is described who was living with her parents and sisters (23, 21) and a 28-year- old half-sister. Her half-sister had four prior abortions, her 23-year-old sister had three abortions and her 21-year-old sister one abortion. Ellen was the family's "good girl," academic and likable and seemed to be mothering her mother and sisters. Ellen conceived out of wedlock and had an abortion. Three months later she was pregnant again. The week after her abortion, Ellen had found her father in bed with her step-sister and discovered that her 23-year-old sister had been aware of the incestuous relationship for 12 years. Ellen was angry, disillusioned and felt betrayed. She felt that the incest had given her permission to stop being a "good girl" and trying to maintain an image of a "good family." She and her boyfriend decided to face the pain of the first abortion, live together and have their baby. Ed. Note: The repeated utilization of abortion appeared to help keep the incest a secret.

3.45.11 "Risk to Offspring of Incest," C.O. Carter, *The Lancet* 1(7487): 436, February 25,1967.

There is a four times greater risk of parents sharing a recessive gene between first- degree relatives compared to first cousins.

3.45.12 "Effects of consanguineous marriages on morbidity and precocious mortality: genetic counseling," N Freire-Maia, *Am J Med Gen* 18(3): 401-406

The excess risks of morbidity and precocious mortality for the offspring of incestuous matings and of matings of uncles-nieces and aunts-nephews, first cousins once removed, and second cousins have been estimated as 32%, 18%, 9%, 5%, and 2% respectively based on certain assumptions discussed in the article.

3.45.13 "A Study of Children in Incestuous Matings," Eva Seemanora, *Human Heredity* 21(2): 108-128 (1971).

Prenatal, neonatal and infant mortality are higher in incestuous unions; also there is an increased incidence of mental retardation and congenital malformation.

3.45.14 "Father-Daughter Incest-Treatment of the Family," M. Kennedy, and B.M. Cormier, *Laval Medical* 40(2): 946-950(1969).

Incest is basically a family pathology and by treating it as such there is evidence that there may be gain for all concerned when the family cooperates in treatment.

3.46 Second and Third Trimester Abortion

3.46.1 "Why Do Women Have Abortions," ? A Torres and JD Forrest, *Family Planning Perspectives* 20(4): 169, 1988.

An Alan Guttmacher Institute survey in 1987 who obtained abortions at 16 gestational weeks or later are significantly more likely to be teenagers under the age of 18, black women, unemployed women, or women covered by Medicaid. Abortions at 16 gestational weeks or more were more apt to be performed if the reason was possible fetal health problems, if the woman's parents wanted her to have an abortion, or if the pregnancy resulted from rape or incest. Women were significantly less likely to have an abortion at 16 gestational weeks or later if they were age 30 or older, if they had no religious affiliation, if they were having health problems, or if their husband or partner wanted them to have an abortion.

3.46.2 "Induced Terminations of Pregnancy: Reporting States, 1988," KD Kochenek, National Center for Health Statistics, *Monthly Vital Statistics Report* 39(12) Supplement, April 30, 1991

Twenty-five percent of young women age 14 had abortions at 13 gestational weeks or greater compared to 19% of women age 16, 13.8% of women age 18, and 11.2% of women age 20-24.

3.46.3   "Emotional Patterns Related to Delay in Decision to Seek Legal Abortion," N Kaltreider, *Cal Med* 118:23, 1973.

Women who have abortions in the second trimester are more likely to use the word " baby" to describe what is in her womb compared to women who have abortions in the first trimester who are more likely to use words such as " this pregnancy" or " this condition."

3.46.4   "Abortion Surveillance-United States, 1996," Koonin et al, *MMWR* 48/No.SS-4, July 30, 1999

11.0% of U.S. white women had abortions at 13 gestational weeks or more compared to 14.2% of black women, and 12.3% of Hispanic women.

3.46.5   "Psychodynamic aspects of delayed abortion decisions," JA Cancelmo et al, *Br J Medical Psychology* 65:333, 1992.

A study of New York City women found that abortion at later gestational ages was significantly associated with a greater disturbance of the basic sense of self due to gender/sexual conflict and lower levels of internalized striving or ambition.

3.46.6   "Delayed Abortion in an Area of Easy Accessibility," WA Burr, KF Schulz, *JAMA* 244 (1): 44, 1980.

Women with moral objections to abortion were more likely to have a late abortion compared to an early abortion. These moral conflicts included opposition of the woman to abortion as well as conflicted decisions.

3.46.7   *Psycho-Social Stress Following Abortion,* Anne Speckhard, (Kansas City, MO: Sheed&Ward, 1987)

A study of women with long term stress reactions following induced abortion had an overrepresentation of women who had abortions in the second trimester.

3.46.8   *Post Abortion Trauma: 9 Steps to Recovery,* Jeanette Vought, (Grand Rapids: Zondervan, 1991)

A religiously based postabortion recovery group had an overrepresentation of women with second or third trimester abortions.

3.46.9   "Psycho-Social Aspects of Late Term Abortions," Thomas Strahan, *Association for Interdisciplinary Research in Values and Social Change Research Bulletin* 14(4): 108, Jan/Feb 2000

Review Article

3.46.10 "Very and moderate preterm births: are the risk factors different?," Pierre-Yves Ancel et al, *Br J Obstet Gynaecol* 106: 1162-1170, Nov, 1999.

A study of preterm birth in 15 European countries found that among women with a previous second trimester abortion there was a 3.67 increased relative risk for very preterm birth (22-32 gestational weeks) and a 2.33 increased relative risk for moderate preterm birth (33-36 gestational weeks). Among women with a previous first trimester abortion there was a 1.86 increased relative risk for very preterm birth and a 1.58 increased risk for moderate preterm birth.

3.46.11 "Induced Abortion and Subsequent Pregnancy Duration," W Zhou et al, *Obstet Gynecol* 94:948-953, 1999.

A Danish study using national registries found that one evacuation had an overall increased relative risk of 2.27 for preterm birth compared to 1.82 for one vacuum aspiration abortion. Two evacuations had an overall increased relative risk of 12.55 for preterm birth compared to 2.45 overall increased relative risk for two vacuum aspirations. Ed Note: evacuations would most likely occur in the second trimester, while vacuum aspirations would occur in the first trimester.

4   Social Effects and Implications of Abortion

4.1   Outcome - Refused Abortions

4.1.1   "Therapeutic Abortion on Psychiatric Grounds," SJ Drower and ES Nash, *South Africa Medical Journal* 54:604-608, 1978.

A South African study of women who were seeking abortion on psychiatric grounds followed up women who were refused abortion as well as women who were granted abortion for 12-18 months. Those who had abortions were more likely to be under psychiatric treatment, admitted to increased use of alcohol, tobacco, or tranquilizers, had experienced adverse personality changes, and had greater social isolation compared to women who had been refused abortion and had a variety of other pregnancy outcomes.

4.1.2   "Abortion Denied - Outcome of Mothers and Babies," (editorial), Carlos Del Campo, *Canadian Medical Association Journal* 130(4): 361-362 ,1984.

Summarizes various studies including those related to the outcome of refused abortions and concludes that abortion is not the answer to social ills.

4.1.3   "Women Refused Second Trimester Abortion: Correlates with Pregnancy Outcome," N. Binkin, C. Mhango, W. Cates, B. Slovis, M. Freeman, *American Journal of Obstetrics and Gynecology*, Feb. 1,1983, pp. 279-284.

United States study reported that 80 percent of the women had their babies.

4.1.4   "One Hundred and Twenty Children Born Alter Application or Therapeutic Abortion Refused,"
         H. Forssman and I. Thuwe, *Acta Psychiatrica Scandinavica* 42:48-59(1966).

         This study attempted to ascertain the mental health, social adjustment and educational level of 120
         children up to age 21. The study concluded that unwanted children did not have the advantage of
         a secure family life, had more psychiatric care, more often displayed anti-social behavior and did
         less well in school than controls. However, there were other confounding variables. For example,
         26.7 percent of the unwanted children were born out of wedlock, compared with 7.5 percent of
         the control children.

4.1.5   "Children Born Following Refused Abortion," Wanda Franz, *Association for Interdisciplinary
         Research Newsletter* 2(4):1-6, Fall 1989

         Data does not support the conclusion that 'unwanted' children should be aborted.

4.1.6   "The Swedish Children Born to Women Denied Abortion Study: A Radical Criticism," P.
         Cameron and Tichenor, *Psychological Reports* 39:391-394(1976).

         (Concludes that re-examination of the data advanced in the light of differences in social class and
         proneness toward psychiatric consultation indicates that children issuing from a denied abortion
         turn out much as children in general.

4.1.7   "Follow-Up Study of Children Born to Women Denied Abortion," Z. Matejcek, *Abortion:
         Medical Progress and Social Implications,* Pitman, (London: Ciba Foundation Symposium 115,
         1985) 136-148.

         Comments of the author:

         In child psychology and psychiatry the opinion is generally accepted that an unwanted pregnancy
         can have a very negative influence on the development of the child. However, the published work
         on this subject is extremely sparse. (Concluded from 1970 study): Although the differences
         between unwanted and control children were not dramatic, they were consistent and tended to
         support the major hypothesis that the development of children born to women denied abortion
         would be more problem prone.

         Unwanted pregnancy represents, in the life history of the child, something of an "aggravating
         circumstance," i.e., a certain risk that may or may not materialize in a particular situation in life.
         (Concluded from 1977 study):

         Differences in school achievement in ratings of the child's personality and parental attitudes were
         more pronounced. (Some questionable aspects of the study-later 38 percent of the mothers denied
         they ever wanted to get rid of the child; many now said they were very grateful abortion was
         denied; others said they hated the commission; parents were paid to participate; school problems
         could be alcohol-related, which was not considered; 20 percent divorce rate of unwanted group is
         a possible confounding factor.

4.1.8   Pregnancy Resolution Decisions: What If Abortions Were Banned?," J. Murphy, B. Symington, S. Jacobson, Journal of Reproductive Medicine 28 (II): 789-797 (1983)

Availability of another person to help with an unplanned child was most closely associated with the decision to carry the baby to term or abort it.

4.2   Sex Selection Abortion

4.2.1   "Attitudes Toward Abortion as a Means of Sex Selection," Richard N. Feil, G Largey and M. Miller, *Journal of Psychology*, 116:269-272(1984).

Acceptance of abortion as a means of sex selection varied widely among students at Mansfield University in New England. Religiosity based on church attendance proved to be the most dominant variable. Thirty-two percent of those who attended church once a month or less were accepting/compared with those who attended more often [8.5 percent]. Overall, about 18 percent of the students showed acceptance of amniocentesis followed by abortion for purposes of sex selection. Attitudes toward other sex-testing methods were also studied.

4.2.2   "Some Social Implications of Sex Choice Technology," L. Fidell, D. Hoffman and P. Keith Spiegel, *Psychology of Women Quarterly*, 4:32-41(1979).

In a California State University at Northridge study of 770 undergraduates, 85 percent wanted male first-born children; 73 percent wanted a second-born girl; 60 percent said they would probably not use sex choice methods; 29 percent said they probably would; and 11 percent said they would use them to guarantee the second child was of the opposite sex to the first.

4.2.3   "Guidelines for the Ethical, Social and Legal Issues in Prenatal Diagnosis," T Powledge and J. C. Fletcher, *New England Journal of Medicine,* 300:168-172(1979).

"Although we strongly oppose any movement aimed at making diagnosis of sex and selective abortion a part of ordinary medical practice and family planning, we recommend that no legal restrictions be placed on the ascertainment of fetal sex.... We think most couples should not seek the information however."

4.2.4   "A Medical View," Haig Kazazian, Jr., *Hastings Center Report*, 10:17-20(1980).

Responses to John Fletcher: John Fletcher argues cogently that if the Supreme Court has given women the right to choose whether or not a pregnancy is carried to term, sex selection is merely an extension of that right.... [But] wholesale acceptance of Fletcher's view on this issue could indirectly be disastrous for legal abortion in this country.

4.2.5   "Gender Ethics," Gertrud Lenzer, *Hastings Center Report*, 10:17-20(1980).

Responses to John Fletcher: Surely it can hardly be the legal moral intent of the Supreme Court's position to guarantee women the right of self-determination for the purpose of discriminating against their own kind by doing away with the fetuses of their own sex or by choosing male children as firstborns by means of newly developed preconceptive technology.

4.2.6   "Negative and Positive Rights," James F. Childress, *Hastings Center Report*, 10:17-20 (1980).

Responses to John Fletcher: Contrary to Fletcher, the Supreme Court did not make "the conscience of the individual woman the sole arbiter of the reasons." Even if this claim holds for *noninterference* it does not hold for *assistance*.

4.2.7   "The Supreme Court and Sex Choice," Margaret O'Brien Steinfels, *Hastings Center Report*, 10:17-20(1980).

Responses to John Fletcher: Gender should not be turned into a disease subject to medical "cure"; one should not foster cultural and social prejudice that values one sex over the other; one should not confirm the prejudice that sex is the governing factor in behavior, status and vocation.

4.2.8   "Preselecting the Sex of Offspring: Technologies. Attitudes and Implications," S. Hartley and L. Pietraczyk, *Soc. Biol.* 26:232-246(1979).

In northern California, 2,138 respondents indicated widespread acceptance of ongoing biomedical research to perfect preselection methods and of making these procedures available to potential parents. Almost half agreed that they might want to use such techniques. Variation in levels of agreement were assessed by sex, race, marital status, child-parity, religious affiliation and attendance, level of education, class and general attitudes toward medical and scientific leaders. The implications of the general acceptability of sex selection go far beyond the freedom of parental choice to such matters to socialization patterns of first son, second daughter ordering, sex role inflexibilities, sex ratio imbalances, and include possibilities for curtailing rapid population growth.

4.2.9   "Ethics of Testing a Baby's Sex," *U.S.A. Today*, October 14,1987.

One-third of the medical geneticists in the U.S. are willing to order prenatal tests to determine a child's sex, even if it meant the parents might abort a fetus that wasn't the sex they wanted. Dr. John C. Fletcher of the University of Virginia School of Medicine, who conducted the study, said, "Giving prenatal diagnosis for sex choice is morally objectionable."

4.2.10   "What Happens When We Get the Manchild Pill?," Colin Campbell, *Psychology Today*, 10(8):86-89 (1976).

Clearly sex control could shake up the human race to its roots. "It is hard to find a scientist in this field who doubts that a cheap, carefree and reliable method of sex control will become available. If large numbers of parents began having boys as eldest children, certain sex role types might harden forever."

4.2.11   "The Slippery Slope of Science," A. Etzioni, *Science*, 183, pp. 1041(1974).

Sex pre-determination may lead to policies of eugenics.

4.2.12   "Sex Determination: Its Impact on Fertility," G. Markle and C. Nam, *Social Biology* 18:73-83(1971).

A review of the literature suggests that people favor sex choice so that they may have smaller families.

4.2.13   "Abortion for "Wrong" Fetal Sex: An Ethical-Legal Dilemma," J. Elliott, *Medical News,* 242:1455-1456(1979)

4.2.14   "Social Acceptance of New Techniques of Child Conception," R.L. Matteson, and G. Terranova, *Journal of Social Psychology* 101:225-229(1977).

4.2.15   "Sex Preselection in the United States: Some Implications," Charles F. Westoff and Ronald R. Rindfuss, *Science,* 184(4127):633-636, May 10,1974

4.2.16   "An Abuse of Prenatal Diagnosis," M. Stenchever, *JAMA*, 221:408(1972).

4.3   Genetic Engineering

4.3.1   "A Support Group for Couples Who Have Terminated a Pregnancy after Prenatal Diagnosis: Recurrent Themes and Observations," L. Suslak, A. Scherer, G. Rodriguez, *J. Genetic Counseling* 4(3): 169,1995

The impact of terminating a pregnancy for a birth defect is a devastating and isolating experience; devastating because the dream of parenthood, of family life and of giving love and nurture is gone. Isolating because in our society there is no formal recognition or acceptable mourning period for grief.

4.3.2   "The Return of Eugenics," Richard John Neuhaus, *Commentary,* 86:15, April, 1988

The reach of the eugenic vision is to eliminate the limits and risks in what was once deemed natural.

4.3.3   "Patient Response to Genetic Amniocentesis," Goldstein and Hyun, *Journal of Perinatology* 5(1):9-12, Winter 1985

Twenty-six out of 107 respondents commenting on abortion said they would consider abortion if results of amniocentesis had shown abnormalities. Despite this response, the authors, based upon other data, concluded that amniocentesis is likely a live-saving procedure.

4.3.4   "CVS for first-trimester fetal diagnosis," Brambiti and Oldrini, *Contemporary OB/GYN* 25(5):94-104, May 1985

Chronic villus sampling (CVS) in the first 250 cases resulted in 22 genetic-induced abortions, 3 non-genetic-induced abortions, 10 fetal losses (4.4%); 11, pre-term deliveries (4.9%); 214 full-term deliveries. Complications included 4 threatened abortion, 42 (18.6%) vaginal bleeding, 7 malformations, 14 intrauterine growth retardation (6.2%). The authors conclude that the sampling technique is safe.

4.3.5   "Pregnancy Termination for Genetic Indications: The Impact on Families. R," Furlong and R. Black, *Social Work in Health Care* 10(1): 17, Fall 1984

In a study of 26 families at Yale New Haven Hospital in 1979-1982, in which mothers underwent abortion because of a serious defect in the unborn child, it represented a difficult and painful chapter of their lives. Fathers were particularly adversely impacted. Nineteen out of 22 children in the families studied had mild to severe reactions based upon observations of the parents.

4.3.6   "Sequelae and Support After Termination of Pregnancy for Fetal Malformation," J. Lloyd and K.M. Laurence, *British Medical Journal* 290:907-909, March 1985.

Some 77% of the women studied experienced an acute grief reaction. Some 46% still remained symptomatic after six months, some requiring psychiatric support. Several would have liked burial or some recognition of death. Several had problems severe enough to influence reproductive behavior.

4.3.7   "The Psychological Sequelae of Abortion Performed for a Genetic Indication, B," Blumberg,M. Golbus and K. Hanson, *Am. J. of Obstet and Gynecol* 122(7):799-808, August, 1975.

Stresses attendant to selective termination produce undesirable marital consequences that threatened marital stability.

4.4   Deterioration of Economic and Social Conditions Following Abortion

One reason advanced for legalized abortion is that it is necessary for the economic and social advancement of women. However, several studies have found that abortion, and particularly repeat abortion, is related to a poorer economic and worsened social condition of women. Overall, 60% of U.S. women who have an abortion will have a repeat abortion by age 30.

4.4.1   "Contraceptive Practice and Repeat Induced Abortion: An Epidemiological Investigation," MJ Shephard and MB Bracken, *Journal of Biosocial Science* 11:289, 1979.

A U. S. study of low income women found that women with repeat abortions were more likely to be divorced, and be on welfare compared to women with first abortions.

4.4.2   "Association of Induced Abortion with Subsequent Pregnancy Loss," AA Levin et al, *JAMA* 243(24): 2495, June 27, 1980.

Women entering Boston Hospital for Women with a history of one or two prior abortions, were more likely to be a welfare recipient (26%-27%) compared to women with no prior abortion. (16.9%)

4.4.3   "Repeat Abortion in Denmark,"Osler et al, *Danish Medical Bulletin* 39(1): 89, 1992.

Danish women repeating abortion were more likely to be unemployed, less likely to have a partner, and were more likely to live alone compared to women with first abortions.

4.4.4   "The First Abortion-And the Last? A Study of the Personality Factors Underlying Repeated Failure of Contraception," P Niemela et al, *Int'l J Gynaecol Obstet* 19:193, 1981

Finnish women seeking a second abortion had less net household income, poorer housing, weaker relationships with their partner, and were poorer at building up the socioeconomic aspect of their lives than women with first abortions.

4.4.5   "Repeat Abortion: A Comparative Study," M Tornbom et al, *J Psychosomatic Obstet Gynecol* 17:208, 1996.

Swedish women applying for a repeat abortion were more likely to have had contact with the social service system, were less satisfied with their partner relationship, and had a more unstable relationship compared to women with a first abortion or women carrying to term.

4.4.6   "The influence of social class on parity and psychological reactions in women coming in for induced abortion," B Hamark et al, *Acta Obstet Gynecol Scand* 74(4): 302-306, 1995

Among women living in Gotenberg, Sweden and seeking a first trimester abortion, previous abortion experience was more likely among women living in lower socioeconomic districts in the city.

4.4.7   "Psychosocial Correlates and Antecedents of Abortion: An Exploratory Study," F. Costa et al, *Population and Environment* 9:3, 1987

A long term study of primarily Anglo women found that women with an abortion history were more likely to exhibit multiple problem behavior, have lower occupational prestige, be similar in educational attainment, and have only slightly higher personal income compared to women with no abortion history.

4.5   Abortion and Race or Poverty

4.5.1   "The African-American Cancer Crisis, Part I: The Problem," L.A. Clayton, W.M. Byrd, *J. of*

Health Care for the Poor and Underserved 4(2): 83,1993

Contemporary African-Americans have the highest age-adjusted rates of cancer incidence and mortality of any racial or ethnic group in the United States.

4.5.2   "Early Adult Psychological Consequences for Males of Adolescent Pregnancy and Its Resolution," M. Buchanan, C. Robbins, *J. Youth and Adolescence* 19(4): 413,1990

In a Texas study of 2522 young men who were first surveyed as 7th grade students in 1971,15% had been involved in a non-marital pregnancy by age 21. 56% of black men had girlfriends who had the child but did not marry or cohabitate, while 28% married and had the child while 16% were ended by abortion. White adolescent males tended to end non-marital adolescent pregnancies by abortion (58%) and 34% chose to marry or cohabitate. Although numbers were small, 55% of Hispanic men married or cohabitated as a result of an adolescent pregnancy. Men whose girlfriends had abortions were more distressed than the men whose girlfriends carried the pregnancy to term.

4.5.3   "A Case Study of Race Differences Among Late Abortion Patients," J. Lynxwiler, M. Wilson, *Women & Health* 21(4): 43,1994

A study of 240 women who had second trimester abortions in a private womens clinic in a large southern city in 1988-1989 found that black women who delayed abortion had lower incomes, were more likely to live with their family of orientation, less likely to live alone, be more religious, more likely to have children, less likely to have pro-choice attitudes and less likely to have support for the abortion decision compared to white women who delayed abortion.

4.5.4   "Abortion Patients in 1994-1995: Characteristics and Contraceptive Use," SK Henshaw, K. Kost, *Family Planning Perspectives* 28(4): 141, July/August 1996.

In a national survey of U.S. women who obtained induced abortions in 1994-1995 61.3% were reported to be white, 31.1% black, 7.6% other races and 20.2% Hispanic. Because of over-lap the total exceeds 100%.

4.5.5   "The Characteristics and Prior Contraceptive Use of U.S. Abortion Patients," SK Henshaw, J. Silverman, *Family Planning Perspectives* 20(4)158-168, July/Aug. 1988.

In a 1987 study of 9,480 women who obtained abortions at 103 clinics, hospital and doctor's offices, 12.8% were Hispanic vs. 8.4% Hispanic (all women); 31.4% were non-white vs. 16.7% non-white generally.

4.5.6   "Abortion Surveillance, United States. 1988," L.M. Koonin, K.D. Kochanek, J.C. Smith, M. Ramick, *MMWR*, V. 140, No. SS-1, June, 1991, pp 15-42.

In 1988 the Centers For Disease Control reported 1,371,285 legal abortions in the U.S.; 35.6% of the abortions were by black women and other women of color. Black or other women of color were more likely to have abortions at a later stage of gestation than white women (14.5 v. 12.0),

(8.0 vs. 5.8) and (5.9 vs. 4.0) at 11-12 weeks, 13-15 weeks and 16-20 weeks gestation respectively.

4.5.7   "Why Do Women Have Abortions?," A. Torres, J.D. Forrest, *Family Planning Perspectives*, 20(4):169-176, July/Aug. 1988.

A 1987 Survey by the Alan Guttmacher Institute of 38 abortion facilities across the U.S. found substantive differences in abortion decision by race. For example, black women were less likely (25%) to have elected to have an abortion in order to keep others from knowing they were have sex or had become pregnant than whites (33%) and other women (Asian, Native American, Hispanic) (40%). White women (26%) were more likely than black women (17-18%) to say they were influenced by their partner's desire for them to have an abortion.

4.5.8   "Fears of Genocide Among Black Americans as Related to Age, Sex and Region," C. Turner and W.A. Darity, *American Journal of Public Health*, 63(12): 1029-1034, December 1973.

This study conducted in Philadelphia and Charlotte, North Carolina concluded that black Americans, especially young, black males, are suspicious that genocide is the aim of family planning programs controlled by whites. Black women are more positively inclined to use birth control than black men.

4.5.9   "Unmarried Black Adolescent Father's Attitudes Toward Abortion. Contraception and Sexuality: A Preliminary Report," Leo E. Hendricks, *Journal Adolescent Health Care* 2: 199-203(1982).

In a study of attitudes of unmarried black adolescent fathers in Tulsa, Chicago and Columbus, Ohio, 77 to 95 percent agreed with the statement, "If I got a girl pregnant, I would not want her to have an abortion because it's wrong." From 44 to 66 percent answered false to the statement, "Birth control is for girls only."

4.5.10 "Contraceptive Needs and Practices Among Women Attending an Inner-city STD Clinic," D. Upchurch, M. Fanner, D. Glasser and E. Hook *American Journal Public Health*, 77(11): 1427-1430, November 1987.

In a Baltimore study of contraceptive use among black women, 46 percent were not using contraception. Substantial numbers had formerly used contraception but had discontinued use. Fifty-one percent indicated an interest in receiving contraceptive services in a STD clinic setting.

4.5.11 "Delivery or Abortion in Inner-City Adolescents," Susan A. Fischman, *American Journal Orthopsychiatry*, 47(1):127-133, January 1977.

Adolescent sexual behavior does not automatically change as the ink dries on new, liberal laws. Birth control methods and legal abortions have been ignored by many, and young unwed girls are increasingly expressing their desire to have babies. Deliverers tended to enjoy a greater degree of emotional support from their mothers. The girl's relationship with her boyfriend was an important factor in the decision-making process-the more stable and long-term the relationship, the lower the abortion incidence. The deliverer's boyfriend was more likely to be working full time as opposed to the aborter's boyfriend, who was apt to be attending school full or part-time. Aborters were more likely to be attending school at their appropriate grade level, while deliverers' had a higher probability of having discontinued school. The pregnancy per se was not the primary reason for school discontinuance and frequently occurred after the girl had left school. Very few of the deliverers planned to marry in the near future. Deliverers attached greater importance to religion. Welfare status of nearly half of the deliverers was not viewed as a deterrent to childbearing. Mere availability of contraceptives was not a deterrent to pregnancy. The decision to become a teenage mother was not affected by such global factors as improved contraception, delayed marriage, changes in roles of women, and general concerns with population and environment.

4.5.12   "The Social and Economic Correlates of Pregnancy Resolution Among Adolescents in New York City, by Race and Ethnicity: A Multivariate Analysis," Theodore Joyce, *AmJ. Public Health* 78(6):626-631, June, 1988.

Availability of abortion had little association with outcome among various ethnic groups in New York City. For blacks, white, and Puerto Rican, the unmarried women least likely to seek abortions and nulliparous, are receiving Medicaid, have no previous abortions and had low levels of schooling. Teenagers who have experienced 1 prior abortion are approximately 4 times more likely to terminate a current pregnancy. Young married black women were more likely to abort than comparable Puerto-Rican, Latinos or white women. Married women were much less likely to abort than single women.

4.5.13   "Predicting the Psychological Consequences of Abortion," L.R Shusterman, *Social Science and Medicine*, 13A: 683-689,1979.

A Chicago study interviewed 345 women pre-abortion with follow-up interviews 2-3 weeks post-abortion; 77% were Caucasians, 23% blacks. Black women claimed the least intimate and least positive relationships with their male partners compared to whites or Orientals. Oriental women were most likely to inform the father whereas blacks were least likely to inform him.

4.5.14   "Race, Motherhood and Abortion," Candace Clark, Ph.D. Thesis, Columbia Univ. (1979) *Dissertation Abstracts Intl* 40(10), April, 1980 Order no. 8008711.

A study of women in the New York area (1973-1976) found that black mothers were much less likely than white mothers to have planned their pregnancies and were much more likely to have terminated unplanned pregnancies. White mothers were no more likely than blacks to hold negative attitudes toward abortion. Many mothers who had opposed having abortions subsequently terminated pregnancies. Data suggested medical personnel may act as barriers to birth or abortion. Findings support a social structural, rather than attitudinal or values interpretation of racial differences in pregnancy outcome among mothers. Ed Note: This study is evidence of racism among facilities where decisions are made for birth or abortion.

4.5.15　*The Connecticut Mutual Life Report on American Values in the '80s: The Impact of Belief,* Commissioned by Connecticut Mutual Life Insurance Co., (Hartford, Connecticut: Factors Affecting Perceived Morality of Abortion, 1981) 92.

In response to the question, "Do you believe abortion is morally wrong, or is it not a moral issue?" 64 percent of whites thought it morally wrong, 73 percent of blacks, 74 percent of people with annual income under $12/000, 64 percent of people with annual income of $12,00- $25,000, and 56 percent of people with annual incomes above $25/000:64 percent male, 67 percent female.

4.5.16　"Abortion Attitudes in Poverty Level Blacks," C.E. Vincent, C.A. Haney, and C.M. Cochrane *Seminars in Psychiatry* 2:309-317(1970),

In a study by the Bowman-Gray Medical School on poverty level blacks, 79 percent of 776 black females, 86 percent of 500 of their sex partners, and 70 percent of 215 low- to middle-income black females were found to be "not in favor of abortions under any circumstances."

4.5.17　"Abortion, Poverty and Black Genocide," Erma Clardy Craven, *Abortion and Social Justice*, ed. T. Hilgers and D. Horan, Thaxton, (Virginia: Sun Life, 1972,1980) 231-243.

Except for the privilege of aborting herself, the black woman and her family must fight for every other economic and social privilege. The quality of life for the poor, the black and the oppressed will not be served by destroying their children. Those who openly propose abortion as a solution to almost any problem openly deny that it has racial implications, yet a social worker in recent testimony before the Minnesota State legislature cited the case where the parents of a white pregnant teenager, learning the father was black, changed their minds from adoption to abortion. The social worker used this incident as an example of why abortion should be available on demand.

4.5.18　*Men and Abortion: Lessons. Losses and Love,* Arthur Shostak and Gary McLouth, (New York: Praeger, 1984).

The authors interviewed 1000 men who accompanied women to abortion clinics. Substantially more black men than white men opposed the abortion.

4.5.19　"Legal abortion mortality in the United States: 1972 to 1982," H.K. Atrash, H.T. MacKay, N. J. Binkin, C.J.R. Hogue, *AmJ. Obstet Gynecol.* 156:605-612,1987.

Based on data from the Centers For Disease Control the rate of mortality from legal abortions and abortion related deaths from 1977 to 1982 was 0.6% per 100,000 abortion procedures for white women and 1.8 per 100,000 abortions from women who were black or other races.

4.5.20　"Deaths From Second Trimester Abortion by Dilatation and Evacuation: Causes, Prevention, Facalitus," W. Cates, Jr., D.A. Grimes, *J. Am. College Obstetricians and Gynecologists* 58(4):401, Oct. 1981.

Among the 18 deaths of U.S. Women from 1972 through 1978 by dilation and evacuation, 11 were black women.

4.5.21 "The Father of the Infant of the Unwed Mother," Dorothy Hollingsworth, K. Thompson, J.A. Carlson and Jackson, University of Kentucky Med. Center, Lexington (1975). Abstract printed in *Pediatric Research* 9:260(1975).

In a study of 411 consecutive pregnancies in women ages 12-18 years, information was collected from mothers on social status, education, income, and relationship with father of infant. The population was unusual [46 percent white, 54 percent black], from low socioeconomic families (mean annual income $4/200]. Primary support was from parental earnings in 60 percent of whites and 48 percent blacks. Striking racial differences were: [1] 44 percent of black fathers were in school vs. 14 percent of whites; [2] unemployment was 24 percent in whites vs. 9 percent for blacks; [3] before conception, 86 percent of fathers in both groups had a close relationship with the mother. By first maternal clinic visit [mean 5.6 months gestation], 36 percent white fathers had abandoned the patient vs. 18 percent blacks; 63 percent black fathers continued dating or planned marriage vs. 34 percent of whites; [4] blacks were more concerned with infant plans: 73 percent of black fathers requested mother to keep child vs. 41 percent of whites; black fathers and/or their families offered infant support significantly more often than whites [70 percent vs. 40 percent]. Post partum, 59 percent of black fathers maintained a close relationship with mother and infant compared with only 36 percent of whites.

4.5.22 "Rising Incidence of Breast Cancer Among Young Women in Washington State," E. White, J.R. Daling, T.L. Norsted and J. Chu, *Journal of the National Cancer Institute* 79(2):239-243, August 1987

Although on the basis of small numbers, the risk for breast cancer among black women aged 25-44 years doubled from 1974-77 to 1982-84 in the state of Washington compared with a 22% increase for white women of the same age. It was noted that black women have a higher rate of induced abortion than white women which may be a contributing factor to the increased incidence.

4.5.23 "Breast Cancer Risk Factors in African-American Women: The Howard University Tumor Registry Experience," A.E. Laing, F.M. Demenais, R. Williams, V.W. Chen, G.E. Bonney, J. *National Medical Association* 85(12): 931-939, Dec. 1993.

In a Howard University case control study of African-American women seen at their hospital from 1978-1987, the multiple logistic estimates of the odds ratio for breast cancer among women under 40 years of age, between 41-49 years and over 50 years was 1.5, 2.8, and 4.7 respectively among women with a history of induced abortions compared to women with no history of induced abortions.

4.5.24 "Akron Pregnancy Services Survey-," 126 Self-Reported Responses to Questionnaires Completed by African-American Women, November, 1988-August, 1994

A long- term study of young African-American women receiving a variety of services at Akron

Pregnancy Services in Akron, Ohio and who reported one or more prior induced abortions found that 81% had one or more psychological complaints including guilt (60%), crying/depression (55%), regret/remorse(49%), inability to forgive self (35%), anger/rage (26%), desire to get pregnant again (23%), lower self-esteem (21%), despair/ helplessness (17%), failure to make decisions (15%), drug/alcohol abuse (6%).; 75% said they would not have their abortion again; 28% said they desired further post abortion support , and 41% said the relationship with the father of the aborted baby soon ended after the abortion.

4.5.25 "Cocaine Use During Pregnancy: Prevalence and Correlates," D.A. Frank, H. Amaro, H. Baucher, R. Hingson, S. Parker, H. Reece and R. Vinci, *Pediatrics* 82(6):888-895, December 1988

A study of 697 Boston inner-city women during 1984 to determine the extent of cocaine use during pregnancy found that a history of two prior abortions doubled the rate of cocaine use (19% vs. 9%) and a history of three or more abortions tripled the risk of cocaine use (9% vs. 3%) compared with non-cocaine users. Some 62% of the cocaine users were North American blacks, 4% were identified as other blacks, 47% of the non-cocaine users were North American blacks and 19% were identified as other blacks.

4.5.26 "Drug Use Among Adolescent Mothers: Profile of Risk," H. Amaro, B. Zuckerman and H. Cabral, *Pediatrics* 84:144-150, July 1989.

A study of 253 inner-city Boston adolescents served at Boston City Hospital during 1984-86 found that a history of a prior elected abortion increased by twice (33.0% vs. 16.3%) the likelihood that the adolescent mother was using alcohol, marijuana or cocaine. Some 67.9% of the drug users were American blacks, 8.9% were foreign-born blacks; 44% of the non-users were American blacks, 14.9% of the non-users were foreign-born blacks.

4.5.27 "Emotional Distress Patterns Among Women Having First or Repeat Abortions," E. Freeman, K. Rickels, G.R. Huggins, C. Garcia and J. Polin, *Obstetrics and Gynecology* 55(5): 630, May 1980

Some 413 women between the ages of 14-40 who underwent first trimester abortions at the University of Pennsylvania in 1977-78 were rated on emotional symptoms on pre-abortion and post-abortion tests. Some 35% of the women were repeating abortions. Seventy percent of the women undergoing a first abortion were black and 93% of the women undergoing a repeat abortion were black. Post-abortion scores of emotional distress of repeat abortion patients compared with women who had a first-time abortion were significantly higher on interpersonal sensitivity, paranoid ideation, phobic anxiety and sleep disturbance.

4.5.28 "Association of Drug Abuse and Child Abuse," Jaudes et al, *Child Abuse and Neglect* 19:1065, 1995.

An urban medical center which served a black population on the south side of Chicago studied children who were exposed to drugs in utero and found that the risk of subsequent child abuse or neglect increased 80% among children whose mothers had previously planned abortions.

4.5.29   "Violence during Pregnancy and Substance Abuse," H Amaro et al, *American Journal Public Health* 80(5): 575, May, 1990.

A predominantly, poor, urban, minority group of women attending clinics at Boston City Hospital who had prior elective abortion were 68% more likely to be a victim of violence during pregnancy compared to women with no abortion history.

4.5.30   "Contraceptive Practice and Repeat Induced Abortion: An Epidemiological Investigation," M Shephard and M Bracken, *Journal of Biosocial Science* 11:289, 1979.

Black women with repeat abortions were more likely to be on welfare compared to black women with one abortion.

4.5.31   "Induced Abortion and Congenital Malformations in Offspring of Subsequent Pregnancies," MB Bracken and TR Holford, *Am J Epidemiology* 109(4): 425, 1979.

Black women with prior induced abortion were more likely than white women with prior induced abortion to have subsequently delivered a malformed child.

4.5.32   "Risk Factors Accounting for Racial Differences in the Rate of Premature Birth," E Lieberman et al, *New England Journal of Medicine* 317:743-748, 1987.

Black women at the Boston Hospital for Women who delivered had a 91% increased risk of premature birth where there was a history of two or more abortions.

4.5.33   "Ectopic Pregnancy in the United States. 1970-1986," H. Lawson, H. Atrash, A. Saftlas and E. Finch, CDC Surveillance Summaries, *MMWR* 1989, 38(SS-2):1-10, September 1989.

In 1986 the rate of ectopic pregnancy per 1,000 pregnancies was 12.4 for white women and 20.1 for black and other minority races. In 1986 there were 36 reported deaths from ectopic pregnancy in the U.S. 17 white and 19 black and other minority races. Teenagers of black and other minority races have a rate of death from ectopic pregnancy almost six times higher than that for white women of the same age group.

4.5.34   "Ectopic Pregnancy Concurrent with Induced Abortion: Incidence and Mortality," H.K Atrash, H.T. MacKay, C.J.R. Hogue, *Am J. Obstet Gynecol* 162:726-730, 1990.

Among 24 U.S. women identified from 1972 through 1985 , who underwent an induced abortion and died as a result of concurrent ectopic pregnancy, 58.3% were black women or other women of color.

4.5.35   "Induced Terminations of Pregnancy: Reporting States. 1985-1986," Kenneth Kochanek, National Center for Health Statistics, *Monthly Vital Statistics Report* 34(4), Supplement 37(12), April 28,1989

Data received from Colorado, Kansas, Missouri, Montana, New York, Oregon, Rhode Island,

South Carolina, Tennessee, Utah, Vermont, Virginia. Some 43.7% of white women and 59.4% of black women in the reporting states had a repeat abortion in 1986. Black women who had abortions tended to be older than white women who had abortions regardless of marital status. Married women had fewer than one induced abortion for every 10 live births while unmarried women had nine induced abortions for every 10 live births. Among married women, the abortion rate was nearly three times as high for black as for white women. However, among unmarried women the ratio was reversed. For white unmarried women the abortion rate was two- and-a-half times that for black unmarried women.

4.6   Abortion and Religion

(see also Abortion and Decline of Religious Involvement)

4.6.1   "A Therapeutic Approach to Reduce Postabortion Grief in University Women," S.C. Tentoni, J. *American College Health* 44: 35, July, 1995

Women who considered themselves to be extremely pro-life and religious and who had undergone elective abortion experienced tremendous guilt and grief 4-6 months after the abortion.

4.6.2   "Post-Abortion Perceptions: A Comparison of Self-Identified Distressed and Non-Distressed Populations," G. Kam Congleton, L.G. Calhoun, *The Intl J. Social Psychiatry* 39(4): 255-265,1993.

Women reporting distress were more often currently affiliated with conservative churches and reported a lower degree of social support and confidence in the abortion decision. They were also more likely to recall experiencing feelings of loss immediately post-abortion.

4.6.3   "Abortion Patients in 1994-1995: Characteristics and Contraceptive Use, S.K," Henshaw, K. Kost, *Family Planning Perspectives* 28(4): 140, July/August 1996

In an Alan Guttmacher Institute National Survey of 9985 U.S. women obtaining abortions in 1994-1995 Catholics were found to be as likely as women in the general population to have an induced abortion, while Protestants were only 69% as likely and Evangelicals or born-again Christians were only 39% as likely.

4.6.4   "Characteristics of Pregnant Women Who Report Previous Induced Abortions," S. Harlap and A. Davies, *Bulletin World Health Organization* 52:149(1975).

Women who reported abortions were less likely to be strict regarding religious observance. Orthodox Jewish women who observed the tradition of going to the ritual bath after each menstruation had an abortion rate of 1.1 percent. Those who observed part of the ritual had a rate of 3.8 percent. Non-observant women had a rate of 12.7 percent.

4.6.5   "Delivery or Abortion in Inner-City Adolescents," Susan F. Fischman, *American Journal of*

Orthopsychiatry 47(1)127-133, January 1977.

Black women who delivered attached greater importance to religion than those who aborted.

4.6.6 "Psychological Problems of Abortion for the Unwed Teenage Girl," Cynthia D. Martin, *Genetic Psychology Monographs* 88:23-110(1973).

Among teenagers undergoing abortion for mental health reasons, 60% had strong post-abortion guilt. A substantial number changed their moral and religious convictions following pregnancy and abortion including feeling differently about sex, abortions or killing, changes in formal religious faiths, and changed feelings about their view of God and what was sinful.

4.6.7 "Psychological Sequelae of Therapeutic Abortion," Judith Wallerstein, *Archives of General Psychiatry* 27:828-832, Dec, 1972.

In a study of unmarried women seeking abortion for mental health reasons. Catholic women were more concerned than other women with protecting their families from knowledge of their pregnancy and abortion. This secrecy remained a continuing source of guilt and difficulty following the abortion.

4.6.8 *The Connecticut Mutual Life Report on American Values in the '80s: The Impact of Belief,* Commissioned by Connecticut Mutual Life Insurance Co., (Hartford, Connecticut: Factors Affecting Perceived Morality of Abortion, 1981) 92.

In answer to the question "Do you believe abortion is morally wrong, or is it not a moral issue?", 65 percent of the general public thought it morally wrong, 43 percent with lowest level of religious commitment, 58 percent with low level of religious commitment, 75 percent with moderate level of religious commitment, 78 percent with high level of religious commitment, and 85 percent with the highest level of religious commitment.

4.6.9 "Post-abortion Dysphoria and Religion," M. Tamburrino, K. Franco, N. Campbell, J. Pentz, C. Evans and S. Jurs, *Southern Medical Journal* 83(7):736-738, July 1990.

In a study of a patient led post-abortion support group 1-15 years following abortion, 46% of the women stated they had changed to a Fundamentalist or Evangelical church. Women members of these groups scored significantly lower on the MCMI inventory in areas of passive-aggressive, ethanol abuse and avoidance.

4.6.10 *The Psycho-Social Aspects of Stress Following Abortion,* Anne Catherine Speckhard, (Kansas City: Sheed and Ward, 1987).

Religious beliefs that included a concept of a forgiving God were often engaged as a means of coping with guilt following abortion. It was an unexpected result that joining a social system with conservative religious beliefs regarding abortion would serve as a coping mechanism for many subjects.

4.6.11   "Justifiable Abortion," Eugene Quay, *Georgetown Law Journal*, 49(395) (1961).

Summarizes early laws on the history of abortion and statements of various religions opposing abortion.

4.6.12   *Abortion and the Early Church*, Christian, Jewish and Pagan Attitudes in the GrecoRoman World, Michael German, (Downers Grove, Illinois: Inter-varsity Press, 1982).

4.6.13   "Abortion, the Bible & the Church. Survey of 150 Denominational Views," T.J. Bosgra, Hawaii Right to Life Educational Foundation, P.O. Box 10129, Honolulu, Hawaii 96816 (1976,1980).

4.6.14   "Women Exploited. The Other Victims of Abortion," Paula Ervin, *Our Sunday Visitor*, Inc., 200 Noll Plaza, Huntington, Indiana (1985).

In a survey of Women Exploited by Abortion, the author reports: "the vast majority of the women had no true religious affiliation. Some belonged half-heartedly to a church. [But] their grapplings with body and soul, flesh and spirit, came some time after the abortion experience. For some it came years afterward" [p. 142]. Insofar as they have come to the feet of Christ, weeping with Magdalene, they have found a sense of peace and self-worth. This does not happen in a day. Some lives have been broken for so long-have wandered down so many twisted side paths-that clergy and support groups will have to join forces to repair the damage. Many professional counselors tend to trivialize guilt. This angers the woman and deepens her sense of isolation, [p.141].

4.6.15   "Post-Abortion Syndrome and the Whole Person," James Burtchaell, Healing Visions Conference, University of Notre Dame, July 1987.

Abortion was defined as a sin in need of forgiveness. A need to recover the meaning of the word sin was underscored. Sin was described as a deterioration of reflection and consent of the will. Sin may often be committed casually, frivolously or impulsively. Sin is both a result and a cause of deteriorating behavior.

4.6.16   *Abortion's Second Victim*, Pam Korbel, (Wheaton, Illinois: Victor Books/ a Division of Scripture Press, 1986).

This book, written by a woman who had an abortion in 1971, offers women torn apart by the aftermath of abortion emotional healing and forgiveness through the peace that only God can give.

4.6.17   "After Abortion Helpline-Soft Data From Calls," Joan C. Pendergast, presented to Annual Meeting of the Association of Interdisciplinary Research, June 1987.

Providence, Rhode Island ministry advertised "Troubled About Abortion" in predominantly Catholic [65 percent] area. From November 21,1985 to March 13/1987,164 calls were received;

103 women after abortion; 16 men before and after abortion; and 45 others. Seventy-five percent of the callers who gave a religious affiliation were Roman Catholic. Most women expressed guilt, depression, loss, confusion, regret, sorrow, relationship changes, anxiety, loneliness, isolation. Callers were often secretive, not trusting anyone with their double scandal, i.e., getting pregnant and then having an abortion.

4.6.18 "The Use of Theological Classics in Teaching Medical Ethics," Fred Rosner, Queens Hospital Center, affiliation of the Long Island Jewish Medical Center (letter). *Journal of the American Medical Association* 258(2):204, July 10,1987,

Modem medicine has moved into new areas in which great moral issues are involved. Organ transplantation, hemodialysis, genetic engineering, abortion, contraception, euthanasia and drug addiction raise serious moral issues. In those areas religion offers a message and an opinion. It emphatically insists that the norms of ethical opinion may be governed neither by the accepted notions of public opinion nor by the whims of the individual conscience. Moral values are not matters of subjective choice or personal preference. Right and wrong, good and evil are absolute values that transcend the capricious variations of time, place and environment as well as human intuition or expediency, [emphasis added])

4.6.19 *Toward a Psychology of Being,* Abraham Maslow, (Princeton: D. Van Nostrand Co., 1962).

"Intrinsic conscience" is the necessity of being true to one's inner self, and not denying it out of weakness or for special advantage.

4.6.20 *Conscience and Guilt,* James A. Knight (N.Y.: Appleton Century-Crofts, 1969).

The bond between the principle and the act is conscience. There is something wrong with psychology's emphasis on "adjustment" rather than "goodness." Real guilt follows in the wake of wrongdoing, seen and accepted as such by the doer, who seeks expiation and makes restitution.

4.7 Decline of Religious Involvement After Abortion

4.7.1 "Characteristics of Pregnant Women Who Reported Previous Induced Abortions," S Harlap and A Davies, *Bulletin World Health Organization* 52:149, 1975.

Orthodox Jewish women who strictly observed the ritual bath after menstruation had a lower incidence of abortion compared to women who observed part of the ritual or compared to non-observant women.

4.7.2 "Psychosocial Correlates and Antecedents of Abortion: An Exploratory Study," F Costa et al, *Population and Environment* 9L1): 3, 1987.

Women who had an abortion attended church less often and were less religious compared to women without a history of abortion.

4.7.3   *Post-Abortion Trauma: 9 Steps to Recovery,* Jeanette Vought (Grand Rapids: Zondervan, 1991)

Many women in a religiously-based postabortion recovery group said they felt alienated from God following their abortion and that God would not forgive them.

4.7.4   "The Repeat Abortion Patient," Judith Leach, *Family Planning Perspectives* 9(1):37, 1977

Women repeating abortion were more likely to report no religious affiliation compared to women aborting for the first time.

4.7.5   "Repeat Aborters-First Aborters, A Social-Psychiatric Comparison," L Jacobsson et al, *Social Psychiatry* 11:75, 1976

Pregnant women carrying to term were more likely to report they were religious (25.5%) compared to women seeking a first abortion (12.0%) or women repeating abortion (2.2%).

5   **Physical Effects of Abortion**

5.1   Abortion Technique and Its Relationship to Adverse Physical Effects

5.1.1   "Pregnancy Termination: Techniques. Risks and Complications and Their Management," Robert Castadot, *Fertility and Sterility*, 45(1):5-16, January 1986.

General review of abortion technology.

5.1.2   *Abortion Practice,* Warren M. Hern (Boulder, CO: Aplengo Graphics, Inc., 1990)

Ed Note: Although somewhat dated, this still remains the leading text on abortion technique.

5.1.3   "Pregnancy Termination," PG Stubblefield in *Obstetrics. Normal & Problem Pregnancies,* Third Edition ed. Steven G Gabbe, Jennifer R. Niebel and Joe L Simpson (New York: Churchill Livingston, 1996) 1249-1278

5.1.4   *Williams Obstetrics,* 20th Edition ed. Cunningham, MacDonald, Gant, Leveno, Gisstrap, Hankins, Clark, (Stamford, CT: Appleton&Lange, 1997) Chapter 26, Abortion pp. 595-605

5.1.5   "Second-Trimester Abortion by Dilation and Evacuation: An analysis of 11.747 Cases," W.F. Peterson, F.N. Berry, M.R. Grace, C. L. Gulbranson, *Obstet Gynecol* 62:185, 1983.

The use of laminaria in second trimester abortion reduced the incidence of cervical laceration. The use of tetracycline before abortion reduced the incidence of fever (38 degrees Centigrade for 2 or more days). The use of vasopressin mixed with lidocaine reduce the incidence of blood loss following abortion.

5.1.6   *Induced Abortion,* A World Review, C. Tietze, (New York: The Population Council, 1983) 83.

Blood loss increases when abortions are performed with general anesthesia, particularly when agents that produce uterine relaxation such as halothane are used. Perforation and cervical laceration occur more frequently with general anesthesia than with local anesthesia. The risk of death from anesthesia-related and other causes is two to four times greater with general anesthesia than with local anesthesia.

5.1.7   "Local versus general anesthesia: Which is safer for performing suction abortions?," D. Grimes, K. Schulz, W. Cates, C. Tyler, *Am. J. Obstet. Gynecol* 135:1030(1979).

Local anesthesia was associated with elevated rates of febrile and convulsive morbidity while general anesthesia was associated with higher rates of hemorrhage, cervical injury and uterine perforation.

5.1.8   "The Effect of Abortion Method on the Outcome of Subsequent Pregnancy," P.E. Slater, A.M. Davies and S. Harlap, *Journal of Reproductive Medicine* 26(3): 123-128, March 1981.

Infants born following a previous induced abortion by dilatation and curettage showed an excess of low birth weight. The greater the degree of dilatation at D&C, the greater damage to the cervix. This in turn produces an increase in low birth weight due to shortened gestation in the next pregnancy. Adverse effects of D&C are applicable only to settings where this procedure is the usual method employed and not to areas where vacuum aspiration is the procedure of choice or where gradual dilatation by use of laminaria is used. If induced abortion is necessary, it should be done as early as possible with the minimum of cervical dilatation.

5.1.9   "Pelvic inflammatory disease following induced first-trimester abortion," Lars Heisterberg, *Danish Medical Bulletin* 35(1):64-75, February 1988.

Induced first-trimester abortion is a procedure which removes the conceptus from the uterine cavity before the end of the twelfth gestational week counted from the first day of the last menstrual period... The surgical field, consisting of the vagina, endocervix, and uterine cavity is contaminated because even meticulous surgical scrub cannot sterilize the endocervix. Consequently, postoperative infection must be expected in a number of women. Citing "Effect of preoperative scrub on the bacterial flora of the endocervix and vagina." N.G. Osborne and R.C. Wright, *Obstetrics and Gynecology* 50:148-151(1977).

5.2   Short Term Complications and Other Aspects of Morbidity

5.2.1   "Somatic Complications and Contraceptive Techniques Following Legal Abortion." G. Fried, E. Ostlund, C. Ullberg, M. Bygdeman, *Acta Obstet Scand.* 68:515-521,1989.

In a study of 1000 women who had abortions in Stockholm, Sweden in 1987, 5.4% were reported to have complications in the form of infection, bleeding or incomplete abortion, fever at over 38 degrees centigrade (1.6%). About one half (2.8%) were re-admitted to the hospital.

5.2.2   "Complications of termination of pregnancy: a retrospective study of admissions to Christchurch Women's Hospital, 1989 and 1990," P. Sykes, *New Zealand Medical Journal* 106: 83-85, March 10,1993.

A 1989-90 New Zealand study found an overall complication rate of 5.8% following induced abortion as measured by readmission of women. This included 2.9% who had retained products of conception. Immediate complications (0.92%) included perforation, hemorrhage and post-operative pain. Delayed complications were lower abdominal pain and vaginal bleeding presumed to be due to endometritis, retained products of conception or both.

5.2.3   "Early Complications After Induced First-Trimester Abortion," L Heisterberg and M Kringelbach, *Acta Obstet Gynecol Scand* 66:201-204, 1987

A Danish study during 1980-85 reported 6.1% of women had postabortion complications requiring hospitalization.

5.2.4   "Induced abortions operations and their early sequelae," P.I. Frank, C.R. Kay, S.S. Wingrave, *J. Royal College General Practitioners* 35: 175, April, 1985

A British study of 6105 women during 1976-79 found that the main factors independently affecting post abortion morbidity were the place of operation, gestation at termination, method of operation, sterilization at the the time of abortion and smoking habits. Morbidity rates were higher for abortion carried out under the National Health Service than in private practice. Overall newly presenting morbidity, as defined in the study, was reported in 16.9% of the patients (1031 patients) in the 21 days following abortion of which 10% (612 patients) was thought to be directly related to the abortion. Major complications as defined in the study were 2.1%.

5.2.5   "Women refused second-trimester abortion: correlates of pregnancy outcome," N. Binkin, C. Mhango, W. Cates, B. Slovis, M. Freeman, *Am.J. Obstet Gynecol* 145:279,1983.

Among 50 women (86% black) who obtained legal abortions in Atlanta, Georgia after being denied abortion at Grady Memorial Hospital in 1978-79, 12% subsequently reported at least one complication including retained placenta, hemorrhage, pelvic infection or cervical or uterine injury when followed-up in 1980-81.

5.2.6   "Morbidity Risk Among Young Adolescents Undergoing Elective Abortion," R.T. Burkman, M.F. Atienza, T.M. King, *Contraception* 30 (2):99-105, Aug. 1984.

In a study at Johns Hopkins Hospital of 399 adolescents (57.4% black) aged 17 or less at the time of their abortion matched to 399 women aged 20-29 years found that adolescents had a statistically significant relative risk of 2.5 of endometritis compared with women aged 20-29 (7%

vs. 2.7%); 1.25% vs. 0.5% had cervical lacerations and 1.75% had hemorrhaging greater than 500 cc (same as controls). Approximately 4% of adolescents had preexisting cervical gonorrhea compared with 2.7% of women aged 20-29.

5.2.7 "A New Problem in Adolescent Gynecology," M Bulfin, *Southern Medical Journal* 72(8): 967-968, Aug 1979.

Fifty-four teenage patients were seen with significant complications after legal abortion. None felt they had been afforded any meaningful information about the potential dangers of the abortion operation. Perforation of the uterus, peritonitis, pelvic pain, pelvic abscesses, bleeding and cramping, cervical lacerations, severe hemorrhage and adverse psychological and psychiatric sequelae were noted in various case reports.

5.2.8 "Pregnancy Complications Following Legally Induced Abortion," E. Obel, *Acta Obstet. Gynecol. Scand.*, 58: 485-490 (1979).

Bleeding before 28 weeks of gestation and retention of placenta or placental tissue occurred more frequently after an abortion than in a control group matched for age, parity and socio-economic status.

5.2.9 "Late Sequelae of Induced Abortion: Complications and Outcome of Pregnancy and Labor," S. Harlap and A.M. Davies, *American Journal of Epidemiology,* 102(3): 217-224 (1975).

Seven hundred fifty-two mothers who were interviewed during a subsequent pregnancy, and who reported one or more induced abortions in the past, were more likely to report bleeding in each of the first three months of present pregnancy. They were subsequently less likely to have a normal delivery, and more of them needed a manual removal of the placenta or other intervention in the third stage of labor. A disturbing finding in this study is the excess of malformations in the births following earlier induced abortions.

5.2.10 "Intrauterine Adhesions Secondary to Elective Abortion," C. March and R. Israel, *Obstetrics and Gynecology,* 48 (4): 422-424 October 1976.

Amenorrhea and/or infertility secondary to intrauterine adhesions (Asherman's syndrome) following elective abortion is a significant complication.

5.2.11 "Increased Reporting of Menstrual Symptoms Among Women Who Used Induced Abortion," L. Roht, M. Former, H. Aoyama and E. Fonner, *American Journal of Obstetrics Gynecology,* 127(4): 356-362 February 15,1977.

D&C technique of abortion appears to create more menstrual disturbances - i.e., menorrhagia and lengthy or painful menses than vacuum aspiration. The broader array of excess symptoms reported by Japanese women suggests a psychic component as well. Japanese women who desire abortion will frequently travel to a different city or neighborhood to avoid friends or acquaintances. Japanese women apparently under report their prior abortion experience in interviews, compared with questionnaires answered anonymously and in the privacy of their homes.

5.2.12   "Morbidity and Mortality from Second Trimester Abortions," D. Grimes and K. Schulz, *Journal of Reproductive Medicine*, 30(7): 505-514 July 1985.

Little information exists concerning the potential late sequelae of second-trimester abortion.

5.3   Immediate Physical Complications

5.3.1   There is no specific definition for abortion complications. The authors of a particular study basically define the term for themselves. The Center for Disease Control has reported that they found about 100 complications from abortion, but the CDC has not ever published a complete list. Some would be rare, others not life-threatening. As high as 30 different immediate complications have ben ascertained from various studies.

5.3.2   "Factors Associated with Immediate Abortion Complications," LE Ferris et al, *Can Med Assoc J* 154:1677, June 1, 1996.

A retrospective study of induced abortion at Ontario general hospitals in 1992-1993 reported 0.7% immediate complications. Immediate complications were defined as retained product of conception, hemorrhage, laceration of the cervix, perforation of the uterus and other or unspecified complications along with a small number of infections.

5.3.3   "Elective Abortion: Complications Seen in a Free-Standing Clinic," G.J. L. Wuiff, Jr. and S. M. Freiman, *Obstetric and Gynecology* 49(3): 351-357, March, 1977.

A study at Reproductive Health Services in St. Louis, Missouri during 1973-76 found an incidence of 1.54% of immediate complications following elective first trimester abortion.

5.3.4   "Complications of First-Trimester Abortion: A Report of 170.000 Cases," E Hakim-Elahi, H.M. Tovell, M.S. Burnhill, *Obstet Gynecol* 76:129, 1990.

Planned Parenthood of New York City reported an immediate complication rate from induced abortion of 0.905% on 170,000 women from 1971-1987.

5.3.5   "Joint Program for the Study of Abortion, (JPSA): Early medical complications of legal abortion," C. Tietze and Lewis, *Studies in Family Planning*, 3:97(1971).

Among immediate complications, hemorrhage, laceration of the cervix and perforation totaled 1.2 percent at eight weeks gestation and 3.6 percent at 15 weeks or longer.

5.3.6   "The risk of serious complications from induced abortion: Do personal characteristics make a difference," ? JW Buehler et al, *Am J Obstet Gynecol* 153:14-20, 1985.

Serious complications were significantly higher where there were previous induced abortions, 12 weeks or greater gestation, advancing gestational age, and one or more previous delivery.

5.4   Cervical Injuries

5.4.1   "Measures to Prevent Cervical Injuries During Suction Curettage Abortion," K. Schulz, D. Grimes and W. Cates, *The Lancet*, May 28,1983, pp. 1182-1184.

In a study of 15/438 women who had suction curettage abortions at about 12 weeks gestation or less from 1975 to 1978, cervical injuries requiring suturing occurred in approximately one out of 100 abortions. Cervical injury is one of the most frequent complications of suction curettage abortion, yet little is known about its risk factors or prevention. Most published reports lack an objective case definition of cervical injury. Reported rate of cervical injury ranges from 0.01 to 1.6 per 100 abortions. In addition to overt injury to the cervix during suction curettage, covert trauma is also important. Micro fractures of the cervix may occur during forceful dilation of the cervix, which may lead to persistent structural changes, cervical incompetence, premature delivery, and pregnancy complications.

5.4.2   "The Risks Associated with Teenage Abortion," W. Cates, K. Schultz, D. Grimes, *New England Journal of Medicine*, 309(11):612-624, September 15,1983.

There is increased risk of cervical injury during suction curettage abortions obtained by teenagers. These findings cause concern because cervical injury in initial unplanned pregnancies may predispose young women to adverse outcomes in future planned pregnancies.

5.4.3   "Pregnancy Termination: Techniques. Risks, and Complications and Their Management," Robert Castadot, *Fertility and Sterility*, 45(1): 5-16(1986).

The use of laminaria tents reduces the risk of cervical laceration of trauma, mostly in the nulliparous patient [citing various studies.] Uterine perforation and cervical laceration are best prevented by adequate training of the operator, avoidance of excessive force and recognition of the direction of the cervical canal by prior sounding. Laparoscopy is very helpful in assessing the perforation, the bleeding involved, and other possible lesions such as bladder perforation, but it cannot rule out bowel perforation. Cervical lacerations should be sutured even if bleeding is minimal.

5.4.4   "Delayed Reproductive Complications After Induced Abortion," K. Dalaker, S.M. Lichtenberg and G. Okland, *Acta Obstet. Gynaecol. Scand.* 58:491-494(1979).

A Norwegian study of 619 women by questionnaire in 1976 found that, among those not pregnant previously, 25.5% of the post-abortion women compared to 13.2% of post-delivery women (matched for age and parity) had post-abortion complications. Complications were cervical incompetence, pre-term delivery, ectopic pregnancy and sterility. Among all groups regardless of parity, total complications in the abortion group was 24.3% vs. 20.2% in the post-delivery women.

5.5   Perforated Uterus

5.5.1   "Management of Uterine Perforations in Connection with Legal Abortions," G. Lindell, F. Flam, *Acta Obstet. Gynecol. Scand.* 74: 373-375,1995.

A Swedish study found that about one-third of uterine perforations occurred at the end of a first trimester suction abortion when using a blunt curette or polyp forceps. It was stated that it was probably wise to refrain from this "security check" in many instances.

5.5.2   "Management of Uterine Perforation Complicating First-Trimester Termination of Pregnancy," R. Goldchmit et. al, *Israel J. Med. Sci.* 31: 232-234, 1995.

Recommended the use of laparoscopic surgical equipment in the management of uterine perforations.

5.5.3   "Uterine Perforation During Elective First Trimester Abortions: A 13-year Review," L.H. Chen et. al, Singapore Med. J. 36: 63-67,1995.

A careful assessment of uterine size and position, vigilance in the use of uterine sound and dilators, greater care in the use of suction cannula and experience in vacuum aspiration will decrease the incidence of uterine perforations during elective abortions.

5.5.4   "Facts About Early Abortion," *Planned Parenthood,* July 1985,11-2

"Perforation: Rarely, an instrument may go through the wall of the uterus. The frequency of this event is about 2 per 1,000 cases."

5.5.5   "A Cluster of Uterine Perforations Related to Suction Curettage," S.B. Conger, C.W. Tyler Jr. and J. Pakter, *Obstetrics and Gynecology*, 40(4): 551-555, October 1972.

The low incidence of uterine perforation reported for suction curettage is one of the major reasons for its widespread use. Twelve menstrual weeks of gestation has been traditionally accepted as the upper limit for performing abortions either by suction or sharp curettage. Higher rates of perforation could possibly be explained by the supplemental use of forceps and surgical curette to complete the abortion in cases of advance gestation. This study of 1,668 abortions performed by a single doctor had no perforations at 10 weeks gestation or less, but 96.8 per 1/000 abortions at 15 weeks gestation or more using suction curettage. The doctor appeared to be underestimating the length of gestation in women over 10 weeks from their last menstrual period.

5.5.6   "Uterine Perforation Following Medical Termination of Pregnancy by Vacuum Aspiration," S. Mittal and S.L. Misra, *International J. Gynecol. Obstet.* 23:45-50 (1985)

Thirty-seven cases of uterine perforation were observed out of 9,344 first-trimester elective abortions by vacuum aspiration. Cases with a retroverted uterus had a higher incidence of perforation. Studies were reviewed and were noted to be in the range of 0.2 to 7.0 perforations per 1,000 cases. Present study was 3.7 per 1/000 cases. All cases were multiparous and one-third of the cases had a history of child birth within the last six months -no laparoscopy was employed to observe possible perforation incidence.

5.5.7   "A case-control study of uterine perforations documented at laparoscopy," M. White, H. Ory and L. Goldenberg, *Am. J. Obstet. Gynecol.* 129: 623 (1977).

A case-control analysis of 19 uterine perforations which occured during laparoscopic sterilization had an overall perforation rate of 30.4 per 1,000 procedures. Case women were more likely to combine two of the three characteristics: age over 34, parity (one or more children) and obesity (20% above the ideal body weight for height).

5.5.8   "Uterine Perforation in Connection with Vacuum Aspiration for Legal Abortion," Peter J. Moberg, *International J. Gynaecol. Obstet.* 14:77-80(1976).

Statistically, 0.64 uterine perforations per 1,000 procedures were observed. It concluded that the correct judgment of uterine position and size immediately prior to the operation appears to be of the utmost importance in reducing perforations - no laparoscopy observation of incidence.

5.5.9   "The frequency and management of uterine perforations during first-trimester abortions," S. Kaali, I. Szigetvari and G. Bartfai, *Am. J. Obstet. Gynecol* 161:406-408, August 1989

The rate of uterine perforations was 8 cases in 6,408 women undergoing first-trimester abortions (1.3 per 1,000). Some 706 abortions were also performed at the time of laparoscopic sterilization; 2.8 per 1/000 were reported before laparoscopy. Some 15.6 per 1,000 unsuspected perforations were discovered during direct laparoscopic visualization. This represents a 19.8 per 1,000 rate of uterine perforation. Our data suggests that the true rate of uterine perforations is significantly underestimated.

5.5.10   "Joint Program for the Study of Abortion," C. Tietze and S. Lewit, *Studies in Family Planning* 3:97(1972).

The rate of unrecognized perforations may be three-to-thirty-fold higher than reported.

5.5.11   "Laparoscopy as a diagnostic and therapeutic technique in uterine perforations during first-trimester abortions," N.H. Lauresen and S. Birnbaum, *Am. J. Obstet. Gynecol.* 117:522(1973).

First report of laparoscopy as a diagnostic tool in uterine perforations. The article concluded that in order to prevent uterine perforation it is of extreme importance to perform a pelvic examination prior to the abortion to determine the position of the uterus since a majority of the perforations occur [to] extremely anteflexed or retroflexed uteri.

5.5.12 "Uterine perforations during sterilization by laparoscopy and minilaparotomy," I.C. Chi and P. Feldblum, *Am. J. Obstet. Gynecol.* 139(6): 735, March 15,1981.

Patients with an interval of less than one year between termination of pregnancy and sterilization were 4.8 times more likely to incur a uterine perforation than those with a longer interval.

5.5.13 "Prevention of uterine perforation during curettage abortion," D. Grimes, K. Schuiz and W. Cates, *JAMA* 251:2108-2111(1984).

No mention of laparoscopy.Reported an incidence of 1 per 1,000 cases. (A previous childbirth increases the risk of perforated uterus by 3.4.) (The level of physician training was the strongest single factor identified with incidence of uterine perforation.

5.5.14 "Elective Abortion: Complications Seen in a Free-Standing Clinic," G. Wulff, George Wulff Jr. and S. Michael Freiman, *Obstetrics and Gynecology* 49(3):351, March 1977.

Reported an incidence of 26 documented and 8 suspected cases of perforated uterus in 16/410 cases (approximately 2 per 1,000 cases.) Reported that laparoscopy was very valuable in ascertaining the exact nature of the perforation. (Laparoscopy not used to determine incidence of perforation.)

Pain in Women

5.6 Acute Pain

5.6.1 "Abortion Probably Most Common Gynecologic Procedure in U.S," Richard M. Soderstrom, *Ob. Gyn. News* 20(3): 19, Feb. 1-14,1985.

The likelihood of successful abortion will be improved with adequate paracervical block anesthesia. Pain intolerance in patients can lead to retained products of conception.

5.6.2 *Guidelines for Women's Health Care,* (Washington D.C.: The American College of Obstetricians and Gynecologists, 1996) 174

Abortion is listed as a common cause of acute pelvic pain.

5.6.3 "Pain of First Trimester Abortion: A study of Psychosocial and medical predictors," E. Belanger, R. Melzack, P. Lauzon, *Pain* 36: 339-350,1989.

A Canadian study of pain in women during first trimester abortion by suction curettage under local anesthesia found that severe acute pain similar to the pain of childbirth or from cancer can occur. Pain scores were significantly higher for younger patients aged 13-17 compared to older women. Severe acute pain was more likely to occur if women were anxious before or after the abortion or if they reported depression or had moral or social concerns about abortion.

5.6.4   "A Causal Model of Psychosomatic Reactions to Vacuum Aspiration Abortion," M.B. Bracken, *Social Psychiatry* 13: 135,1978.

Severe acute pain is more likely to occur if the abortionist is inexperienced.

5.6.5   "Physical and Psychological Injury in Women Following Induced Abortion," Lee Gsellman, *Association for Interdisciplinary Research in Values and Social Change* 5(1): 1-8, Sept./Oct.1993

Both immediate and later abdominal pain were reported in a sample of primarily teenage postabortion women.

5.6.6   "Pain of first trimester abortion: It's quantification and relations with other variables," G.M. Smith et. al.. *Am. J. Obstet. Gynecol* 133: 489,1979.

Gynecological characteristics such as uterus retroversion, history of menstrual pain and increased gestational age at the time of abortion were found to increase acute pain from abortion.

5.6.7   "Pain and Distress During Abortion," Nancy Wells, *Health Care for Women Int'l* 12: 293-302,1991.

Abortion was found to produce greater sensory scores than menstrual pain or dental pain.

5.7   Chronic Pain

5.7.1   "Factors Influencing Spontaneous Abortion, Dyspareunia, Dysmenorrhea, and Pelvic Pain," Lars Heisterberg *Obstet. Gynecol.* 81:594,1993.

Pelvic pain is more likely to occur in women with post abortion pelvic inflammatory disease.

5.7.2   "Morbidity following pelvic inflammatory disease," H Buchan et al, *Br J Obstet Gynaecol* 100:558, 1993

Women with a diagnosis of PID were 10 times more likely to be admitted to a hospital for abdominal pain, and four times more likely to be admitted to a hospital for gynecological pain.

5.7.3   "Psychological Profile of dysphoric women post-abortion," K. Franco et. al, *J. American Medical Women's Assn.* 44: 113, July/Aug. 1989.

Long lasting somatoform disorders and physical symptoms such as abdominal pain, headaches and chest pain were reported in women who reported poorly assimilating their abortion experience and were attending a post abortion support group. This was particularly the case where women also reported anniversary reactions.

5.7.4   "Factors Associated with More Intense Labor Pain," Gerd Fridh et. al. *Research in Nursing & Health* 11: 117, 1988.

Post-abortion women were found to have an increased likelihood of severe pain in subsequent childbirth compared to women with other pregnancy outcomes.

5.7.5   "Aftermath of Abortion. Anniversary Depression and Abdominal Pain," J.O. Cavenar Jr., A.A. Maltbie, J.L. Sullivan, *Bulletin of the Menninger Clinic* 42(5): 433-444,1978.

Cases are cited where abdominal cramping was associated with anniversary reaction to abortion due to incomplete or abnormal grieving of the loss of the fetus.

Organ or System Failure

Organ or system failure as a result of induced abortion is very infrequent but nevertheless potentially extremely serious and, in many instances, fatal.

5.8   Cerebrovascular Diseases (Stroke)

5.8.1   "Suicide Deaths Associated with Pregnancy Outcome: A Record Linkage Study of 173,279 Low Income American Women," D Reardon et al, *Clinical Medicine & Health Research* clinmed2001030003v1 (April 25, 2001)

State funded medical insurance records identifying all paid claims for abortion or delivery were linked to the state death certificate registry among low income women in California who had either an induced abortion or delivery in 1989. Compared to women who delivered (1.0), those who aborted had a statistically higher adjusted risk of dying from cerebrovascular diseases (5.46) Ed Note: There is evidence that induced abortion increases the incidence of hypertension in women. This may have been a factor in the considerably higher incidence of deaths from cerebrovascular diseases.

5.9   Circulatory Diseases

5.9.1   "Suicide Deaths Associated with Pregnancy Outcome: A Record Linkage Study of 173,279 Low Income American Women," D Reardon et al, Clinical Medicine & Health Research clinmed/2001030003v1 (April 25, 2001)

Compared to women who delivered (1.0) , those who aborted had a statistically higher adjusted risk of dying from circulatory diseases (2.87)

5.9.2   "Fatal Myocarditis Associated with Abortion in Early Pregnancy," DA Grimes and W Cates, Jr,

Southern Medical Journal 73(2):236, 1980

Describes four cases of abortion-related deaths due to myocarditis.

5.9.3   "Fatal Myocardial Infection Resulting From Conorary Embolism After Abortion: Unusual Cause and Complication of Endocarditis," 29:175, 1997

5.9.4   "Maternal and Fetal Outcomes of Subsequent Pregnancies in Women with Peripartum Cardiomyopathy," U Elkayam et al, *N Eng J Med* 344(21):1567, May 24, 2001

This study found an elevated incidence of prior therapeutic abortion in women with left ventricular dysfunction which was sometimes fatal.

5.10   Disseminated Intravascular Coagulation (DIC)

DIC, or consumptive coagulophy, is caused by trauma or sepsis. It breaks down the various functions of the blood, resulting in defective coagulation with the risk of life-threatening hemorrhage and multiple organ failure.

5.10.1   "Coagulopathy and Induced Abortion Methods," ME Kafrissen et al, *Am J Obstet Gynecol* 147: 344, 1983.

The incidence of coagulopathy associated with first trimester abortion is 8 per 100,000 abortions; with D&E abortions it is 191 per 100,000 abortions; and with saline instillation abortions it is 658 per 100,000 abortions.

5.10.2   "Manmagement of Disseminated Intravascular Coagulophy," ME Richey et al, *Clinical Obstetrics and Gynecology* 38 (3): 514-520, 1995.

Induced Abortion is listed as one of the common causes of consumptive coagulophy.

5.11   Amniotic Fluid Embolism

Amniotic fluid embolism, an unusually catastrophic condition, is a sudden rush of amniotic fluid containing placental or fetal tissue fragments into maternal circulation. Frequently it is fatal. Although it can occur in a first trimester abortion, it is much more likely to occur in a second trimester abortion.

5.11.1   "Fatal pulmonary embolism during legal induced abortion in the United States from 1972 to 1985," HW Lawson et al, *Am J Obstet Gynecol* 162:986, 1990.

Includes deaths from amniotic fluid embolism as well as air embolism and pulmonary embolism.

5.11.2   "Amniotic Fluid Embolism," SL Clark, *Critical Care Clinics* 7(4):877-882, 1991.

" AFE has been reported under many conditions. These include first-trimester curettage abortion, second-trimester abortion with saline, prostaglandin, urea, and hysterotomy."

5.11.3   "Amniotic fluid embolism: Analysis of the national registry," SL Clark et al, *Am J Obstet Gynecol* 172:1158-1169, 1995.

Listing prior elective termination of pregnancy as one of the demographic data for patients with amniotic fluid embolism.

5.12   Pulmonary Embolism

Pulmonary embolism is an obstruction of pulmonary arteries, most frequently by detached fragments of clots from a leg or pelvic vein, especially following an operation or confinement to bed. Pulmonary embolism is known to occur in adolescents or adults following induced abortion. An incidence of 2.2 cases of pulmonary embolism per 10,000 induced abortions has been reported.

5.12.1   "Pulmonary Embolism in Adolescents," D Bernstein et al, *Am J Diseases of Children* 140:667, 1986

5.12.2   "Pulmonary Embolism in a 14 Year Old Following Elective Abortion," R Nudelman et al, *Pediatrics* 68:584, 1981

5.12.3   "Deaths Caused by Pulmonary Thromboembolism After Legally Induced Abortion," AM Kimball et al, *Am J Obstet Gynecol* 132:169, 1978.

5.13   Adult Respiratory Distress Syndrome

5.13.1   *Manual of Obstetrics: Diagnosis and Therapy,* 4 Edition, Kenneth R Niswander and Arthur T Evans (Boston: Little, Brown, 1991) 90

Adult respiratory distress syndrome (ARDS) is diffuse damage to the small cells of the lung accompanied by an excessive accumulation of water in the cells of the lung. It can occur from such etiologies as amniotic fluid embolism, sepsis, overdose or toxicity from various medications or chemicals, or in connection with DIC.

Infection Associated With Abortion

5.14 Septic Abortion

5.14.1 *Infections and Abortion,* Sebastian Faro and Mark Pearlman (New York: Elsevier, 1992) 42

Acute complications from septic abortion include adult respiratory distress syndrome, septic shock, death of woman, renal failure, abscess formation, and septic emboli.

5.14.2 "Postabortion Infection, Bacteremia, and Septic Shock "in *Infectious Diseases of the Female Genital Tract, 3rd Edition,* Ed. Richard L Sweet and Ronald S Gibbs (Baltimore, Wilkins & Wilkins, 1995) 363-378

5.14.3 "Fatal Myocardial Infarction Resulting From Coronary Artery Septic Embolism After Abortion: Unusual Cause and Complications of Endocarditis," Victor Caraballo, *Annals of Emergency Medicine* 29(1): 175, Jan 1997.

"Emergency physicians often encounter patients who have undergone abortions. Such patients are at risk for many infectious and thromboembolic complications."

5.15 Acute Renal Failure from Septic Abortion

5.15.1 "S.R. v. City of Fairmont," 280 S.E. 2d 712 (W. Va. 1981)

A young woman underwent an induced abortion at a private abortion facility. The doctor noted on the medical record that fetal parts were seen following the abortion. It appeared that the woman was discharged without being so advised. She then developed cramps, vaginal bleeding and fever. She went to a local hospital but the personnel there were unsuccessful in diagnosing the exact nature of the problem. She went into shock. Ultimately, she was transferred to a larger medical center where the personnel there were able to save her life. However, before the undelivered fetal parts were removed, she developed acute renal failure arising from the septic abortion. In the absence of a kidney transplant, had to rely upon an ambulatory dialysis machine as a life support system.

5.16 Autoimmune Disease

5.16.1 "Pregnancy outcome and anti-Ro/SSA in autoimmune diseases. a retrospective cohort study," CP Mavragini et al, *Br J Rhewmatol* 37(7): 740-745, 1998.

A Greek study found that anti-Ro/SSA-positive women with systemic lupus erythematosus reported a significantly higher rate (18%) of therapeutic abortions compared to anti-Ro/SSA-negative women (5.6%) and healthy controls (4.6%).

5.16.2   "Etiological aspects of insulin dependent diabetes mellitus: an epidemiological perspective," G
          Dahlquist, *Autoimmunity* 15(1):61-65, 1993.

          The mechanism of beta-cell destruction leading to insulin dependent diabetes is probably a cell
          mediated auto-immune process occurring in genetically susceptible individuals... Risk factors that
          may increase the peripheral need for insulin (infectious diseases, stressful life events, etc) may act
          as promoters of a beta-cell impairment and make the disease clinically overt.

5.16.3   "Stress and auto-immune endocrine diseases," J Leclere and G Weryha, *Hom Res* 31(1-2): 90-93,
          1989.

          Auto-immunity may occur in all endocrine tissues, with a particular prevalence in thyroid and
          pancreatic islets... clinical observation registers frequent stressful life events just before the onset
          of these diseases... recent findings on the close relations between the immune system and central
          nervous system lead to conceive an actual psychoneuro-endrocine-immune axis.

5.16.4   "Fatal myocarditis associated with abortion in early pregnancy," DA Grimes, W Cates, Jr,
          Southern Medical Journal 73(2): 236-238, Feb 1980.

          Four abortion-related deaths from 1975-78 are described which were attributed to myocarditis in
          the first trimester of pregnancy. The authors stated that, " the potential influence of pregnancy or
          abortion on the development or severity of cases of myocarditis is speculative. Since mild cases
          are usually undetected, the incidence of this condition among women of childbearing age is
          unkown. Only 59 women in the U.S. of childbearing age (15-44) were reported to have died from
          acute or subacute myocarditis in 1975." The authors noted that three of the four deaths were
          associated with conditions which have a presumed immunologic mechanism. Ed Note:
          myocarditis is inflammation of the muscular walls of the heart.

5.16.5   "Interplay between environmental factors, articular involvement, and HLA-B-27 in patients with
          psoriatic arthritis," R Scarpa et al, *Annals of Rheumatic Diseases* 51:78-79, 1992.

          An Italian study of the medical records of patients with psoriatic arthritis and rheumatoid arthritis
          were reviewed. 9% of the patients with psoriatic arthritis had an acute disorder, which included
          abortion, immediately preceding the onset of the arthritis. In contrast, only 1% of the patients
          with rheumatoid arthritis recorded an acute event prior to the onset of their arthritis.

5.17   Endometritis

Endometritis is an infection in the inner uterine wall. It sometimes may be called febrile reactions.
If not promptly treated, endometritis can require hostipalization and can impair future fertility.
Endometritis is a major cause of maternal mortality.

5.17.1   "Postabortal Endometritis and Isolation of Chlamydia trachomatis," MB Barbacci et al, *Obstet*

Gynecol 68:686, 1986.

A Johns Hopkins University study found that 10% of chlamydia positive women who underwent a first or second trimester abortion developed endometritis compared to 3.5% for chlamydia negative women.

5.17.1.1 "Morbidity Risk Among Young Adolescents Undergoing Elective Abortion," RT Burkman et al, *Contraception* 30(2): 99, 1984.

A Johns Hopkins University study found that teenagers age 17 or younger were more likely to develop postabortion endometritis (7.0%) compared to women age 20-29 (2.7%).

5.17.1.2 "Postabortal pelvic infection associated with Chlamydia trachomatis infection and the influence of humoral immunity," S Osser and K Persson, *Am J Obstet Gynecol* 150:699, 1984.

A Swedish study found that chlamydia positive women age 13-19 were more likely to develop postabortion endometritis (28%) compared to chlamydia positive women age 20-24 (22.7%) or chlamydia positive women age 25-29 (20%). The same study found that chlamydia negative women aged 13-19 were also more likely to develop postabortion endometritis (9.3%) compared to chlamydia negative women age 20-24 (4.8%) or chlamydia negative women age 25-29 (4.7%).

5.17.1.3 "Preventing febrile complications of suction curettage abortion," T-K Park et al, *Am J Obstet Gynecol* 152:252-255, 1985.

A study of 26,332 women undergoing abortion at five abortion facilities during 1975-1978, found that post-abortion infections as measured by an oral temperature of 38 degrees centigrade for two or more days were significantly lower (relative risk 0.54) among women with one or more previous births compared to women with no previous births.

5.17.1.4 "Postabortal Endometritis in Chlamydia-Negative Women- Association with Preoperative Clinical Signs of Infection," B Hamark and L Forssman, *Gynecol Obstet Invest* 31:102-105, 1991.

Women with clue cells constitute a group at risk for postabortal endometritis.

5.18 Genital Tract Infection

5.18.1 "Trichomonas Vaginalis: A Re-emerging Pathogen," P. Heine, J.A. McGregor, *Clinical Obstetrics and Gynecology* 36(1): 137, March 1993.

Trichomoniasis is the most prevelent non-viral sexually transmitted disease. Worldwide, there are approximately 180 million cases and 2.5 to 3 million infections occurring annually in the United States. There is an association between postabortal infection and trichomonal colonization. Improved understanding of the natural history, pathobiology, diagnosis and treatment of this common protozoa is urgently needed. Practitioners should consider routinely screening and treating women for trichomoniasis before any reproductive tract surgery (chorionic villi sampling, hysterectomy, cesarean section, dilation and curettage and therapeutic abortion).

5.18.2   "Pre-operative Cervical Microbial Flora and Post-Abortion Infection." P.T. Moberg, P. Eneroth, J. Harlin, A. Liung, and C.E. Nord, *Acta Obstet. Gynecol. Scand* 57:415-419. (1978).

One of the important complications of first-trimester abortion by vacuum aspiration is pelvic infection. The incidence of this complication varies widely [0.3-18 percent] due to differences in [1] definition of post-abortion infection; [2] use of prophylactic antibiotic treatment; [3] time of observation. Of 104 women who underwent first-trimester abortions, no patients showed any sign of lower genital tract infection prior to the operation. Nevertheless, 14 percent required postoperative treatment with antibiotics because of mild or severe infection of the upper genital tract. Patients were studied after two months.

5.18.3   "Genital Tract Infection," *Ob. Gyn. News* 20(3):42 February 1-41 1985 (quoting Kenneth Schulz, Division of Sexually Transmitted Disease, Center for Disease Control, Atlanta, Georgia).

An estimated 13,000 women develop postabortal upper genital tract infection which is associated not only with long-term morbidity but also, occasionally, with long-term sequelae such as infertility and ectopic pregnancy.

5.18.4   "Preventing Febrile Complications of Suction Curettage Abortion," F.K. Park, M. Flock, K. Schulz, and D. Grimes, *American Journal of Obstetrics and Gynecology*, 152:252-255, June 1,1985.

Despite the clinical and public health importance of infection, the risk factors for postabortal infection are not well understood. Because of the lack of uniform definitions and diagnostic criteria, rates of infectious complications, including endometritis, salpingitis or peritonitis, are difficult to interpret. Fever can provide a more objective estimate of the incidence of infectious morbidity, yet it is not an ideal indicator of infection. Little information has been published on the effect of parity on abortion complications. In the study, febrile morbidity rate was 0.34 per 100 abortions, with oral temperature greater than 38°C. for two days.

5.18.5   "Observations on Patients Two Years After Legal Abortion," P. Jouppila, A. Kauppila and L. Punto, *International Journal Fertility*, 19:233-239(1974).

Five hundred sixty-two Finnish patients who underwent legal abortions [69 percent by vacuum aspiration] were invited to a follow-up exam two years later. Only 25 percent came to a detailed gynecological exam. The rest either had an unknown address or were unwilling to take part in the discussion of an experience with "negative personal associations." Of the 143 patients examined, 14 percent had some early complications associated with the abortion. There were six cases of endometritis, six cases of heavy bleeding, one cervical rupture and one uterine perforation. A gynecological exam gave rise to suspected cervical insufficiency in 15 women, of which 10 had abortions by vacuum aspiration. Hysterosalpingography suggested tubal pathology in 18 percent. Laparoscopy revealed a normal tubal finding in 50 percent, although the HSG finding had been pathologic. Patients with pathologic tubal findings in laparoscopy [adhesions, nodules and sactoaalpinx formations] had not had early complications on abortion. The author concluded, "The need of new follow-up examination following induced abortion is obvious." This is one of the few studies on longer term effects.

5.18.6 "Morbidity after termination of pregnancy in first-trimester," S. Duthrie, D. Hobson, I.A. Tait, B. Pratt, N. Lowe, P. Sequeira and C. Hargreaves, *Genitourinary Medicine* 63(3): 182-187, June 1987.

Pre-abortion clinical and microbiological tests were undertaken. Post-abortion morbidity was measured in 167 women in Liverpool, England during 1984. Twelve percent had major upper genital tract infection 8-17 days after their abortion. Another 10% later showed clinical signs that suggested minor upper genital tract infection. Abnormal cervical cytology (mostly inflammation) was found in 52% of the overall sample and 79% of the women with chlamydial infection had abnormal cervical cytology. Neither the medical history nor clinical examination before the abortion would have indicated that post-abortion complications were likely to occur. Ed. Note - The findings strongly suggest that it was the abortion procedure that was the primary cause of the post-abortion morbidity.

5.18.7 "Postabortal pelvic infection associated with chlamydia trachomatis infection and the influence of humoral immunity," S. Osser and K. Perrson, *Am. J. Obstetrics and Gynecology* 150:699-703 (1984)

Chlamydia positive women aged 13-19 were more likely to develop post-abortion endometritis (28%) compared to women aged 20-24(22.7%) or women aged 25-29(20%). Chlamydia positive women aged 13-19 were more likely to develop post-abortion salpingitis (21.9%) compared to women aged 20-24 (13.6%).

Pelvic Inflammatory Disease (PID)

5.19 General Background Studies for PID

5.19.1 "Factors Related to Infertility in the U.S.. 1965-1976," William D. Mosher and Sevgi 0. Aral, *Sexually Transmitted Diseases*, 12(3): 117-123, July/September 1985.

The longer sexually active women postpone having their first baby, the greater is their risk of pelvic inflammatory disease and hence primary infertility.

5.19.2 "Chlamydia Trachomatis in Acute Salpingitis," J. Paavonen, E. Vesterinen and K. Aho, *British Journal Venereal Diseases,* 55: 203-206 (1979).

Acute salpingitis is a common disease and seems to be increasing. The clinical diagnosis of acute salpingitis was based on common criteria: pelvic pain of short duration, tender adnexal masses, increased erythrocyte sedimentation rate, and usually fever. The late sequelae of salpingitis are well known: infertility, increased frequency of ectopic pregnancies, and chronic abdominal pain. The risk of spread of cervical infection to the fallopian tubes must be considered in the treatment of cervical chlamydia.

5.19.3 "Chlamydial Infection in Infertile Women," T.R. Moss (letter). *Fertility and Sterility,* 44(4): 559, October 1985.

Chlamydial pelvic inflammatory disease (PID) is an important cause of lost fertility. The challenge must be to prevent the tubal damage by early diagnosis, effective chemotherapy and prevention of reinfection. Fifteen percent of male patients attending this clinic were found to be asymptomatic with chlamydia trachomatis. It is considered a serious clinical omission in the investigation of PID to fail to take specimen from the anterior urethra of the male partner of the female patient.

5.19.4 "Chlamydia Trachomatis Infection in Women," *Farq, Journal of Reproductive Medicine* 30(3):273-278 (Supp), March 1985.

Infants of women with cervical chlamydial colonization have a 60-70 percent risk of being colonized during birth. Approximately 25-50 percent of them develop conjunctivitis, and 10-20 percent develop pneumonia. The patophysiology of Chlamydia trachomatis genital tract infection is not well understood. However, the principal focus of infection appears to be the cervix. Sequelae to acute salpingitis include chronic pelvic pain, hydrosalpinx pyhosalpinx, ectopic pregnancy, infertility, tuboovarian abscess and the Fitz-Hugh-Curtis syndrome.

5.19.5 "Effect of Acute Pelvic Inflammatory Disease on Fertility," L. Westrom, *American Journal of Obstetrics and Gynecology*, 12(5); 707-713, March 1,1975.

Obstruction of the fallopian tube is the most common cause of sterility in women. The only unequivocal proof of preserved tubal function after PID is an intrauterine pregnancy. Reinfection was found to have the strongest effect on fertility after PID. One out of five previously healthy women who fell ill with acute PID had a second infection. The relatively low frequency of sterility (12.8 percent) after one infection increased nearly threefold (to 35.5 percent) after two infections, and six fold (18 out of 24 cases) after three or more infections.

5.19.6 "Pelvic Inflammatory Disease: Etiology. Diagnosis and Treatment," Richard L. Sweet, *Sexually Transmitted Diseases*, 8(4): 308-315 (Supp.) December 1981.

PID caused by sexually transmitted pathogens results in infertility in more than 20 percent of the cases, and the risk of ectopic pregnancy increases six- to tenfold after PID. It is crucial to prevent reinfection by seeking out the sexual partners of women with PID and treating them for sexually transmitted diseases. In this way, the recurrent infections which lead to poor prognosis for fertility can be circumvented.

5.19.7 "Economic Consequences of PID in the U.S," James Curran, *American Journal of Obstetrics Gynecology*, 138 (7): 848 (1980).

In 1978, nearly one million women in the United States suffered from PID and its sequelae. They accounted for more than 2.5 million physician visits, 250,000 hospital admissions and nearly 150,000 surgical procedures. PID associated with sexually transmitted disease often begins in young, single women; manifestations of recurrent disease, sterility, ectopic pregnancy and major surgery occur five to ten years later. It was estimated that the direct annual cost is greater than $600 million, and the total cost for this disease is upwards of $3 billion.

5.19.8 "The Economic Cost of Pelvic Inflammatory Disease," A.E. Washington, P.S. Arno, M.A. Brooks, *Journal of the American Medical Association,* 255(13): 1735-1738, April 4,1986.

This study concluded that the total cost of PID and PID-associated ectopic pregnancy and infertility in the U.S. exceeded $2.6 billion in 1984. By 1990, the estimated cost of PID and its sequelae will total $3.5 billion per year, assuming an annual medical care inflation rate of 5 percent and the constant rate of incidence of PID during this six-year period. The study concludes that these estimated costs of PID and its associated sequelae emphasize the urgent need for effective programs to prevent Pm.

5.19.9 "Incidence, Prevalence and Trends of Acute Pelvic Inflammatory Disease and Its Consequences in Industrialized Countries," L. Westrom, *American Journal Obstetrics Gynecology,* 138: 880-892 (1980).

Despite antibiotic therapy, patients who have had at least one episode of salpingitis have a 21 percent rate of involuntary infertility, as compared with the rate of 3% among the control population.

5.19.10 "Introductory Address: Treatment of Pelvic Inflammatory Disease in View of Etiology and Risk Factors," L. Westrom, *Sexually Transmitted Diseases,* October-December 1984, pp. 437-440.

Clinically, PID can vary from an almost symptom-free disease to a life threatening condition. Sequelae to the disease are common. Ever since the first reports on PID in the literature, a strong correlation has been observed between sexually transmitted disease and PID. In recent studies, up to 75 percent of cases of PID in women less than 25 years of age have been associated with cultural and/or serologic evidence of infection with n. gonorrhea, chlamydia trachomatis, or m. hominis. For any sexually active woman, the risk of acquiring a sexually transmitted disease (STD), and hence of running this high risk of acquiring PID, is proportional to the regional prevalence of the corresponding STD and to the number of sexual partners.

5.20 Abortion-Related Pelvic Inflammatory Disease

5.20.1 "Induced Abortion: Microbiological Screening and Medical Complications," B. Stray-Pederson et. al.. *Infection* 19: 305,1991.

A Scandinavian study found that Pelvic Inflammatory Disease developed significantly more often in untreated chlamydia-positive women (22.7%), mycolpasma hominis-positive women (8.1%) and Group B streptococci-positive women (6.1%) than in women without these microbes (0.5%).

5.20.2   "Bacterial Vaginosis and Anaerobes in Obstetric-Gynecologic Infection," D.A. Eschenbach, *Clinical Infectious Diseases* 16 (Suppl. 4): S282, 1993

Bacterial vaginosis has an important role in the development of postabortion pelvic inflammatory disease.

5.20.3   "Early and Late Onset Pelvic Inflammatory Disease among Women with Cervical Chlamydia trachomatis Infection at the Time of Induced Abortion- A Follow-up Study," J.L. Sorensen et al.. *Infection* 22(4): 242,1994.

A Danish study found that untreated women with chlamydia trachomatis infection at the time of induced abortion had a cumulative risk of 72% of developing early or late pelvic inflammatory disease, if observed for 24 months.

5.20.4   "Delayed Care of Pelvic Inflammatory Disease as a Risk Factor for Impaired Fertility," S.D. Hillis et. al.. *Am. J. Obstet. Gynecol.* 168:1503-1509,1993.

A Centers for Disease Control study found that women who delayed care for pelvic inflammatory disease after onset of symptoms had nearly a threefold increase risk of fertility impairment. Among women who delayed seeking care were women who had a history of a recent induced abortion.

5.20.5   "A Randomized Trial of Prophylactic Doxycycline for Curettage in Incomplete Abortion," J.A. Preito et. al., *Obstet. Gynecol.* 85: 692-696,1995.

Several epidemiologic studies have examined risk factors associated with postabortal pelvic infection. These include: patient less than 20, nulliparity, multiple sex partners, previous PID or gonorrhea, and untreated lower genital tract infections.

5.20.6   "Pelvic Inflammatory Disease Following Induced First-Trimester Abortion. Risk Groups. Prophylaxis and Sequelae," L. Heisterberg, *Danish Medical Bulletin* 35(1): 64-75, February, 1988.

Little is known about the costs of abortion complications and the true incidences of their sequelae. Long term prospective studies with follow-up of women who had abortions are most needed to assess the rate of sequelae after post aborted complications.

5.20.7   "Mobiluncus and Clue cells as Predictors of PID After First-Trimester Abortion," P.G. Larsson, B. Bergman, V. Forsum, J. Platz-Christenson and C. Pahlson, *Acta Obstet Gynaecol Scand.* 68:217-220, (1989).

In a Swedish study of 531 women in 1985-86 a correlation was found between the presence of mobiluncus and clue cells in vaginal discharge and the incidence of PID. Where women had clue cells the incidence of post-abortion PID was 11.8% compared to 3.2% PID when women showed normal epithelium cells.

5.20.8   "Early Complications of Induced Abortion in Primigravidae," K. Dalaker, K. Sundfor and J. Skuland, *Annes Chirurgiae et Gynaecologiae* 70:331-336(1981).

A follow-up examination 4-6 weeks following abortion by vacuum aspiration found 4.8% with retained fetal parts: 11.1% had post-abortion bleeding greater than normal menstrual period, and 4.1 % had pelvic inflammatory disease.

5.20.9   "Therapeutic Abortion," F. Jerve and P. Fylling, *Acta. Obstetric Gynecology Scand.* 57:237 (1978).

Pelvic inflammatory disease is a major complication after therapeutic abortion; readmission rates to hospitals were 4 percent in this study, with pelvic infections and retained products being the main causes.

5.20.10 "Chlamydia Trachomatis in Relation to Infections Following First Trimester Abortions," T. Radberg and L. Hamberger, *Acta. Obstetrida Gynecological* (Supp. 93) 154:478 (1980). (abstract)

In a Swedish study, women with endocervical chlamydial infections were over five times more likely than uninfected women to develop PID within four weeks after a first-trimester induced abortion. (23.4% vs. 4.4%)

5.20.11 "Chlamydia Trachomatis Infections in the United States, What Are They Costing Us?" A. Eugene Washington, R. Johnson, and L. Sanders, Jr. *Journal of the American Medical Association,* 257(15):2070-2072 April 17,1987.

Approximately 30-50 percent of PID episodes are caused by chlamydia trachomatis infection. It is estimated that each year 402,200 episodes of chlamydial PID occur, leading to 1,005,400 outpatient visits 106,900 hospitalizations, 8,050 infertility consultations, 13,900 ectopic pregnancies, and 280 deaths. Other adverse health effects, and estimated direct and indirect costs are discussed. Ed. Note - This report is most significant to the issue of induced abortion as it is implicated in the onset of pelvic inflammatory disease.

5.20.12 "Therapeutic Abortion and Chlamydia Trachomatis Infection," E. Qvigstag, K. Skaug, F. Jerve, I. Vik and J. Ulstrup, *British Journal of Venereal Disease*, 58:182-183(1982).

In a study of 218 women admitted for legal termination of pregnancy in Oslo, Norway, 30 (13.8 percent) had chlamydia trachomatis in the cervix before abortion. Twenty-one of the 30 patients exhibiting chlamydia trachomatis were followed up three months after their abortions. Seven (23.3 percent) had developed PID, six (20 percent) had developed salpingitis, 17(81 percent) showed detectable chlamydial antibodies. Conclusion: Patients harboring chlamydia trachomatis in the cervix at termination of pregnancy are at high risk of developing post-operative infections. Routine screening in the cervix before surgery is essential.

5.20.13 "Chlamydial Serology in Infertile Women by Immunofluorescence, R," Punnonen, P. Terho, V.

Nikkanen and O. Meurman, *Fertility and Sterility*, 31(6): 656-659(1979).

This study showed the distribution of chlamydial antibody titers among infertile women, pregnant women and women exposed to males with STD. Non-sexually promiscuous women have significantly lower percentages of chlamydial antibodies.

5.20.14 *Sexually Transmitted Diseases,* K.K. Holmes, P.A. Mardh, P.F. Sparling, P.J. Wiesner (McGraw-Hill, 1984) 623

Operative procedures such as cervical dilatation, curettage, tubal insufflations and IUD insertions carry a small risk of infectious complications. During the last few decades, the numbers of legal abortions and IUD insertions have reached such proportions that the immediate consequences have influenced the epidemiology of salpingitis.

5.20.15 "Acute Salpingitis: Aspects on aetiology, diagnosis and prognosis," L. Westrom and P-A Mardh in *Genital Infections and their Complications,* D. Danielsson et al. eds. (Stockholm: Almqvist & Wiksell International, 1975,) 157-165.

In some cases iatrogenic procedures, such as legal abortions and insertion of IUD's, can cause an unrecognized infection in the cervix to spread to the uterine tubes.

5.21 Bacterial Vaginosis

Bacterial vaginosis appears to be one of the serious consequences of the sexual revolution and is of considerable concern to public health officials as the following articles indicate. It also appears that a substantial number of women presenting for induced abortion would have bacterial vaginosis.

5.21.1 "Bacterial vaginosis: a threat to reproductive health? Historical perspectives, current knowledge, controversies and research demands," PA Mardh, *Eur J Contracept Reprod Health Care* 5(3): 208-219, Sept 2000.

Bacterial vaginosis is a change in flora, the cause of which is still unknown in the vast majority of instances. Bacterial vaginosis has generally been used to represent any change in vaginal flora resulting in an assumed loss of lactobacilli. However, whether or not such a flora represents the genetically normal state of some women is poorly defined. The present "crude" diagnosis of bacterial vaginosis ought to be refined... Although bacterial vaginosis is generally believed to be an endogenous condition, a number of behavioral factors are involved, such as the use of contraceptive and intimate hygiene products and smoking habits. Although bacterial vaginosis is not considered a true sexually transmitted infection, it is related to sexual activities.

5.21.2 "Association Between Bacterial Vaginosis and Preterm Delivery of a Low Birth Weight Infant," SL Hillier et al, *New England Journal of Medicine* 333:1737-1742, 1995.

Bacterial vaginosis is a condition in which the normal, lactobacillus- predominant vaginal flora is replaced with anaerobic bacteria, Gardnerella vaginalis, and Mycoplasma hominis. Bacteria vaginosis has been associated with preterm delivery, premature of the membranes, infection of the chorion and amnion, histologic chorioamnionitis, and infection of amniotic fluid.); see also "Bacterial Vaginosis and Anaerobes in Obstetric-Gynecologic Infection," DA Eschenbach, *Clinical Infectious Diseases* 16(Suppl 4): S282-S287, 1993.

5.21.3   "Bacterial Vaginosis in Pregnancy: An Approach for the 1990s," MC McCoy et al, *Obstetrical and Gynecological Survey* 50(6): 482, 1995.

Screening for it is suggested because 50% of bacterial vaginosis is asymptomatic. The diagnosis, which is rapid and inexpensive, remains defined by clus cells seen on wet prep, high vaginal pH, and amine odor of vaginal discharge.

5.21.4   "Is bacterial vaginosis a sexually transmitted infection?," MC Morris et al, *Sex Transm Infect* 77(1): 63-68, Feb 2001.

Bacterial vaginosis is associated with some factors related to the acquisition of gonorrhoea and chyamydia trachomatis, see also "Bacterial vaginosis: a public health review," M Morris et al, *BJOC* 108 (5): 439-450, May 2001.

5.21.5   "Vaginal infections in human immunodeficiency virus-infected women," A Helfgott et al, *Am J Obstet Gynecol* 183(2): 347-355, Aug 2000.

There were significant associations between human immunodeficiency virus infections and bacterial vaginosis.

5.21.6   "Preventing adverse sequelae of bacterial vaginosis: public health program and research agenda. CDC Bacterial Vaginosis Working Group," EH Koumans and JS Kendrick, *Sex Transm Dis* 28(5): 292-297, May 2001.

The cause of bacterial vagnosis remains poorly understood. Recent evidence strengthens the association between bacterial vaginosis and serious medical complications. Recent evidence shows that screening and treatment of bacterial vaginosis before abortion reduces pelvic inflammatory disease.

5.21.7   "Universal prophylaxis for chlamydia trachomatis and anaerobic (bacterial) vaginosis in women attending for suction termination of pregnancy: an audit of short-term health gains," AL Blackwell et al, *Int J STD & AIDS* 10(8): 508-513, 1999.

In a British study of 400 women who obtained abortions, 8% had cervical chlamydia trachomatis and 28% had bacterial vaginosis. 53% of the women with preoperative c. trachomatis also had bacterial vaginosis. Among the untreated women with c. trachomatis, 63% developed postabortion upper genital tract infection; When treated with metronidazole suppositories and oral oxytetracycline, 12% developed upper genital tract infection. Ed Note: The incidence of bacterial vaginosis (BV) was much higher than chlamydia trachomatis in this study. The presence of BV at the time of the abortion also appeared to substantially increase the incidence of post abortion upper genital tract infection.

5.21.8   "Mobiluncus and clue cells as predictors of PID after First Trimester Abortion," P-G Larsson et al, *Acta Obstet Gynecol Scand* 68:217, 1989.

A Swedish study found that the presence of bacterial vaginosis and the time of induced abortion increased the incidence of postabortion PID to 11.8% compared to 3.2% when bacterial vaginosis was not present.

5.21.9   "Antibiotic prophylaxis to prevent post-abortal upper genital tract infection with bacterial vagnosis: a randomized controlled trial," T Crowley et al, *BJOG* 108(4): 396-402, 2001

A British study of women undergoing first trimester suction abortion found that bacterial vaginosis was present in 29.3% of women. Treatment with metronidazole resulted in an incidence of 8.5% upper genital tract infection compared to 16% of women treated with a placebo.

5.21.10   "Can Fem Card use facilitate bacterial vaginosis diagnosis on day of abortion to prevent postabortion endometritis?," L Miller, *Obstet Gynecol* 97(4 Suppl 1): S58-S59, April 2001.

A self-collected vaginal swab FemExam test card result to Nugent Gram stain scoring of the same specimen was undertaken to test the hypothesis that bacterial vaginosis (BV) treatment begun on the day of an elective abortion would reduce postabortion endometritis. Of the women tested, 39% tested BV positive using the FemExam test card. Results of the study were incomplete.

5.22   Chlamydia Trachomatis Infection

5.22.1   "The Influence of Sexual and Social Factors on the Risk of Chlamydia Trachomatis Infections: A Population-Based Seriologic Study," M Jonsson et al, *Sexually Transmitted Diseases* 229(355), Nov/ Dec, 1995.

A history of therapeutic abortion was a statistically significant risk factor for prevalence of antibodies to chlamydia trachomatis.

5.22.2   "Chlamydia Trachomatis in Relation to Infections Following First Trimester Abortions," T Radberg and L Hamberger, *Acta Obstricia Gynecological* (Supp. 93)154:478, 1980. (Abstract)

In a Swedish study, women with endocervical chlamydial infections were over five times more likely than uninfected women to develop PID within four weeks after a first-trimester induced abortion (23.4% vs. 4.4%)

5.22.3   "Pelvic Infection After Elective Abortion Associated with Chlamydia Trachomatis," B Moller et al, *Obstetrics and Gynecology* 59(2): 210-213, Feb, 1982.

Women applying for abortion should be examined and treated for gonorrhea and infection with chlamydia trachomatis either before or, at the least, in conjunction with the abortion.

5.22.4 "Criteria for Selective Screening for Chlamydia Trachomatis Infection in Women Attending Family Planning Clinics," H Handsfield et al, *Journal of the Medical Association* 225(13): 1730-1734, April 4, 1986.

Selective screening of sexually active women for chlamydial infection is advocated as a necessary and cost effective measure.

5.22.5 "Significance of Cervical Chlamydia Trachomatis Infection in Post-Abortal Pelvic Inflammatory Disease," L Westergaard et al, *Obstetrics and Gynecology* 60(3): 322-325, Sept, 1982.

The presence of chlamydia in the cervical canal at the time of the abortion in asymptomatic women increases the risk of postabortal PID from 10% (without chlamydia) to 28% (with chlamydia)

5.22.6 "Chlamydia Trachomatis Infection in Sexually Active Adolescents: Prevalence and Risk Factors," Mariam R Chako and JC Lovchik, *Pediatrics* 73 (6), June, 1984.

The prevalence of chlamydial infection in 280 sexually active urban adolescents was 26%: 35% in male adolescents, 27% in pregnant female adolescents, and 23% in non-pregnant female adolescents. Chlamydia was almost three times as prevalent as gonorrhea in the same population. Age, past history of sexual transmitted disease, oral contraceptive use, and concomitant gonorrhea were not significantly associated with chlamydial infection. However, multiple current partners, contact with sexually transmitted disease, genitourinary symptoms, and cervical ectopy were significantly associated with chlamydial infection.

5.22.7 "Favors Barrier Methods Over OCs for Sexually Active Teenagers." Richard Brookman, *Family Practice News* 17, November 1-14, 1987.

About 20 percent of 4,000 patients at an adolescent health clinic in Richmond, Virginia were screened for sexually transmitted diseases. Thirty percent had at least one infection; the most common were gonorrhea and chlamydia. About 12 percent were pregnant/ one quarter of them also had an STD. One reason for the high incidence of infection among adolescents is that at puberty, and perhaps several years after, the squamocolumnar junction is on the outer portion of the cervix. The exposed columnar epithelium is particularly susceptible to gonorrhea and chlamydia if exposure occurs.

5.22.8 "Post-Abortal Endometritis and Isolation of Chlamydia Trachomatis," M. Barbacci, M. Spence, E. Kappus, R. Burkman, L. Rao and T. Quinn, *Obstetrics and Gynecology* 68(5):686-90 November 1986.

In a Johns Hopkins study of 505 women who had an induced abortion, 17.6% had a chlamydia infection. Six of 17 patients with post-abortal endomhetritis were culture positive immediately prior to abortion. Some 10% of c. trachomatis-infected women vs. 3.5% of non-c.trachomatis-infected women had endometritis following induced abortion. The article stated: "It is believed that a factor in the development of endometritis is the induced abortion itself as it has been documented that dilation of the cervical canal and curettage of the uterine cavity can stimulate spread of an unrecognized cervical infection to the uterine cavity.") Citing "Culture and treatment results in endometritis following elective abortion," Burkman et al., *American Journal of Obstetrics and Gynecology* 128: 566 (1977). Ed. Note - Endometritis is inflammation of the uterine wall.

5.22.9   "Genital infections in women undergoing therapeutic abortion," D. Avonts and P. Piot, *Europ. J. Obstet. Gynec. Reprod. Biol.* 20: 53-59 (1985).

In a study of 170 women at the Institute of Tropical Medicine in Belgium, there was found to be a strong correlation between an infection with c. trachomatis before abortion and the appearance of infectious complications after the aspiration curettage. Post-abortion infections were stated to be caused by microorganisms introduced in the uterine cavity during the intervention. In addition, sexually transmitted micro-organisms such as n. gonorrhea and c. trachomatis can colonize the endocervix and cause endometritis or PID (pelvic inflammatory disease) after the aspiration curettage.

5.22.10   "Chlamydial and gonococcal infection in a defined population of women," L. Westrom et. al, *Scand. J. Infect. Dis.* 32: 157 (1982).

The risk of acquiring pelvic inflammatory disease (PID) appears to decrease with increasing age among sexually experienced women. The relative risk for PID in women who were culturally positive from the cervix for n. gonorrhea, c. trachomatis or both, assigning a relative risk of 1.0 in the 15-19 year old age group were 0.7 for women 20-24; 0.4 for women 25-29 and 0.2 for women 30-34. Cited in *Sexually Transmitted Diseases* K.K. Holmes, P-A Mardh et. al (McGraw-Hill, 1989) 598.

5.23   Gonnorhea

5.23.1   "Disseminated Gonococcal Infection," K.K. Kerle et. al., *American Family Physician* 45(1): 209, Jan., 1992.

The most frequent systemic complication of acute, untreated gonorrhea is disseminated infection which develops in 0.5-3% of the more than 700,000 Americans infected with gonorrhea each year. Up to 80% of disseminated gonococcal infection occur in women.

5.23.2   "Untreated Endocervical Gonorrhea and Endometritis Following Elective Abortion," R.T. Burkman, J. Tonascia, M. Atienza and T. King, *American Journal of Obstetrics and Gynecology*, 126: 648-651(1976).

2.7 percent of 4,823 patients had gonorrhea; 14.7 percent of patients with gonorrhea developed endometritis over a two-year period. The authors concluded that there is a potential threefold increase for postabortal endometritis with untreated endocervical gonorrhea, which indicates a need to reevaluate approaches to some patients requesting pregnancy termination.

5.23.3   "Gonorrhea: Update on Diagnosis and Management," Steven D. Colby, *Medical Aspects of Human Sexuality* 22:15-24, Mar. 1988.

In 1986 approximately one million cases of gonorrhea were reported to public health officials in the U.S.; it is estimated that up to 3 million are infected annually. Strains of neisseria gonorrhea are becoming increasingly resistant to a variety of antibiotics. Attempts to develop a vaccine against gonorrhea have not been successful.

5.24   HIV/AIDS

5.24.1   "Deliveries, abortion and HIV-1 infection in Rome, 1989-1994," Damiano D. Abeni et al., *European Journal of Epidemiology,* 13:373-378, 1997.

Significantly higher prevalences of infection [HIV-1] were associated with induced abortion (0.49%) than with delivery (0.18%) (OR: .2.72; 95% CI: 2.29-3.22).

5.24.2   "HIV Infection at Outcome of Pregnancy in the Paris area, France," E. Couturier, Y. Brossard, C. Larsen, M. Larsen, *Lancet* 340:707-709,1992.

A French study in the Paris area and 3 surrounding districts with 46% of the reported AIDS cases in France found that HIV seroprevalence rate in women having a elective abortion was twice that of women who delivered (0.54% v. 0.28%), 2% of women with ectopic pregnancy and 4.8% of women having a therapeutic abortion were HIV seropositive.

5.24.3   "Prevalence of HIV among childbearing women and women having termination of pregnancy: multidisciplinary steering group study," D.S. Goldberg, H. MacKinnon, R. Smith, N.B. Patel, *British Medical Journal* 304:1082-1088, April 25,1992.

A Scottish study in 1988-1990 found that 0.13% of women attending an antenatal clinic and 0.85% of women obtaining abortions had HIV infection.

5.24.4   "Chlamydia Is Getting No Respect," *Medical Tribune* 29(3):1,10-11/17, August 18,1988.

A history of Chlamydia is associated with an enhanced risk of human immunodeficiency infection (HIV). In a study presented at the recent Fourth International Conference on AIDS in Stockholm, researchers followed 500 prostitutes from Nairobi, Africa from 1984-1987. During that time HIV seropositivity rose from 59% to 85% of the women. A sub-group of 124 women were questioned regarding sex practices, history of sexually transmitted diseases, etc. Eighty-three of the members of this sub-group sero-converted. For the sero-converted women, a history of Chlamydia was associated with almost a fourfold increased risk of HIV seroconversion independent of other factors. One reason for the possible relationship between HIV and Chlamydia is that Chlamydia causes an intense inflammation of the cervix. Another possible explanation is that Chlamydia may produce a focus of inflammatory cells that could be infected by the HIV virus.

5.24.5 "The Transmission of AIDS: The Case of the Infected Cell. Tay," A. Levy *JAMA* 259(20):3037-3038, May 27,1988.

In Africa, where heterosexual spread is prominent, transmission appears to be enhanced by concurrent venereal diseases, particularly those caused by Haemophilus ducreyi (chanceroid) and herpes virus, which produce ulceration's in both men and women. Citing several studies. Furthermore, the copious inflammatory genital fluid, containing potentially large numbers of virus-infected cells, may be an added factor increasing HIV transmission. (Resistance to HIV of an intact squamous epithelial lining of the vaginal canal most likely plays an important role in limiting HIV infection in women. (When lesions occur in the vagina or cervix secondary to venereal infections, women can become more susceptible to HIV. Citing three studies.

5.24.6 "Measures to Prevent Cervical Injury During Suction Curettage Abortion," K. Schulz, D. Grimes, W. Cates, *The Lancet*, May 28,1983, p. 1182.

In addition to overt injury to the cervix during suction curettage, covert trauma is also important. Microfractures of the cervix may occur during forceful dilatation of the cervix/which may lead to persistent structural changes, cervical incompetence, premature delivery and pregnancy complications. Citing several studies.

5.24.7 "Pelvic inflammatory disease following induced first-trimester abortion." Lars Heisterberg, *Danish Medical Bulletin* 35(1):64-75, February 1988.

Reviews the current status of studies on the subject. Notes that studies show evidence of elevated risk of post-abortal PID for women with history of PID or c. trachomatis. A recent episode of vaginitis may also be a risk factor.

5.24.8 "HIV/AIDS Prevention and Multiple Risk Behaviors of Gay Male and Runaway Adolescents," Clara Haignere, M. Rotheram-Borus, C. Koopman, P. Cristina, M. Burchfield and A. Morales, Paper presented to the Sixth International Conference on AIDS, San Francisco, June 1990. (Abstract)

In a study by researchers from the New York State Psychiatric Institute and Columbia University on 75 female adolescent runaways in New York City. Suicide attempts and suicide ideation were found to be significantly related to having had an abortion, (p .05). Female runaways who had been pregnant were also more likely to have been in trouble with the law, to use drugs, to engage in frequent unprotected sexual intercourse, and to have had sex with multiple partners in the previous three months. Ed. Note - This study indicates that abortion may increase sexual promiscuity, lessen the desire for self-preservation and increased self-destructive behavior, including the increased risk of HIV/AIDS.

5.24.9 "Impact of the HIV Epidemic on Mortality in Women of Reproductive Age. United States," S.Y. Chu, J.W. Buehler and R.L. Berkelman, *JAMA* 264(2):225-229, July 11,1990

In 1987 the leading cause of death in black women residing in New York and New Jersey was HIV / AIDS. Malignant neoplasms were second. Drug abuse was listed on 27% of the HIV/AIDS death certificates as an associated cause of death. Ed. Note - Laboratory tests at the University of Minnesota have found that HIV grew as much as three times faster in peripheral blood mono nuclear cells exposed to doses of cocaine compared to non-cocaine exposed controls.

5.24.10 "The Effects of Gender and Crack Use on High Risk Behaviors," E. Golden, M. Fullilove, R. Fullilove, R. Lennon,D. Porterfield, S. Schwarcz and G. Bolan, Paper presented at the 6th International Conference on AIDS: San Francisco, June, 1990

The Center for AIDS Prevention Studies in San Francisco found that among black sexually active teenagers (15-19 years) the practice of engaging in the exchanging of sexual favors for drugs and having sex under the influence of drugs or alcohol were significant predictors of pregnancy in female crack users. The total number of drugs used predicted the number of sexually transmitted diseases. It was concluded that crack use may be an important risk factor for HIV infection in young women.

5.24.11 "The Increasing Frequency of Hetero-sexually Acquired AIDS in the United States -1983 -1988," K.K. Holmes, J. Karon and J. Kreiss, *American Journal of Public Health* 80(7):858- 863, July,1990

Drug use, exchange of sex for drugs or money and early onset of sexual activity are increasingly associated with heterosexually transmitted infections, particularly in inner-city populations. It was concluded that promotion of "safe-sex" practices would be especially difficult in this group.

5.24.12 "AIDS and behavioral risk factors in women in inner city Baltimore: A comparison of telephone and face to face surveys," M. Nebot et. al, *J. Epidemiology & Community Health* 48(4): 412-418, Aug. 1994.

A telephone survey found telephone surveys among women aged 17-35 were more likely to report HIV testing, live in subsidized housing, report a previous abortion or surgical sterilization compared to face to face counseling.

5.24.13 "Psychosocial correlates and predictors of AIDS risk behaviors, abortion, and drug use among a community sample of young adult women," J.A. Stein et. al. *Health Psychology* 13(4): 308-318, July, 1994

Risky AIDS behavior was strongly associated with multiple drug use and less social conformity and modestly related to sexual experience and abortion.

5.24.14 "Psychosocial and behavioral factors associated with physical and sexual abuse among HIV infected women," LA Bedimo et al, *Int Conf AIDS, 1998*; 12:219 (abstract no. 14185)

Among women attending a HIV outpatient program in New Orleans, Louisiana, 45% reported ever experiencing sexual abuse, 82% acquired HIV through heterosexual contact. Among those sexually abused, 27% first experienced it before the age of 17. Factors associated with a history of sexual abuse included having a history of abortion (33% vs. 9%)

5.24.15 "HIV-1 infection and reproductive history: a retrospective study among pregnant women: Adidjan, Cote d'Iviire," A Desgrees et al, *Int'l J STD & AIDS* 9:452, 1998

A study of pregnant women in West Africa found that having had an abortion increased the likelihood of HIV-1 particularly among younger women.

5.25   Hepatitis

5.25.1   "Health issues associated with increasing use of "crack" cocaine among female sex workers in London," H Ward et al, *Sex Transm Infect* 76(4):292-293

Thirty-four percent of female sex workers reported using " crack" cocaine in 1995-1996. Crack use was associated with abortion and hepatitis C infection. It is possible that "crack" use facilitates hepatitis C transmission due to oral lesions from smoking.

5.25.2   "A study of the role of the family and other risk factors in HCV transmission," S Brusaferro et al, *Eur J Epidemiol* 15(2): 125-132, 1999

Surgical procedures such as abortion and/or uterine curettage significantly increased the risk of HCV transmission both with univariate and multivariate analysis.

5.25.3   "Risk factors of contamination by hepatitis C virus in the general population," V Merle et al, *Gastroenterol Clin Biol* 23(4): 439-446, 1999 (English Abstract)

Multiple deliveries or abortion significantly increased the risk of infection by hepatitis C virus.

5.25.4   "Hepatitis C virus, hepatitis B virus and human immune infection in pregnant women in North-East Italy: a case-control study," V Baldo et al, *Eur J Epidemiol* 16(1): 87-91, 2000

A history of a previous abortion increased the likelihood of HCV infection in pregnant women, Odds Ratio 2.8

5.26   Use of Antibiotics in Connection With Induced Abortion

5.26.1   "Antibiotic Prophylaxis for Gynecologic Procedures," ACOG Practice Bulletin, No. 23, January, 2001.

The optimal antibiotic and dosing regimens for induced abortion and dilation and curettage remain unclear. Both tetracyclines and nitro-imidazoles provide significant and comparable protection against postabortal pelvic inflammatory disease. Based on good and scientific evidence, it was recommended that " women undergoing surgically induced abortion are candidates for antibiotic prophylaxis."

5.26.2　"Tetracycline resistance determinants: mechanisms of action, regulation of expression, genetic mobility, and distribution," MC Roberts, *FEMS Microbiol Rev* 19(1): 1-24: 1996.

Tetracycline resistant bacteria are found in a wide variety of ecosystems. see also "Tetracycline resistant Chlamydia trachomatis in Toulouse, France," JC Lefevre et al, *Pathol Biol* (Paris) 45(5): 376-378, 1997.

5.26.3　"Antibiotics at the Time of Induced Abortion: The Case for Universal Prophylaxis Based on a Meta-Analysis," G.F. Sawaya, D. Grady, K. Kerlikowske, D.A. Grimes, *Obstet. Gynecol.* 87(5): 884, May, 1996.

A meta-analysis concluded that there is a potentially substantial protective effect in all subgroups of women, even women in low-risk groups if antibiotics are routinely used at the time of induced abortion. It was estimated that if this was done that up to half of all cases of postabortal infections could be prevented.

5.26.4　"Preventing Febrile Complications of Suction Curettage Abortion," T.K. Park, M. Flock, K. Schulz and D. Grimes, *Am. J. Obstetrics and Gynecology* 152:252-255(1985); JPSA-III (1975-1978).

This study evaluated the relative risk of antibiotics, previous deliveries, type of anesthesia, level of physician training and type of suction cannula on the frequency of febrile complications, i .e. 38c temp for 2 days or more. Despite the clinical and public health importance of infection, the risk factors for postabortal infections are not well understood. (Prophylactic antibiotics reduced the rate of febrile complications i.e. 38c temperature for 2 or more days by one-third.)

5.26.5　"Antibiotic prophylaxis to prevent post-abortal upper genital tract infection in women with bacterial vaginosis; randomized controlled trial," T Crowley et al, *BJOG* 108(4): 396-402, 2001.

A British study of women undergoing first trimester suction abortion found that bacterial vaginosis was present in 29.3% of the women. Treatment with metronidazole resulted in an incidence of 8.5% post-abortal upper genital tract infection compared to 16% for women treated with a placebo.

5.26.6　"Universal prophylaxis for chlamydia trachomatis and anaerobic (bacterial) vaginosis in women attending for suction termination of pregnancy: an audit of short-term health gains," AL Blackwell et al, *Int J STD & AIDS* 10(8): 508-513, 1999.

In a British study of 400 women who obtained abortions, 8% had cervical chlamydia trachomatis and 28% had bacterial vaginosis. 53% of the women with preoperative c. trachomatis also had bacterial vaginosis. Among untreated women with c trachomatis, 63% developed upper genital tract infection; when women were treated with metronidazole suppositories and oral oxytetracycline, only 12% developed upper genital tract infection.

5.26.7   "Prophylactic Antibiotics for Curettage Abortion," D. Grimes, K. Schulz and W. Cates, *American Journal of Obstetrics and Gynecology* 150(6):689-694, Nov. 15,1984.

Legal abortion is the most frequently performed gynecologic operation in the United States, with nearly 1.3 million procedures reported in 1980. Curettage procedures were used for 96 percent of these abortions. Opinion is divided as to the advisability of routine use of prophylactic antibiotics for curettage abortion. Nausea and vomiting caused by tetracyclines may preclude administration of these antibiotics before the abortion, but a short course of antibiotic could begin after the procedure. Prophylaxis may help prevent both short-term morbidity and potential late sequelae, such as ectopic pregnancy and infertility.

5.26.8   "A Clinical Double-Blind Study of the Effect of Tinidazole on the Occurrence of Endometritis after First Trimester Legal Abortion," L. Westrom, L. Svensson and P. Wolner-Hanssen, *Scand. Journal Infect. Dis.*, Suppl. 26: 104-109 (1981).

Twelve percent of women who had undergone vacuum aspiration abortion had febrile reactions with rectal temperatures above 38° C. The author observed that a portion of the early febrile reactions after VA are not attributable to infection, at least not those covered by the study. He also observed that acute salpingitis, as confirmed by laparoscopy, is rarely diagnosed during the first week after VA.

5.26.9   "Pelvic Inflammatory Disease Following Induced First-Trimester Abortion Risk Groups, Prophylaxis and Sequelae," L. Heisterberg, *Danish Medical Bulletin*, 35(1): 64-75, February, 1988.

Reviews six studies on antibiotic prophylaxis in induced first trimester abortion; two were clinical controlled trials: 4 cohort studies could be undermined by bias including selection bias such as assigning women at risk to the treatment group. Also, knowing which women receive treatment can influence both the women and the physicians in their recognition of symptoms and diagnosis of infection. Concludes that antibiotic prophylaxis should be used.

5.26.10 "Survey Reveals Noncompliance with Guidelines on Treating PID," *Family Practice News* 17(21): 341 Nov 1-14,1987.

A 1983-84 Seattle survey of 520 physicians and nurses who treated ambulatory patients for PID found that only 23% fully conformed to the Centers for Disease Control guidelines for antibiotic treatment: 63% provided intermediate therapy and 14% provided consistently inadequate therapy.

5.26.11 "Inflammatory Disease and Its Consequences in Industrialized Countries," L. Westrom, *American Journal Obstetrics Gynecology*,138: 880-892 (1980).

Despite antibiotic therapy, patients who have had at least one episode of salpingitis have a 21 percent rate of involuntary infertility/ as compared with the rate of 3% among the control population.

Impact on Later Pregnancies

5.27   Secondary Infertility

5.27.1   "Role of Induced Abortion in Secondary Infertility," J.R. Daling, L.R. Spadoni, I. Emanuel, *Obstet Gynecol* 57: 59,1981.

A case-control study of married couples diagnosed as having secondary infertility at the University of Washington Hospital in 1976-78 found that women with a history of prior induced abortion had a 1.31 relative increased risk of secondary infertility (0.71-2.43, 95% C.I.), which was not statistically significant, compared with controls.

5.27.2   "Induced abortions, miscarriages and tobacco smoking as risk factors for secondary infertility," A. Tzonou, et al, *J. Epidemiology and Comm. Health* 47:36,1993.

In a case-control study by the Harvard Schools of Public Health and the University of Athens, of women in Athens, Greece in 1987-88, the occurrence of either induced abortions or spontaneous abortions independently and significantly increased the risk of subsequent secondary infertility. The logistic progression adjusted relative risks was 2.1 (1.1-4.0, 95% C.I.) for secondary infertility when there was 1 previous abortion and 2.3 (1.0-5.5, 95% C.I.) when there were 2 previous abortions. The adjusted relative risk of tobacco smoking for secondary infertility was 3.0 (1.3-6.8, 95% C.I.) compared to non-smokers. Secondary infertility was defined as [1] patient had a previous conception; [2] patient was married; [3] husband had a normal semen analysis and [4] patient had been trying become pregnant for at least 18 months.

5.27.3   "The effect of induced abortion on subsequent fertility," P Frank et al, *Br J Obstetrics and Gynecology* 100:575, 1993.

In a follow-up analysis of British women who had an induced abortion compared to women whose last pregnancy had a natural outcome, it was found that at the end of 12 months 89% of the abortion group had achieved a pregnancy compared to 93.3% on the non-abortion group which approached statistical significance

5.27.4   "Contraception after abortion and postpartum," H. Vorherr, *Am.J. Obstet. Gynecol.* 117(7):1002, Dec. 1, 1973

A study at the University of New Mexico reported that in 5-10% of healthy nonpostpartum women (apparently post abortion women) anovulary cycles are observed.

5.27.5   "Short and Long-term Results of Pregnancy by Different Methods, E.I," Sotnikova, *Acta Medica Hungarica* 43 (2): 139-143 (1986).

A Russian study of 560 women undergoing abortion by curettage, prostaglandin and vacuum aspiration found that one-third of the women had serious ovarian dysfunction 3-5 years post-abortion. Ovarian dysfunction was six times more observed than genital inflammations. Post-abortion complications were more frequent in women with a late menarche and with a history of genital inflammation. Instrumental abortion has more short-term complications (12%) than the other methods.

5.28   Uterine Fibroids

5.28.1   "Risk factors for uterine fibroids among women undergoing tubal sterilization," CR Chen et al, *Am J Epidemiol* 153(1): 20-26, 2001.

Parous women were at reduced risk for uterine fibroids while elective abortion did not reduce the risk for uterine fibroids compared to nulliparous women.

5.28.2   "Risk factors for uterine fibroids: reduced risk associated with oral contraceptives," RK Ross et al, *British Medical Journal* 293:359, August 9, 1986.

The risk of fibroids decreased consistently with increasing number of term pregnancies. There was no reduction in risk with incomplete pregnancies (induced abortion or spontaneous abortion) but a slight, but not significant increase in risk of fibroids.

5.29   Gestational Trophoblastic Disease

Gestational trophbloastic neoplasia includes complete hydatidiform mole, invasive mole, and choriocacinoma. Choriocarcinoma is malignant and therefore is considered a form of cancer. According to a 1986 U.S. study the incidence of choriocarcinoma is about 1 in 24,000 pregnancies. The incidence of molar pregnancy is reported to be 1 per 1500 live births and it is potentially life threatening. According to pregnancy-related deaths of U.S. women compiled by the CDC for 1987-90, 6 women died from molar pregnancy.

5.29.1   "Risk Factors for Gestational Tropoblastic Neoplasia," ML Messerli et al, *Am J Obstet Gynecol* 153:294, 1985.

A case-control study of gynecologic and reproductive risk factors for gestational trophoblastic neoplasia among Baltimore area women from 1975-1982 found that there was a higher mean incidence of induced abortions or spontaneous abortions among cases compared to controls, while women having at least one term pregnancy or one live birth provided a protective effect.

5.29.2   "A Case-Control Study from the People's Republic of China," LA Brinton et al, *Am J Obstet*

Gynecol 161:121, 1989.

A case-control study of Chinese women with complete hydatidiform mole found that a history of a term birth was associated with a statistically significant reduced risk of 0.6 , while a history of one induced abortion had a nonsignificant increased relative risk of 1.2, and a history of two or more induced abortions had a statistically significant increased risk of 2.8, compared to women with no history of induced abortion.

5.29.3   "Risk factors for complete molar pregnancy from a case-control study," RS Berkowitz et al, *Am J Obstet Gynecol* 152:1016-1020, 1985.

A Massachusetts study of women with molar pregnancy matched with parous controls without molar pregnancy found that there was a 8-fold increased risk for molar pregnancy when the prior pregnancy was an induced abortion.

5.29.4   "Case-Control Study of Gestational Choriocarcinoma," JD Buckley et al, *Cancer Research* 48:1004-1010, 1981.

A multi-centered study of women with gestational choriocarcinoma matched women by year of pregnancy, age at pregnancy, and geographical residence found that an induced abortion preceding the choriocarcinoma was a risk factor while a live birth was protective against choriocarcinoma. The authors concluded that the most important factor for choriocarcinoma is the nature of the preceding pregnancy.

5.29.5   "Pregnancy Termination, Choricarcinoma Presenting as a Complication of Elective First Trimester Abortion," F.A. Lyon and L.L. Adcock, *Minnesota Medicine*, October, 1980, pp. 733-735.

A case report is presented in which metastatic gestational disease was detected at a routine two-week post abortion examination due to the incomplete removal of fetal remains.

5.29.6   "Choriocarcinoma Following M.T.P," A.S. Gupta, K. Mukherjee, S. Chowdhury, *J. Indian Medical Association* 82(7): 255, July, 1984.

Two cases are presented where choricarcinoma developed in Calcutta, India hospital following induced abortion.

5.30   Hypertension (High-Blood Pressure)

5.30.1   "Pregnancy-Related Mortality in the United States. 1987-1990," C.J. Berg et. al., *Obstetrics and Gynecology* 88:161,1996.

According to data published by the Centers for Disease Control for 1987-1990, 256 U.S. women died from complications due to pregnancy-induced hypertension out of a total number of 1453 pregnancy-related deaths during this period which represented 17.6% of all pregnancy-related deaths.

5.30.2   "The relationship between abortion in the first pregnancy and development of pregnancy-induced hypertension in the subsequent pregnancy," DM Strickland et al., *Am. J. of Obstet. Gynecol.* 154: 146,1986.

In a study of 24,646 women who delivered at Parkland Memorial Hospital during 1977-80, the incidence of pregnancy-induced hypertension was 25.4% in primiaravid women, 22.3% among women whose only previous pregnancy terminated in abortion (either spontaneous or induced), and only 10% among women who carried two or more successive pregnancies to viability. Additional completed pregnancies after the first pregnancy did not confer any additional protective effect. It was concluded that the protective effect from abortion was small compared to a completed pregnancy.

5.30.3   "A Multivariate Analysis of Risk Factors for Preclampsia," B. Eskenazi et. al., *JAMA* 266: 231,1991.

A study of women who gave birth at Northern California Kaiser Permanent Hospital in 1984-85 found that women with a history of therapeutic abortion were 2.16 times more likely to have preclampsia (1.18-3.96, CI 95%) compared to no therapeutic abortion history. In contrast to induced abortion, a previous spontaneous abortion was found to have a protective effect (0.48, 0.24-0.95, CI 95%.)

5.30.4   "Pregnancy-Induced Hypertension in North Carolina," 1988 and 1989, D.A. Savitz, J. Zhang, *Am. J. Public Health* 82 (5): 675,1992.

A study of birth records in North Carolina during 1988-1989 examined the risk for pregnancy-induced hypertension (PIH) and found that the overall risk of PIH was 43.1 per 1000 births. Having had one child (Parity 1) was protective against PIH compared to no children (Parity 0) (0.4, 0.3-0.4, CI 95%). Blacks and whites were found to be a virtually equal risk. Mothers aged 35 or older were at increased risk compared to mothers aged 20-34 (1.6,1.4-1.8, CI 95%).

5.30.5   "Pre-eclampsia in second pregnancy," D.M. Campbell, I. MacGillivray, R. Carr-Hill, *Br. J. Obstet. Gynaecol.* 92: 131, Feb. 1985.

In a comprehensive and well-designed study of 29/851 women in Aberdeen, Scotland with first or second pregnancies, found that the incidence of proteinuric pre-clampsia after early abortion, which was either spontaneous or induced (separately studied) was similar to the population incidence in a first pregnancy (7.6% v. 5.6%). Only a pregnancy of 37 weeks gestation or more was likely to offer protection against pre-eclampsia in a second pregnancy. The incidence of proteinuric pre-eclampsia or mild pre-eclampsia in the next pregnancy after an induced abortion was 7.6% and 26.7% respectively in contrast to 1.9% and 17.0% where there was a viable first pregnancy prior to the second pregnancy.

5.31 Ectopic Pregnancy

5.31.1 "Risk of Ectopic Pregnancy and Previous Induced Abortion," C Tharaux-Deneux et al, *Am J Public Health* 88(3): 401, 1998.

A French case-control study found that among women with no previous ectopic pregnancy, women with one previous induced abortion had a statistically significant increased risk of 1.4, while women with two or more previous induced abortions had a statistically significant increased risk of 1.9 for ectopic pregnancy compared to women with no previous induced abortion. Ed Note: This study is possibly the only one which did not include women with a previous ectopic pregnancy. Previous ectopic pregnancy greatly increases the likelihood of another ectopic pregnancy and is a confounding factor. Failure to control for this variable would tend to make it appear that there was a lesser risk or perhaps no statistically increased risk of ectopic pregnancy from induced abortion.

5.31.2 "Risk Factors for Ectopic Pregnancy. A Population-Based Study," P.A. Marchbanks et. al, *J. American Medical Association* 259(12): 1823, March 25, 1988.

A case-control study at Mayo Clinic from 1935-1982, using univariate analysis found a 2.5 relative risk for ectopic pregnancy from induced abortion (1.02-6.1, 95% CI and a 4.0 relative risk from pelvic inflammatory disease (2.2-7.2, 95% CI. The Multivariate risk from induced abortion was 2.1 (0.8-5.9, 95% CI) and 3.3 (1.6-6.6, 95% CI for pelvic inflammatory disease.)

5.31.3 "An Updated Protocol for Abortion Surveillance With Ultrasound and Immediate Pathology," S.R. Goldstein, M. Danon, C. Watson, *Obstet. Gynecol.* 83: 55-58,1994.

In a study of 674 women who presented for first trimester abortion ultrasonography determined that 2.5% were 13 weeks or more despite bimanual examinations and the last menstrual period suggesting 12 or fewer weeks. The incidence of ectopic pregnancy was 0.58% and tubal pregnancy was 0.29% with an overall incidence of 0.87% using HCG and ultrasonography on-site testing.

5.31.4 "Induced abortions and risk of ectopic pregnancy," F. Parazzini et al. *Human Reproduction* 10(7): 1841,1995.

An Italian case-control study found that the multivariate risk of ectopic pregnancy for any induced abortion was 2.9,1.6-5.3, 95% CI. The risk increased with the number of induced abortions both with obstetric and non-obstetric controls.

5.31.5 "Ectopic Pregnancy Surveillance United States, 1970 - 1987," K. Nederof, H. Lawson, A. Saftlas, H. Atrash and E. Finch, *Morbidity and Mortality Weekly Report* 39(SS-4) December, 1990.

Ectopic pregnancy has risen from 17,800 cases in 1970 to 88,000 hospitalized cases in 1987. From 1970 - 1987 approximately 877,400 cases have been reported among U.S. women 15-44 years. Thirty women were reported to have died from ectopic pregnancy in 1987. Although the cause of ectopic pregnancy is unknown, it has been attributed to alteration in tubal motility, hormonal release and anatomical changes such as scarring. Scarring may be caused by acute and chronic salpingitis.

5.31.6　"Ectopic Pregnancy and Prior Induced Abortion," A.Levin, S. Schoenbaum, P. Stubblefield, S. Zimicki, R. Monson and K. Ryan, *American Journal of Public Health*, 72(3):253-256, March 1982.

This study found a relationship between the number of prior induced abortions and the risk of ectopic pregnancy: the crude relative risk of ectopic pregnancy was 1.6 for women with one prior induced abortion and 4.0 for women with two or more prior induced abortions; however, use of multivariate techniques to control confounding factors reduced the relative risks to 1.3 and 2.6, respectively. The analysis suggests that induced abortion may be one of several risk factors for ectopic pregnancy, particularly for women who have had abortions plus pelvic inflammatory disease or multiple abortions.

5.31.7　"Pathogenesis of Tubal Pregnancy," J. Niles, and J. Clark, *American Journal of Obstetrics and Gynecology,* 105 (8): 1230-1234, December 15,1969.

A pathologic review was made of 436 ectopic pregnancies treated at a hospital over a 10 1/2 year period. Only about 40 percent of the cases studied had a histologic diagnosis of chronic inflammatory disease. Fifty-eight percent of the cases had no demonstrable histologic abnormality to produce an ectopic nidation, suggesting a functional pathogenesis. From the literature, the study noted factors which theoretically and logically could play a more important role in ectopic nidation than that of chronic pelvic inflammatory disease. They are (1) iatrogenic factors, (2) hormonal, (3) retrograde menstruation, (4) functional causes, and (5) the conceptus. Various studies were cited.

5.31.8　"Etiology of Ectopic Pregnancy: A New Concept," Joseph G. Asherman, *Obstetrics and Gynecology*, 16(6):619-624, December 1955.

Out of 325 patients with a history of ectopic pregnancy, 181 had one or more abortions, either spontaneous or induced. Of those, 135 were induced and 67 were spontaneous abortions. Twenty-one of the 181 women had both induced and spontaneous abortions. The study found that functional disturbances of the propelling mechanism of the tubes are to blame rather than pathologic changes in the tubes themselves. The movements of the tubal musculature (an inner circular and an outer longitudinal layer) are as dependent upon the hormonal as upon the nervous system. Any disturbance in the neurodendocrine balance is likely to bring about a change in the normal functioning of the tubes and may result in infertility or tubal pregnancy, depending on the severity of the disturbance. Why are induced abortions twice as damaging as spontaneous ones, when the intervention is the same for both? There is only one difference between the two kinds of abortion, the impact of psychic trauma. Any abortion, whether spontaneous or induced, may be the source of bitter frustration which will deepen with the passage of time if the yearning for motherhood is not satisfied. In induced abortion, however, an additional emotional factor is at work, leading, in the course of time, to a guilt complex. These make the inner tension of such women much higher than those experiencing spontaneous abortion.

5.31.9 "Ectopic Pregnancy and Myoma Uteri: Tetragenic Effects and Maternal characteristics," E. Matsunaga, and K. Shiota, *Teratology* 21: 61-69 (1980).

Fetal malformations were found in 11.6 percent of ectopic pregnancies compared with lesser percentages for controls. Maternal smoking and drinking were cited as causes.

5.31.10 "Induced Abortion and Ectopic Pregnancy in Subsequent Pregnancies," C.S. Chung, R.G. Smith, P.G. Steinoff, and M.P. Mi, *American Journal of Epidemiology* 115(6): 879-887 (1982).

There was a clear association between the presence of post-abortion infection or retained parts and a 5 fold increase in ectopic pregnancy compared to uninfected women.

5.31.11 "Etiology of Cervical Pregnancy," D. Dicker, D. Feldbeg, N. Samuel, J.A. Goldman, *The J. of Reproductive Medicine* 30(1): 25, Jan., 1985.

An association was found between cervical pregnancy and prior induced abortion.

5.31.12 "Ectopic Pregnancy and First Trimester Abortion," L.A. Schonberg, *Obstetrics and Gynecology* 49(1) (Supp): 735, Jan. 1977.

Among a total of 41/753 first trimester abortions done over a 4 year period at two Planned Parenthood Centers in New York City from 1971-1975 only 11 verified cases of ectopic (tubal) pregnancy were discovered; 3 patients had a rupture of their tubal pregnancy immediately following suction curettage, 6 patients had rupture of the tube from 1-19 days after suction curettage. Only two unruptured ectopic gestations were diagnosed. Ed. Note: In 1975 the ectopic pregnancy rate was 7.6 per 1000 pregnancies (live births, induced abortions and ectopic pregnancy). Based on that rate PP should have discovered about 312 ectopic pregnancies.

5.31.13 "Ectopic Pregnancy in Relation to Previous Induced Abortion," T.R. Daling, W.H. Chow, N.S. Weiss, B.J. Metch and R. Suderstrom, *Journal of the American Medical Association*, 253(7): 1005-1008, February 15,1985.

Women who have one induced abortion showed virtually no excess risk of ectopic pregnancy. (RR=1.4). For women with two or more abortions, the relative risk was 1.8. In the author's opinion, it remains unresolved whether having a legal induced abortion imparts an excess risk of ectopic pregnancy. Nonetheless, the results relating to the group of women having two or more abortions (RR of 1.8 and 2.6 in two of the studies) are worrisome.

5.31.14 "Risk Factors For Ectopic Pregnancy: A Case-Control Study in France, with Special Focus on Infectious Factors," J. Coste, N. Job-Spira, H. Fernandez, E. Papiernik, A. Spira, *Am.J. Epidemiology* 133(9): 839, May, 1991.

A case-control study in 1988 in seven Paris area hospitals found a 1.6 relative risk of ectopic pregnancy where there was prior induced abortion (1.1-2.3,95% C.I.). If adjustments were made for age, smoking and pelvic inflammatory disease the association disappeared. Ed. Note: Adjustments for PID and smoking should not have been made as induced abortion is implicated.

5.31.15 "Ectopic Pregnancy Critical Analysis of 139 Cases," M. Faith Kamsheh, *Minnesota Medicine*, February 1983, pp. 83-86.

Between 1975 and 1981, the number of ectopic pregnancies at Fairview Hospital more than doubled. Ectopic pregnancy is responsible for 10 percent of all maternal deaths. Patients who are infertile, did not use birth control, or who have a history of recent abortion or menstrual extraction, of PID, of IUD or recent removal of IUD or a history of previous tubal sterilization, tubal pregnancy, tubal reconstruction, and abdominal surgery have a high index of suspicion.

5.31.16 "Ectopic Pregnancy Case Study," Clinton A. Turner, *Perspectives and Problems in OB/GYN*, January 1985, Published for Stuart Pharmaceuticals by Communications in Med. Div. of Cahners Pub. Co., 475 Park Avenue S., New York, NY 10016.

The most alarming risk factor of all for ectopic pregnancy is a prior history of ectopic pregnancy. The risk of ectopic pregnancy in a patient who has had a prior one is approximately 20 times greater than that of a general population. A previous history of PID or a prior abortion were listed as risk factors for ectopic pregnancy.

5.31.17 "Ectopic Pregnancy - A New Surgical Epidemic," Louis Weinstein, M. Morris, D. Dotters and C.D. Christian, *Obstetrics and Gynecology*, 61(6): 698-701, June 1983

Between March 1972 and September 1981,154 patients were diagnosed for ectopic pregnancy at the University of Arizona. Currently, the incidence of ectopic pregnancy at the University of Arizona is one in 45 live births. 22.7 percent reported one or more previous therapeutic abortions; 14.9 percent reported a history of previous PID. Pelvic inflammatory disease is believed to be the major etiologic factor in the rising rate of ectopic pregnancy.

5.31.18 "Ectopic Pregnancy in the United States: 1970-1983," H. Atrash, *Morbidity and Mortality Weekly Report* 35(22S) Aug. 1986.

70,000 women were hospitalized for ectopic pregnancy in the U.S. in 1983, resulting in 70,000 fetal deaths. Ectopic pregnancy accounted for 12.8 percent of all maternal deaths in the U.S. in 1983. In 1985 black women continued to have a 3.5 times higher risk of death from ectopic pregnancy. Teenage black women have a 6.2 times higher risk than white teenagers.

5.31.19 "A 21-Year Survey of 654 Ectopic Pregnancies," James L. Breen, *American Journal of Obstetrics and Gynecology*, 106(7):1004-1019, April 1,1970

A review of the patients' operations or therapy seemed to substantiate that antecedent inflammatory disease recorded in 185 patients is a prime etiologic factor in ectopic pregnancy. A history of previous antibiotic therapy in 345 patients also implied therapy of pelvic inflammatory disease. A previous ectopic pregnancy in 45 patients (6.9 percent) or a previous tubal ligation in four patients (0.6 percent) may have been potentially edologic.

5.31.20 "An Overview of Infectious Aunts of Salpingitis, Their Biology and Recent Advances in Methods of Detection," P-A Mardh, *American Journal Obstetrics and Gynecology,* 138(7):933-951 Part 2, December 1,1980.

In salpingitis, it is believed that anaerobic bacteria often gain entrance to the tubes as secondary invades from the lower genital tract in patients whose tubes have been damaged with sexually transmitted disease agents. In such secondary infections, both anaerobic and facultatively anaerobic bacteria can be demonstrated. Endogenous tubal infections may occur in hosts whose genital organs have been "compromised" by gynecologic surgery, curettage, legal or illegal abortion, or various diagnostic procedures. In the hospital catchment region of Lund such "iatrogenic" cases constitute approximately 15 percent of all salpingitis patients. See"Epidemiology. Etiology and Prognosis of Acute Salpingitis - a study of 1.457 laparoscopically verified cases," L. Westrom and P-A Mardh, in *Non-gonococcal Urethritis and Related Infections,* D. Hobson and K. Holmes, eds.,(Washington, D.C.: American Society for Microbiology, 1977) 84-90.

5.31.21 "Repeat Ectopic Pregnancy: A Study of 123 Consecutive Cases," Jack G. Hallatt, *American Journal of Obstetrics and Gynecology,* 122(4): 520, June 15,1975.

This study concludes the principal etiology of ectopic pregnancy as healed salpingitis which may have been gonorrheal, post-abortal or puerperal. These infections are readily controlled with antibiotics but fusion of the plical of the endosalpinix is a sequelae. These tubal adhesions subsequently trap the developing embryo.

5.31.22 "Chlamydia Trachomatis Infections in the United States, What Are They Costing Us?" A. Eugene Washington, R.E. Johnson, L.L. Sanders, *Journal of the American Medical Association,* 257(15): 2070-2072, April 17,1987.

It is estimated that each year 402,200 episodes of chlamydial PID occur, leading to 13,900 ectopic pregnancies and 280 deaths.

5.31.23 *Sexually Transmitted Diseases. K.K. Holmes,* P.A. Mardh, P.F. Sparling, O.J. Wiesner (~~~~1984) 630.

Women in the post-salpingitic state have a seven- to tenfold risk for ectopic pregnancy, compared with women who never had the disease.

5.32   Placenta Previa/Aburuptio Placentae/Retained Placenta

5.32.1   "The Association of Placenta Previa with History of Caesarean Delivery and Abortion: A Meta

Analysis," CV Anath et al, *Am J Obstet Gynecol* 177: 1071, 1997.

A review of 12 studies by researchers at the Robert Wood Johnson Medical School found that there was a strong association between a previous induced abortion and a higher risk of placenta previa among U.S. women.

5.32.2 "Placenta Previa in Relation to Induced and Spontaneous Abortion: A Population-Based Study," V.M. Taylor et al., *Obstet. Gynecol.* 82: 88-91,1993

A study of birth certificate data among Washington state white women during 1984-1987 found that women who reported one or more induced abortions were 1.28 times more likely to have a pregnancy complicated by placenta previa which was statistically significant.

5.32.3 "Induced Abortion: A Risk Factor For Placenta Previa," J.M. Barrett, F. H. Boehm, A.P. Killam, *AmJ. Obstet Gynecol* 141:769,1981.

A study at Vanderbilt University in 1979-80 found that 3.8% of the women with a history of induced abortion had placenta previa. If it was the first delivery since an induced first trimester induced abortion, the incidence of placenta previa was 4.6% compared to an overall percentage of 0.9%.

5.32.4 "Long-term sequelae following legally induced abortion," E.B. Obel, *Danish Medical Bulletin* 27(2): 61, April, 1980.

A Danish study compared women who's previous pregnancy was terminated by a legal induced abortion (group 1), with women whose previous pregnancy had ended in a spontaneous abortion or still birth (group 2), women whose previous pregnancy ended in a live birth (group 3), and women with no previous pregnancies. The study found that an induced abortion increases the risk of bleeding in a subsequent pregnancy compared with women with previous deliveries as well as women with no previous pregnancies. Delivery following a legally induced abortion had a greater tendency of retention of placenta or placental tissue than in a woman with no previous pregnancies. A legally induced abortion complicated by pelvic inflammatory disease may reduce a woman's fertility.

5.32.5 "Abruptio placentae and placenta previa: Frequency, perinatal mortality and cigarette smoking," R.L. Naeye, *Obstet Gynecol.* 55:701-704,1980.

Abruptio placentae and placenta previa was greater in women who smoked than in those who had never smoked. Perinatal mortality showed similar differences. Placenta previa became more frequent with age and with number of years smoked. Mothers who stopped smoking had a 23% lower frequency of abruptio placentae and a 33% lower frequency of placenta previa than women who continued to smoke during pregnancy.

5.32.6 "The conservative aggressive management of placenta previa," D.B. Cotton, J.A. Read, R.I.T. Paul, E.J. Quilligan, *AmJ. Obstet.Gynecol.* 137:687,1980.

A California study of 173 cases of placenta previa during 1975-78 found that a history of prior abortion, previous placenta previa or prior cesarean section enhanced the risk of developing placenta previa. The complications associated with placenta previa included fetal malpresentation (breech or transverse lie), cord prolapse and premature rupture of the membranes.

5.32.7 "Late Sequelae of Induced Abortion: Complications and Outcome of Pregnancy and Labor," S. Harlap and M. Davies, *Am. J. Epidemiology* 102(3): 217,1975.

A prospective study of 11,057 pregnancies of West Jerusalem mothers found that 0.3% of women reporting no previous induced abortions had placenta previa compared to 0.8% of women reporting one or more induced abortions according to crude rates. Standardized rates showed no statistical significance (0.4% vs. 0.5%).

5.32.8 "Risk Factors for Abruptio Placentae," M.A. Williams et. al.. *Am. J. Epidemiology* 134: 965-972, 1991

A prior induced abortion was 1.3 times more likely to result in abruptio placente in a subsequent pregnancy compared to no prior induced abortion.

5.32.9 "The Impact of Multiple Induced Abortions on the Outcome of Subsequent Pregnancy," A. Lopes et. al., *Aust NZ Obstet. Gynaecol.* 31(1): 41,1991

In a study of Chinese women with two previous induced abortions and a subgroup of women with three or more previous induced abortions compared to age-matched primigravidas, the incidence of retained placenta was significantly higher among women with two prior induced abortions (2.9%) or three or more prior induced abortions (7.0%) compared with the control group (0.4%). Postpartum hemhorrage was also higher in women with two prior induced abortions (1.6%) or among women with three or more induced abortions (3.5%) compared with controls (0.8%).

5.33 Subsequent Miscarriage, Premature Birth or Low Birth Weight

5.33.1 "Abuse During Pregnancy: Effects on Maternal Complications and Birth Weight in Adult and Teenage Women," B. Parker et al., *Obstet. Gynecol.* 84: 323,1994

A study of poor African-American, Hispanic and white urban female residents from 1990-1993 in Baltimore, Maryland and Houston, Texas found that physical and sexual abuse during pregnancy occured among one in five teens and one in six adult women. Abused women were significantly at risk for pregnancy complications as well as drug or alcohol use.

5.33.2 "Induced Abortion as a Risk Factor for Subsequent Fetal Loss," C Infante-Rivard and R Gauthier, *Epidemiology* 7:540, 1996.

In a Canadian case-control study of fetal losses and prior reproductive history in a Montreal obstetrical care facility during 1987-91, it was found that compared to women with no previous pregnancies (1.0), women with one prior pregnancy and no induced abortions had a non-significant (1.03) increased relative risk; women with two prior pregnancies and no induced abortions had a non-significant (0.71) reduced relative risk; women with one prior pregnancy and one prior induced abortion had a non-significant (1.41) increased relative risk; and women with two prior pregnancies and two prior abortions had a statistically significant (4.43) increased relative risk of fetal loss.)

5.33.3   "Induced Abortion and Subsequent Pregnancy Duration," W Zhou et al, *Obstetrics and Gynecology* 94:948, 1999.

A Danish study using national registries found a statistically significant 1.96 increased relative risk of preterm delivery for women with pregnancy intervals exceeding 12 months with one vacuum aspiration abortion, 2.62 increased relative risk for two vacuum aspiration abortions, and 2.16 for three vacuum aspiration abortions compared to women with other pregnancy outcomes and no induced abortion history.

5.33.4   "Risk factors associated with preterm and early preterm birth, univariate and multivariate analysis of 106,345 singleton births from the 1994 statewide perinatal survey of Bavaria," JA Martius et al, *Eur J Obstet Gynecol Reprod Biol* 80(2): 183-189, 1998.

In a mulitvariate analysis, an increased risk of early preterm birth was associated with previous induced abortion (OR 1.8, 1.57-2.13 ,95% CI)

5.33.5   "A Comparison of Risk Factors for Preterm Labor and Term Small for Gestational Age Birth," JM Lang et al, *Epidemiology* 7:369, 1996.

A study at the Boston Hospital for Women controlled for the effects of 23 factors on preterm labor and fetal growth retardation. Compared to women with no previous induced abortion (1.0) , women with one induced abortion had a non-significant (1.1) increased relative risk of preterm labor; women with two previous induced abortions had a statistically significant increased relative risk of (1.9); and women with three or more induced abortions had a statistically significant increased relative risk of (3.6).

5.33.6   "Very and moderate preterm births: are the risk factors different," ? Pierre-Yves Ancel et al, *Br J Obstet Gynaecol* 106: 1162-1170, 1999.

A case-control study in 15 European countries found that a previous first trimester abortion increased the risk of very preterm births (22-32 weeks) by 86% and increased the risk of moderate preterm births (33-36 weeks) by 58%. A previous second trimester abortion increased the risk of very preterm births by 267% and increased the risk of moderate preterm births by 133% compared to controls (37 weeks or more).

5.33.7   "The epidemiology of pre-term birth," Judith Lumley, *Bailliere's Clinical Obstetrics and Gynaecology* 7(3): 477, Sept. 1993

A study of more than 300,000 first singleton births in Victoria, Australia from 1986-1990 found that 6.5 per 1000 births were 20-27 gestational weeks where the woman had one prior induced abortion compared to 10.3 per 1000 births (two prior induced abortions) and 23.1 per 1000 births (three or more prior induced abortions). The rate of pre-term births at 32-36 gestational weeks was 54.1 per 1000 births where the women had one prior induced abortion, 78.7 per 1000 births where women had two prior induced abortions and 120.1 per 1000 births where women had three or more prior induced abortions. For purposes of analysis women who had experienced both induced and spontaneous abortions were excluded.

5.33.8 "Association of Induced Abortion with Subsequent Pregnancy Loss," A. Levin, S. Schoenbaum, R. Monson, P. Stubblefield, and K. Ryan *Journal of American Medical Association* 243:2495(1980).

This study compared prior pregnancy histories of two groups of women, one having a pregnancy loss up to 28 weeks gestation and the other having a full-term delivery. Women who had two or more prior induced abortions had a twofold to threefold increase in first-trimester spontaneous abortions (miscarriage) between 14 to 20 and 20 to 27 weeks. The increased risk was present for women who had legal induced abortions since 1973. It was not explained by smoking status, history of prior spontaneous loss, prior abortion method, or degree of cervical dilation. No increased risk of pregnancy loss was detected among women with a single induced prior abortion.

5.33.9 "A Comparison of Risk Assessment Models for Term and Preterm Low Birthweight," R Michielutte et al, *Preventive Medicine* 21:98-109, 1992.

A large North Carolina study found that two or more previous induced abortions increased the risk of low birth weight in subsequent birth by 42%; one or more second trimester abortions increased the risk of low birth weight in subsequent birth weight by 78%; a previous live birth reduced the risk of low birth weight compared to no previous live birth.

5.33.10 "The association with multiple induced abortions with subsequent prematurity and spontaneous abortion," L.H. Roht, H. Aoyama, G.E. Leinen, *Acta Obstet Gynaecol, Japan* 23:140-145,1976.

Induced abortion was associated with higher prematurity and spontaneous abortion rates in later pregnancies. Women who had 2 or more abortions had a 2-3 times increased risk of miscarrying a pregnancy.

5.33.11 "Late sequelae of induced abortion in primigravidae," 0. Koller and S.N. Eikhom, *Acta Obstet. Gynecol. Scand*, 56:311 (1977).

The total rates of later abortions and infants with low birth weight below 2500 grams was higher in women with a previous induced abortion than in women whose previous pregnancy ended in a spontaneous abortion or delivery.

5.33.12 "Influence of induced abortion on gestational duration in subsequent pregnancies," J.W. Vander Slikke and P.A. Treffers, *British Medical Journal* I, 270-272 (1978).

A Dutch study compared the outcome of subsequent pregnancies of 265 women who had at least one abortion in a previous pregnancy with the outcome in an age matched group of 265 with no abortion history. 6.4% women with abortion history had deliveries prior to the 32nd week of gestation compared to only 1.2% of the women with no abortion history.

5.33.13 "Late Sequelae of Induced Abortion: Complications and Outcome of Pregnancy and Labor," S. Harlap and M. Davies, *AmJ. Epidemiology* 102(3):217 (1975).

This study found that birthweight less than 2500 grams as well as a birthweight less than 2000 grams were significantly more frequent in an obstetric history of one or more induced abortions than in a group of patients without a history of induced abortion; 6.3% v. 4.7% below 2500 grams and 2.3% v. 1.4% below 2000 grams. The differences in birthweight were found to be due to preterm delivery and not to growth retardation. It was not clear whether the induced abortions in all cases immediately preceded the current pregnancy. Most abortions in this study were thought to have been illegal.

5.33.14 "Delayed reproductive complications after induced abortion," K. Dalaker, S.M. Lictenberg, G. Okland, *Acta Obstel Gynecol Scand.* 58:491-494,1979.

A Norwegian study compared 619 women who had their last pregnancy terminated by abortion to an age and parity matched group of women who continued the pregnancy to delivery. Among those who had not been pregnant previously the complications rate was 25.5% in the abortion group compared to 13.2% in the control which was statistically significant. Complications included first and second trimester abortion (miscarriage), cervical incompetence, pre-term delivery, ectopic pregnancy and sterility. After women had one or two live births there was no statistical significance between the two groups.

5.33.15 "Second-trimester abortion after vaginal termination of pregnancy," C.S.W. Wright, S. Campbell, J. Beazley, *Lancet* 1,1278-1279 (1972).

A British study compared the outcome of the subsequent pregnancy in 91 women who had induced abortions with a control group of 3233 women in which no induced abortions had occurred. In the group with prior induced abortion 9% had second trimester abortions (miscarriage) compared to only 0.9% in the group with no induced abortions.

5.33.16 "Gestation, Birth-Weight and Spontaneous Abortion in Pregnancy After Induced Abortion," Report of the Collaborative Study by World Health Organization Task Force on Sequelae of Abortion. *The Lancet* I, 142-145, January 20,1979.

In a study of 7228 European women from 8 cities the reduction in mean birth-weight associated with cigarette smoking varied from 120-146 grams. Low birth weight in the pregnancy after induced abortion by vacuum aspiration was 5.4% to 6.1% compared with 2.9%-4.7% for prior live birth or 3.7% if no previous pregnancy. Short gestation (258 days) was 4.7%-5.7% in the pregnancy after abortion with vacuum aspiration compared to 2.0%-3.9% for prior live birth or 2.4%-3.0% for no previous pregnancy. No significant differences between groups were found with respect to mid-trimester spontaneous abortions.

5.33.17 "Low Birth Weight in Relation to Multiple Induced Abortions," M.T. Mandelson, C.B. Maden. J.R. Daling, *AmJ. Public Health* 82(3):391-394, March, 1992.

In a Washington State study of 6541 white women who delivered their first child between 1984-87, 4.4% of women with no reported abortions had low birth weight babies (2500 grams or less) compared to 5.7% of women reporting 1 abortion, 7.7% of women reporting 2 abortions, 7.1% of women reporting 3 abortions, and 9.6% of women reporting 4 or more abortions. These differences approached statistical significance.

5.33.18 "Effects of legal termination on subsequent pregnancy," J.A. Richardson and G. Dixon, *British Medical Journal* 1,1303-1304 (1976).

This study observed more first-trimester abortions (miscarriages), second trimester abortions and premature deliveries (less than 37 week amenorrhea) in a group of 211 patients whose previous pregnancy was artificially interrupted than they observed in a parity matched group of 147 women whose previous pregnancy resulted in a spontaneous abortion. Ninety-one of the 211 women became pregnant again within 1 year despite good contraceptive advice.

5.33.19 "A study on the effects of induced abortion on subsequent pregnancy outcome," C. Madore, W.E. Haws, F. Many, A.C. Hexter, *AmJ. Obstet. Gynecol* 139:516-521,1981.

A California case-control study of 2081 women who had one or more induced abortions matched with 4098 controls without a history of abortion found that a prior induced abortion had a relative risk of 1.45 (1.06-1.99, 95% C.I.) of pregnancy failure (ectopic pregnancy, spontaneous abortion, fetal or neonatal death). Smokers had a relative risk of 1.85, (1.11-3.10, 95% C.I.) of pregnancy failure.

5.33.20 "Impact of Abortion on Subsequent Fecundity," Carol J. Hogue, *Clinics in Obstetrics and Gynecology* 13(1): 95, March, 1986

Comments of the author:

Compared to women who have previously delivered the risk of low birth weight is elevated for women delivering for the first time after an induced abortion by vacuum aspiration.

Studies of first-trimester spontaneous abortion following induced abortion have been seriously flawed.

Women who choose to have their first pregnancy terminated by abortion are at no increased risk of failing to conceive at a later date unless the abortion is complicated by infection leading to pelvic inflammatory disease. Women whose first pregnancy is terminated by vacuum aspiration are at no increased risk of subsequent ectopic pregnancy unless the abortion is complicated by pre-existing C. Trachomatis or post-abortion infection.

More research is needed before it is clear whether multiple induced abortions carry an increased risk of adverse pregnancy outcomes.

5.33.21 "Risks of Preterm Delivery and Small For Gestational Age Infants Following Abortion: A Population Study," R. Pickering and J. Forbes, *British Journal of Obstetrics and Gynecology*, 92:1106-1112, Nov. 1985.

Concludes that the relative risk of preterm delivery is significantly increased following abortion. "Late Sequelae of Induced Abortion: Complications and Outcome of Pregnancy and Labor," S. Harlap and A. Davies, *American Journal of Epidemiology*, 102(3):217-224,1975. There was a significant increase in the frequency of low birth weight, compared to births in which the mother has no history of previous abortion.

5.33.22 "Pregnancy Complications Following Legally Induced Abortion," Erik Obel, *Acta Obstet. Gynecol. Scand.*, 58: 485-490(1979).

The study could not demonstrate an increased frequency of low birth weight among women whose previous pregnancy had been terminated by legal abortion, but did find that the rate of deliveries before 37 weeks gestation increased with the number of induced abortions.

5.33.23 "Prospective Study of Spontaneous Fetal Losses After Induced Abortions," S Harlap, P. Shioho, S. Ramcharan, H. Berendes, and F. Pellegrin *New England Journal of Medicine*, 301(13):677-681, September 27,1979.

The relative risk of spontaneous fetal losses after induced abortion increased with the number of previous induced abortions and was not explained by the distribution of demographic and social variables.

5.33.24 "Habitual Abortion, Causes, Prevention and Management," William D. Schlaff, *The Female Patient*, 12:45-61 March, 1987.

A number of reproductive tract infections have been suggested as possible causes of recurrent [spontaneous] abortion. Unfortunately, there seems to be no clear causative association between most of these infections and reported miscarriages. It is often difficult to differentiate the effect of an infection on the fetus from the maternal effect. Furthermore, studies examining the impact of infections on fetal wastage are frequently confounded by the presence of many other variables. Habitual abortion has been noted in approximately 15 percent of patients with intrauterine synexhiae [Asherman's syndrome]. This syndrome may be produced by intrauterine infection, puerperal dilatation and curettage or abortion.

5.33.25 *World Health Organization, Special Program of Research, Development and Research Training in Human Reproduction: Seventh Annual Report.* (Geneva: WHO, November 1978).

A repeat abortion is associated with a two- to two and a half-fold increase in the rate of low birth weight and short gestation when compared with either one abortion or one live birth. Women were matched with women who had the same operative procedure. Cases and controls were matched also for age, smoking, institution and duration of gestation at entry into the study. See "Repeat Abortions Increase Risk of Miscarriage, Premature Birth and Low Birth-weight Babies" Family Planning Perspectives 11(1): 39- 40, Jan/Feb 1979

5.34   Neonatal Infection

5.34.1   "Reproductive history and the risk of neonatal sepsis," M. Germain, M.A. Krohn, J.R. Daling, Pediatric and Perinatal Epidemiology 9: 48-58,1995.

Induced abortion was associated with a statistically significant risk of neonatal sepsis in a subsequent pregnancy. The authors suggested that the procedures involved in induced abortion might produce a latent, sub-clinical infection until the next pregnancy, and then is transmitted to the newborn. Neonatal sepsis although it occurs in 1-10 cases per 1000 live births has a case fatality rate of 50-75% and is complicated by meningitis in 20-30% of cases and surviving children frequently have neurological defects.

5.35   Intraamniotic Infection

5.35.1   "Prior pregnancy outcome and the risk of intraamniotic infection in the following pregnancy," MA Krohn et al, *Am J Obstet Gynecol* 178: 381-385, 1998.

A Washington state study of hospital records found that the risk of intraamniotic infection was 4 times higher when the prior pregnancy outcome was an elective abortion compared to a prior birth of more than 20 weeks gestation.

5.36   Subsequent Fetal Malformation/Birth Defects

5.36.1   "The Relationship Between Idiopathic Mental Retardation and Maternal Smoking During Pregnancy," C.D. Drew et. al. *Pediatrics* 97(4): 547, April, 1996.

A study by researchers at Emory University suggested that maternal smoking may be a preventable cause of mental retardation in children.

5.36.2   "A Population-Based Study of Gastroschisis: Demographic, Pregnancy, and Lifestyle Risk Factors," C P. Torfs et all.. *Teratology* 50: 44-53,1994

Urivariate analysis found a statistically significant risk of 1.96 of gastroschisis (an abdominal wall defect in newborns) where the mother had one or more elective abortions which was reduced to a 1.59 non-significant risk when adjusted for other reproductive variables.

5.36.3   "Hispanic Origin and Neural Tube Defects in Houston/Harris County. Texas, II Risk Factors."

M.A. Canfield et al. *Am. J. Epidemiology* 143(1): 12,1996

In a study of Hispanic women, any previous pregnancy termination or fetal loss was significantly associated with anencephaly in subsequent births in a final logistic regression model, 2.48,1.20-5.10, CI 95%). In contrast, with one or more live births in comparison with no previous births, there was a slight non-significant decrease in risk. The authors stated that " one of the factors for increased risk for anencephaly among Hispanic women might be elective pregnancy termination")

5.36.4   "Search for maternal factors associated with malformed human embryos: a prospective study," E. Matsunaga and K. Shiota, *Teratology* 21:323-331,1980.

3,474 malformed embryos from induced abortion were subjected to morphologic examination. 1.7% were malformed if there was no maternal genital bleeding; 4.9% were malformed with maternal genital bleeding; 15.8% were malformed if threatened abortion. Mothers of low parity showed an increased frequency of malformed embryos.

5.36.5   "Adverse effects on offspring of maternal alcohol abuse during pregnancy," Ouellette et al, *New England Journal of Medicine* 297:528-530,1977.

A 1974-75 study at Boston City Hospital found that infants born to heavy drinkers had more than twice the congenital abnormality (32%) compared to abstainers (9%) or light drinkers (14%).

5.36.6   "Late Sequelae of Induced Abortion: Complications and Outcome of Pregnancy and Labor," S. Harlap and A.M. Davies, *Am J. Epidemiology* 102(3): 217,1975.

A prospective study of 11,057 West Jerusalem mothers interviewed during pregnancy found that those who reported one or more prior induced abortions in the past were more likely to report bleeding in the 1st, 2nd. and 3rd. months of their pregnancy compared with women reporting no previously induced abortions. Women with prior abortions were less likely to have a normal delivery. In births following induced abortions, the relative risk of early neonatal death was doubled, while late neonatal deaths showed a 3 to 4 fold increase. Major and minor malformations were increased in the abortion group.

5.36.7   "Induced abortion and subsequent congenital malformations in offspring of subsequent pregnancies," M.B. Bracken, T.R. Holford, *Am.J. Epidemiology* 109(4):425-432,1979.

A Connecticut case-control study during 1974-76 found that mothers with prior induced abortions had odds ratios above 1.0 with respect to the following specific congenital malformations of subsequently born children: Inquinal Hernia (OR 1.4, P=0.24); Anencephaly (OR 1.3, P=0.62); Poly-syndactyly (OR 2.7, P=0.02;); Downs (OR 1.5, P=0.46). Overall, white women delivering babies with congenital malformations were significantly *less* likely to report having had a previously induce abortion (OR 0.7, P=0.01) while black women who delivered were significantly *more* likely to have experienced a past induced abortion (OR 1.7, P=0.04).

5.36.8   "Ectopic Pregnancy and Myoma Uteric: Teratogenic Effects and Maternal Characteristics," E.

Matsunaga and K. Shiota, *Teratology* 21:61-69,1980.

In a Japanese study of 3614 well preserved human embryos derived from artificial termination of pregnancy, the frequency of malformed embryos recovered from ectopic pregnancies was 11.6% compared to 6.2% recovered from myomatous pregnancies and 3.3% from normally implanted pregnancies not complicated by myomas. Ed. Note: myoma means a benign neoplasm of the muscular tissue.

Cancer Risk Associated With Abortion

5.37   General Studies

5.37.1   "Depressed Mood And Development of Cancer," R.W. Linkins and G.W. Comstock, *Am.J. Epidemiology* 132(5): 962,1990.

A study was undertaken by researchers at Johns Hopkins University to determine whether premorbid depressed mood is associated with the development of cancer. Scores on the Center for Epidemiologic Studies Depression Scale were available for 2264 participants in a mental health study conducted in 1971-74 in Washington County, Maryland who were still free of cancer 2-4 years later. Over a 12 year follow-up period from 1975-87,169 cancers were diagnosed among these persons. Although there was only a slight association of depressed mood with subsequent cancer among the total study population, the association was much stronger among cigarette smokers. Compared with the risk seen in never smokers without depressed mood, those with a depressed mood at the highest level of smoking (25 or more cigarettes per day) had a 4.5 relative riskfor total cancer incidence, 2.9 for sites not associated with smoking (including breast cancer) and 18.5 for cancer at sites associated with smoking.

5.37.2   "Psychological Distress After Initial Treatment of Breast Cancer, Assessment of Potential Risk Factors," E. Maunsell, J. Brission, L. Deschenes, *Cancer* 70(1): 120, July 1,1992.

A Canadian study during 1984 among women with newly diagnosed breast cancer in Quebec City Hospital found that the number of stressful life events before diagnosis appeared to be strong indicators of the risk of psychological distress. High levels of psychological distress were present on 63% of the women with a history of depression compared to only 14.3% of those with no depression history.

Breast Cancer

The American Cancer Society estimates that there will be 178,700 new invasive cases of breast cancer in women in 1998 and an estimated 43,500 women will die from breast cancer in 1998. One out of eight U.S. women will have breast cancer in their lifetime. The five year survival rate for U.S. white females is 86%. The five year survival rate for African-American females with breast cancer is 70%.

5.38 Protective Effect of "Early Childbirth"

Between 45-50% of U.S. women undergo induced abortion of their first pregnancy each year. It is well established that an early full-term childbirth has a protective effect against breast cancer in women. Breast feeding has also been demonstrated to have a modest protective effect against breast cancer. An increasing number of term births also protects against breast cancer. As the following studies indicate, all of these factors are independent protective factors against breast cancer

5.38.1 "Age at First Birth and Breast Cancer Risk," B MacMahon et al, *Bulletin of the World Health Organization* 43:209, 1970.

An international collaborative study of 250,000 women on breast cancer and reproductive experience was carried out in seven areas throughout the world. It was estimated that women having their first child under age 18 have only about one-third the breast cancer risk of those whose first birth is delayed until age 35 or more. The researchers also stated that " data suggested an increased risk associated with abortion contrary to the reduction in risk associated with full-term births."

5.38.2 "Age at Any Birth and Breast Cancer Risk," D Trichopoulos et al, *Int'l J Cancer* 31:701, 1983.

Data gathered from an international-case control study of breast cancer and age at birth found that there was a 3.5% increase of risk for every one year increase of age at first birth. Age at subsequent births had an independent and smaller effect of a 0.9% increase of risk for every year increase of age at any birth.

5.38.3 "Effect of Family History , Body-Fat Distribution, and Reproductive Factors on the Risk of Postmenopausal Breast Cancer," TA Sellers et al, *New England Journal of Medicine* 326:1323, 1992.

A 1986 survey of Iowa women found that the age-adjusted relative increased risk associated with late age at first pregnancy i.e. 30 years of age or more was 5.75(3.15-10.49, CI 95%) for women with a family history of breast cancer, and 2.04 (1.31-3.17, CI 95%) for women without such a family history.

5.38.4 "Exogenous Estrogens and Other Factors in the Epidemiology of Breast Cancer," JL Kelsey et al, *Journal of the National Cancer Institute* 67(2):327, 1981.

In a hospital-based case-control study of Connecticut women with newly diagnosed breast cancer in 1977-79, it was found that higher than average risks were found among women who had never given birth to a child, women with an early age at menarche, women who had given birth to their first child at a relatively late age, women with previous benign breast disease, and women with a history of breast cancer in a sister or mother.

5.38.5 "The Independent Associations of Parity, Age at First Full Term Pregnancy of Breast and Duration of Breast Feeding with the Risk of Breast Cancer," PM Layde et al, *J Clin Epidemiol* 42(10:963, 1989.

In a case-control study involving eight population-based cancer registries in the United States, it was found that the age at first full-term pregnancy exerted a strong influence on the risk of breast cancer. Parity and duration of breast feeding also had a strong influence on the risk of breast cancer.

5.38.6 "A Prospective Study of Reproductive Factors and Breast Cancer," I. Parity, G Kvale et al, *Am J Epidemiology* 126(5): 831, 1987.

A large prospective study of Norwegian women found a strong and highly significant inverse association between the number of full-term pregnancies and the risk of breast cancer . There were increasing protective effects among women with as high as fifteen children.

5.38.7 "A case-control study of parity, age at first full-term pregnancy, breast feeding and breast cancer in Taiwanese women," FM Lai et al, *Proc Nat'l Sci Counc Repub China* B:20(3):71, 1996.

A case-control study of Taiwanese women found that women having had more than three full-term pregnancies, were younger than age 30 at first full-term pregnancy, and breast feeding for more than 3 years, had significantly protective effects against breast cancer. The effect of the number of full-term pregnancies on the risk of breast cancer was independent of the age at first full-term pregnancy. Also, the effect of age at first full-term pregnancy and the number of full term pregnancies was also independent of the effect of breast feeding.

5.38.8 "Lactation and A Reduced Risk of Premenopausal Breast Cancer," PA Newcomb et al, *New England Journal of Medicine* 330:81, 1994.

Patients less than 75 years old identified from various statewide tumor registries were compared to controls who did not have breast cancer. It was found that premenopausal women who had lactated when compared with women who were parous but never lactated had a statistically significant reduced risk of breast cancer. However, there was no reduced risk in postmenopausal women who had lactated.

5.38.9 *Canonical Variates in Post Abortion Syndrome,* HP Vaughan, (Portsmouth NH: Institute for Pregnancy Loss, 1990)

In a study of 232 women seen at crisis pregnancy centers with self-reported post abortion syndrome an average of 11 years following their abortion, 67.5% had one or more children following their abortion, 9.6% had no children, and 22.8% had not tried to have children. Nineteen percent of the women had aborted their only pregnancy.

5.38.10 "Abortion and breast cancer risk in seven countries," K.B. Michels et. al.. *Cancer Causes and Control* 6: 75-82,1995

A study by researchers at the Harvard School of Public Health found that among parous women, those with a history of abortion exhibited a 29% increased risk if the incomplete pregnancy occurred before first birth (1.16-1.36, 95% CI) Spontaneous and induced abortions were grouped together.

5.39 Induced Abortion as an Independent Risk Factor For Breast Cancer

5.39.1 "Abortion and the Risk of Breast Cancer: A Case-Control Study in Greece," L. Lipworth et. al., *Intl J. Cancer* 61: 181-184,1995.

Using parous women with no history of abortion as the baseline, an induced abortion before a first full-term pregnancy was 2.06 times more likely to result in breast cancer compared with controls (1.45-2.90, CI 95%).

5.39.2 "Carcinoma of the breast associated with pregnancy," R.M. King et. al, *Surg. Gynecol. Obstet.* 160: 228-232,1985.

In a series of 63 pregnant patients at the Mayo Clinic, a 5-year survival of 43% was reported in the interrupted pregnancy group compared to 59% in the full-term pregnancy group. 86% of the 17 patients with Stage I disease who delivered survived.

5.39.3 "Breast Cancer and Pregnancy: the ultimate challenge," R.M. Clark, T. Chua, *Clin. Oncology* 1:11-18,1989.

Abortion during pregnancy may be deleterious to survival from breast cancer.

5.39.4 "Familial Risk of Breast Cancer and Abortion," N. Andrieu et. al.. *Cancer Detection and Prevention*, 18(1): 51-55,1994.

A French Study found that the risk of breast cancer associated with a family history of breast cancer increased with the number of abortions, induced as well as spontaneous, in a study of 495 breast cancer cases and 785 controls aged 20-56 years. For women who had undergone at least two abortions, the risk associated with a family history did not seem to depend on the type of abortion.

5.39.5 "Familial risk, abortion and their interactive effect on the risk of breast cancer-a combined analysis of six case-control studies," N. Andrieu et. al., *Br. J. Cancer* 72(3): 744-751, Sept., 1995.

Data obtained from France, Australia and Russia found that the relative risk conferred by a family history of breast cancer increased with the number of abortions (1.8 for no abortion, 1.9 for one abortion, and 2.8 for two or more. The familial risk was highest for those who had an abortion before first childbirth (1.9 for abortion after first childbirth and 2.7 for abortion before first childbirth).

5.39.6 "Breast Cancer Incidence and Mortality-United States, 1992," *MMWR* 45 (39): 833, October 4,1996.

In 1996, a total of 184,3000 new cases of and 44,300 deaths from invasive breast cancer are projected among women. In 1992, 43,063 U.S. women died from breast cancer. The death rate for white women was 26.0 per 100,000 women. The death rate for black women was 31.2 per 100,000 women.

5.39.7 "Induced abortion as an independent risk factor for breast cancer: a comprehensive review and meta-analysis," J. Brind et al, *J. Epidemiology and Community Health* 50: 481-496,1996.

A meta-analysis of 28 published reports which included specific data on induced abortion and breast cancer incidence concluded that there was an independent risk of 30-50% for breast cancer as a result of induced abortion. Slightly higher risks for breast cancer among women with multiple abortions compared to one abortion were found in 7 of 10 studies. The authors stated that " a crucial distinction in the assessment of the real magnitude of breast cancer risk attributable specifically to induced abortion, is the ability to distinguish this from the known increased risk attributable to a delay in the first full term pregnancy by any means. From the point of view of women considering abortion, parous women would be subject only to the independent effect of induced abortion, whereas nulliparous women would be subject to both the risk enhancing effects of the abortion, depending on their age at time of abortion, and if and when they subsequently have any children."The authors also stated that " induced abortion may independently increase risk via the tumor promoting effect of considerably raised estradiol (estrogen) concentrations of early pregnancy, while denying a woman the differentiating effect of the hormonal milieu of late pregnancy. This differentiating effect is presumably the mechanism by which an early completed pregnancy confers permanent protection against breast cancer. In addition, induced abortion may enhance the estrogen mediated proliferation of normal but primitive cells, resulting in the presence of more cells which are vulnerable to subsequent primary carcinogenesis."

5.39.8 "Risk of Breast Cancer Among Young Women: Relationship to Induced Abortion," J. R. Daling et. al., *J. of the National Cancer Institute* 86(21): 1584, Nov. 2,1994.

Among women who had been pregnant at least once, the overall risk of breast cancer among women who had experienced an induced abortion was 50% higher which was statistically significant. Highest risks were noted when the abortions occurred among women younger than 18 years, particularly after 8 weeks gestation, or at 30 years or older.

5.39.9 "Reproductive and lifestyle risk factors for breast cancer in African-American Women," (Abstract) A.E. Laing et al , *Genetic Epidemiology* 11: 285-310,1994.

Data on lifestyle and reproductive variables were collected on 202 African-American women with breast cancer at Howard University Hospital and Washington Hospital Center between September 1989 and December, 1993. 70% of the cases had at least one unaffected sister to serve as a control. Conditional logistic regression analysis was conducted on 138 pairs of case-sister controls. Significant increases in risk for breast cancer were found to be conferred by experiencing induced abortions (OR= 2.44, p= 0.05).

5.39.10 "Exposure, susceptibility and breast cancer risk: A hypothesis regarding exogenous carcinogens, breast tissue development, the social gradients including black/white differences in breast cancer incidence," Nancy Kreiger, *Breast Cancer Research and Treatment* 13:205,1989.

It is well known that a second major round of breast tissue growth occurs during the first trimester of a woman's first pregnancy; that full development of this tissue into secretory cells requires a full-term pregnancy, that pregnancy promotes the vascularization of breast tissue, and that a woman's breast is qualitatively transformed by her first full-term pregnancy, resulting in a much higher ratio of differentiated to undifferentiated cells--If a woman's first pregnancy resulted in a first trimester abortion, the dramatic rise in undifferentiated cells that takes place during the first trimester would not be followed by the marked differentiation occurring during the second and third trimesters. The consequent sharp rise in the number of vulnerable cells would thus elevate the breast cancer risk.

5.39.11 "Her-2/neu and INT2 Proto-oncognene Amplification in Malignant Breast Tumors in Relation to Reproductive Factors and Exposure to Exogenous Hormones," H. Olsson, A. Borg, M. Ferno, J. Ranstam, H. Sigurdsson, *J. National Cancer Inst.* 83(20):1483, Oct. 16,1991.

In a study of genetic markers in premenopausal breast tumors, it was found that tumors from patients with any abortions before a first full-term pregnancy were 26 times more likely to show amplification for the INT2 gene which was an indication of faster tumor growth and lower survival.

5.39.12 "Breast Cancer and Pregnancy: The Ultimate Challenge," R.M. Clark, T. Chua, *Clin Oncology A Journal Of The Royal College of Radiologists,* 1:11-18 (1989).

In a Canadian study of 154 pregnant women with breast cancer, 20% of the 116 patients who carried their children to term were ultimately cured of their cancer, 40% of the 13 patients who spontaneously aborted were cured, but none of the 21 patients who had a "therapeutic" abortion survived. It was concluded that a "therapeutic" abortion did not confer any benefit and may reduce survival.

5.39.13 "Proliferation and DNA Ploidy in Malignant Breast Tumors in Relation to Early Oral Contraceptive Use and Early Abortions," H. Olsson, J. Ranstam, B. Baldetorp, S. Ewers, M. Ferno, D. Killander and H. Sigurdsson, *Cancer* 67:1285-1290(1991).

In a Swedish study at University Hospital, Lund, tumor tissue was analyzed indicating a higher rate of tumor cell proliferation for 175 premenopausal breast cancer patients. A history of early abortions was associated with a 49% higher S-phase fraction. A higher percentage of DNA aneuploid tumors was seen for patients with an early induced or spontaneous abortion (68% vs. 54%). Abortions (spontaneous or induced) before the first full-term pregnancy also were associated with a higher SPF compared with other young patients (under 20 years of age) with

211

breast cancer (P=0.03).

5.39.14 "Rising Incidence of Breast Cancer Among Young Women in Washington," State/ E. White/ J.R. Daling, T.L. Norsted and J. Chu, *Journal of the National Cancer Institute* 79(2): 293-243, August 1987.

A study of 1/869 cases of breast cancer in Washington state women (ages 25-) found that the incidence of breast cancer increased 22% between 1974-77 and 1982-84. The estimated annual increase was 2.5%. The risk for black women doubled based on small numbers. Conclusion: One reason for the increase may be the dramatic exposure to induced abortion... Black women have a higher abortion rate than white women.

5.39.15 "Breast Cancer Risk Factors in African-American Women: The Howard University Tumor Registry Experience," A.E. Laing, F.M. Demenais/ R. Williams, V.W. Chen, G.E. Bonney, *J. National Medical Association* 85(12): 931-939, Dec. 1993.

In a Howard University case control study of African-American women seen at their hospital from 1978-1987, the multiple logistic estimates of the odds ratio for breast cancer among women under 40 years of age, between 41-49 years and over 50 years was 1.5, 2.8, and 4.7 respectively among women with a history of induced abortions compared to women with no history of induced abortions.

5.39.16 "The epidemiology of breast cancer as it relates to menarche, pregnancy, and menopause," M.C. Pike, B.E. Henderson and J.T. Casagrande in *Hormones and Breast Cancer.* M.C. Pike, P.K. Siiteri and C.W. Welsch, eds. (Cold Harbor N.Y.: Cold Harbor Pub. Co., 1981)

A means is proposed to explain the international variance in breast cancer. Early Menarche and the length of menstrual life prior to first pregnancy are particularly important risk factors. Three intervals of time are defined: menarche to first full-term pregnancy; first full-term pregnancy to menopause; and menopause to current age. The incidence of a given cancer at a particular time is a function of time. An equation was developed which can account for approximately 85% of the international variation in breast cancer. (Quoted from *Diagnosis and Management of Breast Cancer,* Marc E. Lippman, Alien Lichter and David Danforth (Philadelphia: W.B. Saunders Co., 1988)

5.39.17 "Age at First Birth and Breast Cancer Risk," B. MacMahon, P. Cole, T.M. Lin, C. Lowe, A. Mirra, B. Ravnihar, E. Salber, V. Valaoras and S. Yuasa, *Bulletin of the World Health Organization* 43: 209-221(1970).

An international collaborative study of breast cancer and reproductive experience was carried out in seven areas of the world. It was estimated that women having their first child under age 18 have only about one-third the breast cancer risk of those whose first birth is delayed until the age 35 or more.) (Data suggested an increased risk associated with abortion contrary to the reduction in risk associated with full-term births.)

5.39.18 "Susceptibility of the mammary gland to carcinogenesis II. Pregnancy interruption as a risk factor for tumor incidence," J. Russo and I.H. Russo, *American Journal of Pathology* 100: 497 (1980)

Researchers studied pregnancy interruption as a risk factor in mammary tumor incidence in rats and found that pregnancy and lactation prior to chemically induced carcinogen administration protected the mammary gland from developing carcinomas and benign lesions. However, once pregnancy had been interrupted the protective effect was eliminated and animals were at the same risk as virgin animals treated with the carcinogen.

5.39.19 "Early Abortion and Breast Cancer Risk among Women under Age 40," H.L Howe, R.T. Senie, H. Bzduch and P. Herzfeld, *International J. of Epidemiology* 18(2):300-304 (1989).

Some 1/451 women with breast cancer were matched with population controls by year of birth and by residence using zip codes in upstate New York Those with a history of induced abortion as determined by fetal death records had a 1.9 odds ratio compared with controls.

5.39.20 "Oral Contraceptive Use and Early Abortion as Risk Factors for Breast cancer in Young Women," M.C. Pike, B.E. Henderson, J.T. Casagrande, I. Rosario and G. Gray, *British Journal of Cancer* 43: 72 (1981).

In a study of 163 white women less than 33 years of age in the Los Angeles area, a first-trimester abortion before a first full-term pregnancy was associated with a 2.4-fold increase in risk of breast cancer.

5.39.21 "Occurrence of Breast Cancer in Relation to Diet and Reproductive History: A Case-Control Study in Fukuoka, Japan," T. Hirohata, T. Shigematsu, A.M.Y. Nomura, *National Cancer Institute Monograph* 69:187,1985.

Two hundred and twelve female breast cancer patients among populations having low risk, intermediate risk and high risk were matched by sex and within 5 years of the same age with a hospital control of women who had no cancer and no benign breast disease as well as a neighborhood control randomly chosen from electoral listings. Among cases as compared to controls, a history of induced abortion had a 1.19 relative risk, which increased to 1.52 after adjustment by multiple logistic regression. Natural or spontaneous abortion had a 1.53 unadjusted relative risk ,which increased to 1.91 once adjusted by multiple logistic regression.

5.39.22 "Breast Cancer in Premenopausal and Postmenopausal Women," K. Stavraky and S. Emmons, *Journal National Cancer Institute* 53(3):647, Sept., 1974.

In a case-control study of premenopausal and postmenopausal women with breast cancer admitted to the Ontario Cancer Foundation, London, Canada during 1967-71 were compared to women admitted to the same clinic during the same period with benign and malignant sites other than breast. Compared with control patients, postmenopausal breast cancer patients had an excess of women who had at least one abortion (37% v. 27%).

5.39.23 "Risk of breast cancer in relation to reproductive factors in Denmark," M Ewertz and S.W. Duffy, *British J. Cancer* 58:99,1988.

All Danish women less than 70 years of age diagnosed with breast cancer in 1983-84 identified from the files of the Danish Breast Cancer Cooperative and the Danish Cancer registry , were compared with an age stratified sample of women drawn from the general population. Women whose first pregnancy was terminated by spontaneous or induced abortion before 28 weeks gestation had a 1.43 relative risk (1.10-1.84, 95% C.I.) of breast cancer compared to women whose first pregnancy was carried to term. Never pregnant women had a 1.47 relative risk (1.14-1.90, 95% C.I.) compared to women whose first pregnancy was carried to term.

Based upon small numbers, women with no full term pregnancies and one induced abortion had a 3.86 relative risk (1.08-13.6, 95% C.I.) for breast cancer compared with nulliparous women who had no abortion history. Again, based upon small numbers women who had no full term pregnancies and one first trimester spontaneous abortion had a 2.63 relative risk (0.83-8.32, 95% C.I.) compared to nulliparous women who had no abortion history. It was concluded that pregnancies have to be carried to term to offer the protective effect against breast cancer.

5.40 Cervical Cancer

Human papillomavirus infection (HPV) has been identified as the cause of cervical cancer. A contributing factor for cervical cancer is smoking. It is known that postabortion women will smoke more cigarettes than women with other reproductive outcomes. Thus, induced abortion may have an indirect role in the development of cervical cancer.

5.40.1 "Induced Abortion in Taiwan," P.D. Dong, R.S. Lin, *J. Royal Soc. Health* 100-108, April, 1995

In a study of 17,047 women in Taipei, Taiwan who attended family planning services centers in 1991-1992 55% of the women had a normal Pap smear, 44% had an atypical finding and only 0.9% had dysplasia. A significantly positive trend was found between those women having had increasing numbers of induced abortions and the incidence of cervical dysplasia (P<0.01)

5.40.2 "Papillomavirus Infection Among Abortion Applicants and Patients at a Sexually Transmitted Disease Clinic," P.A. Csango et. al.. *Sexually Transmitted Diseases* 19(3): 149, May/June 1992.

A Norwegian study found that 6.1% of induced abortion applicants had human papillomavirus (HPV) infection. The proportion of high-risk HPV was 89.7%. HPV appears to be a risk factor for cervical cancer.

5.40.3 "Induced abortion as cancer risk factor: a review of epidemiological evidence," Larissa I. Remennick, *J. Epidemiol Community Health* 44(4): 259-264, Dec. 1990.

This article reviewed several studies on women in the Soviet Union and surrounding areas. It was reported that the majority of cervical cancers in Armenia were registered in three cities where induced abortion rates have been high. Where induced abortion rates have been lower in other regions, cervical cancer incidence has also been lower. Similarly, induced abortion and cervical cancer is high in migrant women, while cervical cancer and induced abortion is low in indigenous women. The author suggested that mechanisms of induced abortion influence on cervical carcinogenessis may be multiple. The first mode of action may be via general endocrine stress in the reproductive system resulting from termination of pregnancy related processes. Another is through mechanical trauma and possible infection associated with the dilation and curettage or incomplete evacuation of the embryo and placenta. Chronic inflammatory lesions may arise in cervical tissue on the site of this trauma, as well as cell abnormalities. In the course of time, the latter may undergo malignant transformation and/or facilitate the action of exogenous carcinogenic agents.

5.40.4   "Human Papillomaviris Infection and Other Risk Factors For Cervical Neoplasia: A Case-Control Study," E.A. Morrison, G. Ho, S.H. Vermund, G.L. Goldberg, A.S. Kadish, *Int'l Journal of Cancer* 49:6-13,1991.

A case-control study of inner city women in a Bronx, New York hospital during 1986-88 found that infection with human papillomaviris (HPV) was the major risk factor for cervical squamous intraepithelial lesions.

5.40.5   "Cigarette Smoking and Dysphasia and Carcinoma In Situ of the Uterine Cervix," E. Trevathan, P. Layde, L.A. Webster, J.B. Adams, *J. American Medical Association* 250(4): 499, July 22-29,1983.

A case-control study among black women in Atlanta, Georgia aged 17-55 from 1980-81 compared women attending a dysphasia clinic with those attending a family planning clinic at the same hospital who had at least two normal pap smears. Cigarette smoking was significantly associated with carcinoma in situ, severe dysphasia, and mild-moderate dysphasia (relative risks, 3.6, 3.3 and 2.4 respectively). Cumulative exposure to cigarette smoking, as measured by pack-years smoked was strongly related to the risk of these conditions. Women with 12 or more pack-years of exposure had relative risks of 12.7,10.2 and 4.3 respectively, for the three conditions. Ed. Note: Women with induced abortions are known to have higher smoking rates than women with other pregnancy outcomes.

5.40.6   "Editorial Commentary: Smoking and Cervical Cancer-Current Status," L.A. Brinton, *Am. J. Epidemiology* 131(6): 958,1990.

Smoking may act as a late stage carcinogen. Given the well- recognized continuum of disease from dysplasia to carcinoma in situ to invasive cancer. Further investigations are needed to address the effects of smoking on the natural history of cervical neoplasia.

5.40.7   "Effect of Cigarette Smoking on Cervical Epithelial Immunity: A mechanism for Neoplastic Change?," S.E. Barton, D. Jenkins, J. Cuzick, *The Lancet*, September 17,1988, p. 652-654.

Cigarette smoking was associated with a significant and dose-dependent decrease in the concentration of Langerhans' cells, the most prominent type of antigen-presenting cell in normal cervical epithelium. This reduction in the number Langerhans' cells available to detect and present viral antigens to T lymphocytes may facilitate the establishment and persistence of local viral infection. This could increase the likelihood of a virally induced neoplastic transformation, as has been proposed for HPV. These findings of a local immunological effect of smoking on cervical epithelium may explain the means by which cigarette smoking contribute to the development of cervical neoplasia. Citing "The wart virus and genital neoplasia: a casual or causal association." A. Singer, D.J. McCance, *Br.J. Obstet. Gynaecol.* 92:1083,1986.

5.40.8   "HPV co-factors related to the development of cervical cancer: results from a population-based study in Costa Rica," A Hildesheim et al, *Br J Cancer* 84(9):1219-1216, May, 2001.

Women who smoked 6 or more cigarettes per day had a 2.7 increase in relative risk for human papillomaviris or cervical cancer compared to non-smokers.

5.40.9   "Smoking, diet, pregnancy and oral contraceptive use as risk factors for cervical intra-epithelial neoplasia in relation to human papillomavirus infection," L Kjellberg et al, *Br J. Cancer* 82(7):1332-1338, April, 2000.

After taking HPV into account, smoking appeared to be the most significant environmental factor for cervical neoplasia.

5.40.10 "Reproductive patterns and cancer incidence in women: a population-based correlation study in the USSR," L.I Remennick, *Int'l. J. Epidemiology* 18: 498, 1989.

A correlation study in the USSR based on official abortion statistics and regional cancer incidence data for the period 1959-1985 showed a significant contribution of induced abortion to the variance of cervical cancer. The correlation between cervical cancer age adjusted incidence rates for women in 70 areas of Russia was 0.77 according to parametric tests and also 0.77 according to Spearman non-parametric rank criteria.

5.40.11 "Oral Contraceptive Use and Breast or Cervical Cancer: Preliminary Results of A French Case-Control Study," M.G. Le, A Bachelot, F. Doyon, A. Kramar, C. Hill in *Hormones and Sexual Factors in Human Cancer Aetiology*, Eds. J.P. Wolff, J.S. Scott, (New York: Excerpta Medica, 1984) 139-147.

A French case-control study during 1982-84 in 8 hospital centers in France of women age 45 or less with histologically verified cervical cancer compared cases with two control subjects with respect to the hospital center, date of interview (within 4 months) and age (within 2 years). Eighty-four cases of cervical cancer were compared with 83 control subjects with nonmaligant diseases and 43 control subjects with nongynecological cancer using logistic miltifactoral regression methods. The relative risk for women with cervical cancer and one abortion was 2.3 (P-value 0.001) compared to women with no abortion. The relative risk for cervical cancer for women with 2 or more abortions compared to women with no abortion was 4.92 (P-value 0.001). The study did not state whether the abortions were spontaneous or induced.

5.40.12 "Oral Contraceptives and Cervical Carcinoma in Situ in Chile," R. Molina, D.B. Thomas, A. Dabancens, *Cancer Research* 48:1011-1015, Feb. 15,1988.

A case-control study of cervical carcinoma in situ was conducted by a standard questionnaire among 133 women aged 15-50 years between 1979-85 in Santiego, Chile. The 254 controls were 2 women in the same 5 year age group as the corresponding case and who also had a normal Pap smear closest in time to the abnormal smear that led to the carcinoma in situ diagnosis. Several sexual variables were associated with an increased risk of carcinoma in situ. These included history of prior miscarriages, any prior aborted pregnancy, including spontaneous and induced abortions, total number of pregnancies, number of sexual partners and age at first sexual intercourse, The relative risk for carcinoma in situ for women with a history of any abortion (spontaneous or induced) compared to women with no abortion history was 1.85 (1.20-2.86, 95% C.I.). The relative risk for carcinoma in situ for a woman with an induced abortion was 1.38 (0.84-2.27, 95% C.I.) compared to women with no induced abortion history.

5.40.13 "Risk factors for adenocarcinoma of the cervix: A case-control study," F. Parazzini, C. LaVecchia, E. Negri, M. Fasoli, G. Cecchetti, *Br. J. Cancer* 57:201,1988.

A case-control study of 39 cases of cervical adenocarcinoma were compared to 409 controls admitted to area hospitals in the Milan, Italy area during 1981-86 for surgical or other traumatic injury. The median age for both cases and controls was 53 years. A history of one or more induced abortions has a relative risk of 2.5 (1.2-5.3, 95% C.I.) for cervical adenocarcinoma compared to women with no induced abortion history using Mantel-Haenszel estimates adjusted for age and age at first birth and parity. The Mantel-Haenszel estimates of relative risk adjusted for age at first intercourse were 3.7 (1.6-8.2, 95% C.I.) for a woman with a history of one or more induced abortions compared to a woman with no history of induced abortion.

5.40.14 "Reproductive factors and the risk of invasive and intraepithelial cervical neoplasia," F. Parazzini, C. LaVecchia, E. Negri, G. Ceccheti, L. Fedele, *Br. J. Cancer* 59:805-809, 1989.

A case-control study by researchers in Milan Italy of 528 cases of invasive cancer was compared with 456 control subjects hospitalized for acute conditions unrelated to any of the established or suspected risk factors for cervical cancer. Relative risks for invasive cervical cancer for women with one induced abortion compared to women with no induced abortion history were 1.89,1.60 and 1.69 based upon Mantel-Haenszel (M-H) estimates adjusted for age, M-H estimates adjusted for age and age at first intercourse, respectively. For women with a history of two or more induced abortions compared with women with no induced abortion history the M-H estimates of risk were 2.38, 2.41 and 1.44 based upon the same adjustments in the same order as above.

When relative risks for induced abortion were subjected to multiple logistic regression equations including adjustments for age, marital status education, age at first intercourse, number of sexual partners, history of Pap smears, smoking habits, oral contraceptive use number of live births, and age at first birth, the relative risk computed by multiple logistic regression ranged from 1.26-1.39 for women with one or more induced abortions compared to women reporting no induced abortion with no significant trend shown with increasing number of induced abortions.

5.40.15 "Epidemiological Study of Carcinoma in Situ of the Cervix," I. Fujimoto, H. Nemoto, K. Kuduka, *The Journal of Reproductive Medicine* 30(7): 535, July 1985.

During 1950-79, 1248 women with carcinoma in situ of the cervix were treated in the Department of Gynecology at the Cancer Institute Hospital in Tokyo, Japan. Cases were compared with noncancer controls admitted to the outpatient clinic of the same hospital at the same time. 69.4% of the cases vs. 55.9% of the controls reported an abortion ,which was statistically significant. The rate of repeated abortions was higher in the cases than the controls with seven the highest number among the cases.

5.40.16 "Characteristics of Women with Dysplasia or Carcinoma in Situ of the Cervix Uteri," R.W.C. Harris, L.A. Brinton, R.H. Cowdel, D. Skegg, *Br. J. Cancer* 42:359, 1980.

A British case-control study compared women with abnormal cervical smears with a control group. Women were classified as having severe dysplasia, mild dysplasia, carcinoma in situ or normal histology. Women with mild dysplasia, severe dysplasia and carcinoma in situ were more likely to report having had a pregnancy terminated but it was statistically significant for mild dysplasia only. (22.7% v. 6.2%) Relative risk 2.76 (1.1-6.8, 95% C.I.)

5.40.17 "Marital and Coital Factors in Cervical Cancer," C.E. Martin, *Am. J. Public Health* 57(5): 803, May, 1967.

A retrospective study of 40 Jewish women in the New York City area during 1960-63 and diagnosed as having invasive or in situ squamous cell carcinoma were compared to 36 Jewish women with a recent hysterectomy and known to be free from uterine cancer. 42.5% of cases vs. 16.7% of controls reported an induced abortion which was statistically significant. Other significant factors for cervical cancer included two or more coital partners, first coitus before age 20, extramarital affairs, coitus with a non-Jew.

5.40.18 "Epidemiology of Cancers of the Uterine Cervix and Corpus, Breast and Ovary in Israel and New York City," H.L. Stewart, L.J. Dunham, J. Casper, *J. of the National Cancer Institute* 37(1); 1-96,1966.

In a case-control study of New York City and Israeli women, the age at first intercourse and age at termination of pregnancy were found to be strongly related to each other. The median ages of termination of first and last pregnancy were consistently lower for patients with cancer of the cervix than for control patients in each ethnic group, p.35.)

5.40.19 *Aborted Women: Silent No More*, David C. Reardon, (Chicago: Loyola Press, 1987).

This work includes personal testimonies from two women describing cervical cancer following induced abortion. In the sample of 252 women surveyed approximately 10 years following their abortion, 4% reported cervical cancer which they attributed to their induced abortion.

5.40.20 "Epidemiologic Study of Carcinoma in Situ of the Cervix," I. Fujimoto, H. Nemoto, K. Fuduka, S. Masubuchi, *J. of Reproductive Medicine* 30(7): 535, July 1985.

In a study of 1,248 cases of carcinoma in situ of the cervix in Tokyo, the women in the cancer group had a significantly greater number of abortions than the control group. It was concluded that the cervical repair process after abortion seems to be too important to disregard as a factor in the development of carcinoma in situ.

5.40.21 "Pap Screening for Teenagers: A life-saving Precaution," Mark Spitzer and Burton A. Krumholz, *Contemporary OB/GYN* 31(1):3341, January 1988;

Dysplasia of the cervix is increasing among adolescents. Sexually active teenagers, especially those who become pregnant, are at high risk for developing cervical dysplasia and, ultimately, cervical cancer.

5.40.22 "Abnormal Cervical Cytology in Sexually Active Adolescents," Joseph F. Russo and Damell Jones, *Journal of Adolescent Health Care* 5: 269-271(1984).

Pap smears on 1,207 sexually active adolescents in a public health department of eastern North Carolina turned up 11% with abnormal findings. Seventy-two percent of those women evaluated by colposcopy with directed biopsies had cervical intraepithelial neoplasia.

5.41 Ovarian Cancer

5.41.1 "Incomplete Pregnancies and Ovarian Cancer Risk," E. Negri et. al., *Gynecologic Oncology* 47: 234-238,1992.

An Italian case-control study found an inverse relationship between the total number of incomplete pregnancies and ovarian cancer risk which was 0.7 for one voluntary abortion and 0.8 for two or more voluntary abortions.

5.41.2 "Determinants of Ovarian Cancer Risk I. Reproductive Experiences and Family," History, D. Cramer, G. Hutchinson, W. Welch, R. Scully and K. Ryan, *Journal of the National Cancer Institute* 71(4): 711-716, October 1983.

In a study of 215 white females in the greater Boston area during 1978-81, pregnancy exerted a strong protective effect against ovarian cancer, which increased with the number of live-born children.

5.41.3 "An Epidemiologic Study of the Relationship of Reproductive Experience to Cancer of the Ovary," D.J. Joly, A. Lillenfeld, E. Diamond and I. Bross, *American Journal of Epidemiology* 99(3): 190-209 (1974).

Ovarian cancer cases had a larger proportion of women who had never been pregnant or had no more than two pregnancies, as compared with controls. The relative risk of ovarian cancer increases as the number of pregnancies decreases.

5.41.4   "The Woman at Risk for Developing Ovarian Cancer," L. McGowan, L. Parent, W. Lednar and H. Morris, *Gynecologic Oncology* 7: 325-344 (1979).

In a case-control study of women in the Washington D.C. area during 1974-77, nulligravidas were 2.45 times more likely to develop malignant ovarian tumors and 2.9 times more likely to develop carcinomas of low malignant potential than women who were pregnant three or more times. The risk of ovarian cancer was greatly reduced among women who had at least one pregnancy. Women with ovarian cancer did not have more spontaneous abortions, still births or defective children than their controls.

5.41.5   ""Incessant Ovulation" and Ovarian Cancer," J.T. Casgrande, M.C. Pike, R.K. Ross, E.W. Louie, S. Royard and B.E. Henderson, *The Lancet*, July 28,1979, pp. 170-173

The risk of ovarian cancer is clearly decreased directly by factors that suppress ovulation.

5.41.6   "Events of Reproductive Life and the Incidence of Epithelial Ovarian Cancer," H. Risch, N. Weiss, J.L. Lyon, J. Daling and J. Liff, *American Journal of Epidemiology* 117(2): 128-139 (1983).

Women with ovarian cancer reported fewer full-term pregnancies, fewer miscarriages and less total time breastfeeding than controls.

5.41.7   "Does Pregnancy Protect Against Ovarian Cancer?," V. Beral, P. Fraser and C. Chilvers, *The Lancet*, May 20,1978, pp. 1083-1087.

A study by English epidemiologists found that there was a clear inverse relationship between completed family size and the death of women from ovarian cancer among women in England and Wales. They reported that, " the findings suggest that pregnancy- or some component of the childbearing process-protects directly against ovarian cancer. This protection seems to persist throughout life." The authors of the study stated that, "ovarian cancer is rare in populations that do not practice birth control. How pregnancy protects against ovarian cancer is unclear. If suppression of ovulation is the key factor, then breast-feeding, which suppresses ovulation, should reduce the risk of ovarian cancer. A pregnancy of short gestation, i.e., one that ended as an abortion, should confer less protection against ovarian cancer than a full-term pregnancy."

5.41.8   "Risk factors for ovarian cancer-a case control study," M Booth et al, Br J Cancer 60:592, 1989 (During 1978-1983, a hospital-based study of 235 British women with histologically diagnosed epithelial ovarian cancer was compared to 451 women hospitalized for other reasons. Childbirth was found to be more protective against epithelial ovarian cancer than incomplete pregnancies.)

5.41.9   "Incomplete pregnancies and risk of ovarian cancer, Washington, United States," M-T Chen et al, *Cancer Causes and Control* 7:415, 1996.

In a study of 322 white female residents aged 20-79 diagnosed with invasive or borderline ovarian cancer in three counties in Washington state in 1986-88, compared to 426 women randomly selected from the same counties, the number of births increasingly reduced the risk of ovarian cancer compared to no births. When the analysis was restricted to ever- pregnant women, a prior induced or spontaneous abortion (evaluated separately) was found not to be associated with the incidence of ovarian tumors, and was decreased only slightly in nulliparous women. It was concluded that, " it is possible that if incomplete pregnancies do affect the risk of ovarian cancer, their impact might be too small to be identified through epidemiologic studies."

5.41.10 "Epithelial Ovarian Cancer and the Ability to Conceive," A.S. Whittemore, M.L. Wu, R. S. Paffenbarger, Jr., D.L Sarles, J.B. Kampert, *Cancer Research* 49: 4047, July 15,1989.

In a case-control study of women in the San Francisco Bay area during 1983-85, ovarian cancer patients were more likely to be nulliparous (20.7%) compared to hospital controls (17.1%) or general population controls (10.0%). Ovarian cancer patients also had fewer number of term pregnancies (2.2) compared to hospital or general population controls (2.5) and had the same number of abortions (0.6) compared to controls.

5.41.11 "Personal and Environmental Characteristics Related to Elithelial Ovarian Cancer. I Reproductive and Menstrual Events and Oral Contraceptive Use," M.L. Wu, A.S. Whittemore, R.S. Paffenbarger, Jr., D.L. Sarles, *Am. J. Epidemiology* 128(6):1216,1988.

In two case-control studies in the San Francisco Bay area during 1974-77 and 1983-85, women having epithelial ovarian cancer had a similar number of reported abortions as controls. It was not specified whether the abortions were spontaneous or induced. Cases were more likely than controls to have been nulliparous.

5.41.12 "Reproductive. Genetic and Dietary Risk Factors for Ovarian Cancer," M. Mori, I. Harabuchi, H. Miyake, J. T. Cassagrande, B.E. Henderson, *Am.J. Epidemiology* 128(4): 771,1988.

A case-control study in Hokkaido, Japan during 1980-86 found that ovarian cancer risk was increased in single women, and in women with a family history of breast, uterine or ovarian cancer in a mother or sister. The risk was decreased in women who had experienced a live birth (OR 0.2, 0.1-0.6, 95% C.I.), an induced abortion (OR 0.5, 0.3-0.9, 95% C.I.), or in women who had permanent sterilization by tubal ligation (OR 0.4, 0.1-0.8, 95% C.I). Each of the reproductive factors remained significant when adjusted for each other using logistic regression analysis. The odds ratio for ovarian cancer decreased significantly with increasing number of live births. Compared with nulliparous subjects, women with 1 or 2 children had a third of the risk of ovarian cancer, women with 3-4 children had one-fourth the risk, and women with 5 or more children had 1/20th the risk.

5.41.13 "Case-Control Study of Borderline Ovarian Tumors: Reproductive History and Exposure to Exogenous Female Hormones," B.L. Harlow, N.S. Weiss, G.L. Roth, J. Chu, J.R. Daling, *Cancer Research* 48: 5849, October 15,1988.

In a case-control study of women in three urban counties in Washington State during 1980-85, the risk of ovarian tumors among women who had given birth to 1 or 2 children and to 3 or more children was 0.7 and 0.4 respectively compared to that of nulliparous women. After adjusting for parity, a history of lactation reduced risk of ovarian cancer by 50%. After adjusting for age and gravidity (from 1 to 4), a similar number of cases and controls reported an induced abortion although it was not statistically significant. More cases than controls reported a history of a prior miscarriage.

5.41.14   "Parity, age at first childbirth, and risk of ovarian cancer," H-O Adami et al, *The Lancet* 344, November 5, 1994 p.1250-1254.

A case-control study of Swedish women born between 1925 and 1960 diagnosed 3486 cases of invasive ovarian cancers including 2992 epithelial, 300 stromal, 149 germ-cell, and 15 not classifiable plus 510 tumors of borderline malignant potential up until 1984. After simultaneous adjustment for parity and age at first birth, increasing parity was associated with a pronounced consistent decrease in relative risk of all invasive cancers, but a less consistent decrease for borderline tumors.

5.41.15   "Reproductive and Other Factors and Risk of Epithelial Ovarian Cancer: An Australian Case-Control Study," D Purdie et al, *Int'l Journal of Cancer* 62:678, 1995.

824 cases of women diagnosed with epithelial ovarian cancer in Queensland, New South Wales and Victoria, Australia between 1990-1993 were compared to 860 controls drawn at random from the electoral roll and stratified by age and geographic region. A reduced risk of ovarian cancer was found to be associated with increasing parity, but there were no associations between the development of ovarian cancer and the number of incomplete pregnancies.)

5.42   Endometrial Cancer

5.42.1   "Epidemiology and Primary Prevention of Cancers of the Breast, Endometrium, and Ovary," JL Kelsey and AS Whittemore, *Ann Epidemiol* 4:89-95, 1994.

Most of the risk factors indemnified for endometrial cancer involve exposure to estrogen with insufficient cyclic exposure to progesterone, and this explanation is generally accepted as a major etiologic pathway for the development of endometrial cancer.

5.42.2   "Is the Risk of Cancer of the Corpus Uteri Reduced by a Recent Pregnancy? A Prospective Study of 765,756 Norwegian women," G Albrektsen et al, *Int'l J Cancer* 61:485, 1995.

A study of 765,756 Norwegian women representing 9,307,118 person years in the age interval of 30-56 years was undertaken using various registries. Compared to women with one full term pregnancy, nulliparous women had an increased risk of endometrial carcinoma. There was a reduced risk of endometrial carcinoma with an increasing number of full term pregnancies. The risk of endometrial carcinoma increased with increasing time since last birth. The reduction in risk among parous women compared to nulliparous women diminished with increasing time since last birth. The researchers concluded that, " our results support the hypothesis that the reduction in risk of endometrial carcinoma associated with a pregnancy is related to a mechanical shed of malignant or pre-malignant cells at each delivery."

5.42.3　"A Case-Control Study of Endometrial Cancer in Relation to Reproductive, Somatometric, and Life-Style Variables," A Kalandidi et al, *Oncology* 53:354, 1996.

A hospital-based case control study of cancer of the endometrium was conducted in Athens, Greece from 1992-94 by researchers at the University of Athens Medical School and the Harvard School of Public Health. It was found that the risk of endometrial cancer decreased with the number of live births but did not decrease with one miscarriage or one induced abortion.

5.42.4　"Reproductive, menstrual, and medical risk factors for endometrial cancer: Results from a case-control study," LA Brinton et al, *Am J Obstet Gynecol* 167:1317, 1992.

During 1987-90, a study was undertaken of 405 cases of newly diagnosed cancer of the uterine corpus in women between the ages of 20-74 years which were obtained from seven hospitals throughout the United States. Populations controls were matched for age, race, and location of residence obtained by random dialing techniques. The mean age of the cases at interview was 59.2 years compared to 58.0 for controls. Compared to women with no term births, the relative risk of endometrial cancer was significantly reduced with an increasing number of live births. The risk of endometrial cancer was the same for women reporting a prior induced abortion compared to women reporting not ever having an induced abortion. Women having one or two or more miscarriages had virtually the same risk as women reporting no miscarriages. It was concluded that the protective effect was limited to term births.

5.42.5　"Risk Factors for Endometrial Cancer," B. MacMahon, *Gynecol. Oncol.* 2: 122, 1974.

A case-control study of Boston area women found that nulliparity produces a twofold risk for endometrial cancer compared to women with one child, and a threefold risk compared to women with five children.

5.42.6　"The epidemiology of endometrial cancer in young women," B.E. Henderson, M.C. Pike, T. Mack, I. Rosario, *Br. J. Cancer* 47: 749,1983.

A case-control study of women age 45 years or less at diagnosis in Los Angeles County during 1972-79 found that increasing parity was strongly assodated with decreased risk for endometrial cancer. RR was 0.12 for women with three children compared to nulliparous women. Incomplete pregnancies (spontaneous and induced abortions) were associated with a slight decrease in risk (data not shown). 5.6 incomplete pregnancies were estimated to be equivalent to one full term pregnancy in terms of risk reduction but the decrease was not statistically significant.

5.42.7　"Reproductive Factors and Risk of Cancer of the Uterine Corpus: A Prospective Study," G. Kvale, I. Heuch, G. Ursin, *Cancer Research* 48: 6217,1988.

A prospective study of 62,079 Norwegian women diagnosed 420 cases of cancer of the uterine corpus from 1961-80. The risk of endometrial cancer decreased significantly with increasing parity. In parous women the odds ratio for those with 3 or more abortions vs. women not reporting abortion was 1.03 (0.58-1.82, 95% CI) after adjustment for parity, age at first birth in addition to demographic variables (unspecified).

5.42.8 "A Case-Control Study of Cancer of the Endometrium," J.L. Kelsey, V.A. LiVoIsi, T.R. Holford, D.B. Fischer, *Am. J. Epidemiology* 116(2): 1982.

A study of the epidemiology of endometrial cancer in women aged 47-74 in Connecticut from 1977-79, found that nulliparity and few pregnancies increased the risk of endometrial cancer.

5.42.9 "Epidemiology of Endometrial Cancer," M. Elwood, P. Cole, K.J. Roghman, S.D. Kaplan, *J. National Cancer Inst.* 59(4): 1055,1977.

In a study of Boston area women during 1965-69, married women with 1 or 2 children had a 0.6 relative risk of endometrial cancer, and women with 3 or 4 children had a 0.3 relative risk compared to married women who were nulliparous. No significant differences were noted between women with a history of stillbirth or miscarriage compared to women with no history of stillbirth or miscarriage.

5.43 Lung Cancer

Cigarette smoking is by far the most important important risk factor for lung cancer. The American Cancer Society estimated that 67,000 U.S. women will die from lung cancer in 1998. About 1 in 18 U.S. women will develop invasive lung and bronchus cancers in their lifetime. The 5- year survival rate for lung cancer is only 14%. In 1958-60, the rate of death from lung cancer of U.S. females was 5.5 per 100,000; By 1971-73, it had increased to 12.7 per 100,000; By 1991-93, it had risen to 32.9 per 100,000 and in 1994 was 42 per 100,000.

5.43.1 "Pregnancy Decision Making as a Significant Life Event: A Commitment Approach," J Lydon et al, *Journal of Personality and Social Psychology* 71(1): 141-151, 1996.

Women who were continuing their pregnancies to term reduced their smoking during pregnancy, while those who aborted did not reduce their smoking over time.

5.43.2 "Psychological responses following medical abortion (using mifepristone and gemepost) and surgical vacuum aspiration," R Henshaw et al, *Acta Obstet Gynecol Scand* 73:812-818, 1994.

Postabortion anxiety scores at 16 days follow-up correlated with the number of cigarettes smoked, with the most anxious women having the heaviest smoking habits.

5.43.3 "Reproductive Patterns and Cancer Incidence in Women: A Population-Based Correlation Study in the USSR," L.I. Remennick, *Int'l Journal Epidemiology* 18(3): 498,1989.

A set of statistical tests was applied to assess associations between reproductive variables, including abortion, and lung cancer incidence among various regions in the USSR. A linear correlation coefficient of 0.42 was obtained with respect to lung cancer and abortion rate. A partial correlation coefficient of 0.36 was obtained with respect to lung cancer and abortion rate. (P=0.05). It was concluded that lung cancer was likely related to smoking.

5.43.4   "Stress and Smoking," *Medical Times* 114(2): 44, 1986.

A study at the University of New Hampshire linked high levels of social stress with high cigarette consumption and respiratory cancer deaths. One of the stress indicators was abortion. A stronger stress-lung cancer connection was found among women than among men although smoking and lung cancer death rates are higher in men. The researchers noted that many of the indicators used to measure stress, such as divorce and abortions could have a greater effect on women than men.

5.43.5   "Lung Cancer and Smoking Trends in the United States over the Past 25 Years," L. Garfinkel, E. Silverberg, CA-A *Cancer Journal for Clinicians* 41(3): 137, May/June, 1991.

According to the figures for the latest available year (1987) women smokers are at least 10.8 times more likely to die from lung cancer than women non-smokers.

5.43.6   "Smoking and women's health," *ACOG educational bulletin,* No 249, September, 1997, *Int'l Journal of Gynecology & Obstetrics* 60:71-82, 1997.

Since 1987, lung cancer has been the leading cause of cancer deaths among women. Women who smoke are 12 times more likely to die from lung cancer than those who never smoked. Citing *American Cancer Society. Cancer facts and figures.* (Atlanta: ACS, 1997) 5008

5.43.7   "Association of Induced Abortion with Subsequent Pregnancy Loss," Levin, *JAMA* 243: 2495, June 27,1980.

A study of women patients entering Boston Hospital for Women during 1976-78 found that 31.7% smoked if there was no history of abortion, compared to 40.3% (one abortion) and 51.7% (two or more abortions).

5.43.8   "Outcome of first Delivery After 2nd Trimester Two-Stage Induced Abortion: A Historical Cohort Study," Meirick and Nygren, *Acta., Obstet, Gynecol Scand.* 63(1): 45,1984.

A Swedish study conducted during 1970-78 found that 37% of the women reporting prior abortion smoked 10 or more cigarettes per day compared to only 21.1% for parity matched controls and 18.9% for Swedish women generally. Heavier smoking was more pronounced among women with a history of abortion than for women with no history of abortion.

5.43.9   "Low Birth Weight in Relation to Multiple Induced Abortions," M.T. Mandleson, C.B. Madden, J.R. Daling, *Am. J. Public Health* 82(3):391, March 1992.

A study of 6,541 white women in major urban counties of Washington state who delivered during

1984-87 found that only 18.0% smoked during pregnancy if women reported no prior abortion compared to 28.1% (one abortion) or 41.6% (four or more prior abortions).

5.44 Colon and Rectal Cancer

5.44.1   "Is the Incidence of Colorectal Cancer Related to Reproduction? A Prospective Study of 63.000 Women," G. Kvale, I. Heuch, *Int'l J. Cancer* 47: 390,1991.

A Norwegian study of 63,090 women survey in 1956-59 and followed through 1980 found 581 cases of colon cancer and 250 cases of rectal cancer. High parity was not associated with reduced risk. Women who had two or more abortions compared to women with no abortions had an increased risk of both colon and rectal cancer ranging from 1.16-1.72 based upon logistic regression analysis taking into account date from al levels of the variables studied. The association was significant for rectal cancer only.

5.44.2   "Large Bowel Cancer in Relation to Reproductive and Hormonal Factors. A Case-Control Study," J. D. Potter, A..J. McMichael, *J. National Cancer Institute* 71(4): 703, October, 1983.

An Australian case-control study in 1979-80 of 99 cases of colon cancer and 56 rectal cancer compared to 311 controls found that colon cancer cases had more failed pregnancies, fewer live births (2.00 and fewer full-term pregnancies (2.1) compared to controls (2.6). Rectal cancer cases had almost the same number of live births (2.4) and full-term pregnancies (2.5) compared to controls (2.6).

5.44.3   "Incidence of Cancer of the Large Bowel in Women in Relation to Reproductive and Hormonal Factors," N.S. Weiss, J.R. Daling, W.H. Chow, *J. National Cancer Institute* 67(1): 57, July, 1981.

A study of women in Washington state from 1976-77 found that, on the average, women with colon cancer had given birth to fewer children than controls. Compared to nulliparous women, the incidence of colon cancer among women with 1 or 2 children was reduced 30% and among women with 3 or more children was reduced by 50%. The occurrence of pregnancy that was not full term did not differ between cases and controls.

5.44.4   "Age at First Pregnancy and Risk of Colorectal Cancer: A Case-Control Study," G.R. Howe, K.J. Craib, A.B. Miller, *J. National Cancer Institute* 74(6): 1155, June, 1985.

A Canadian study of women from Toronto and Calgary in 1976-78 found a strong protective effect of early age at first pregnancy for both colon and rectal cancers with little or no effect noted for the total number of pregnancies

5.44.5   "Children, Age at First Birth, and Colorectal Cancer Risk," Data from Melbourne Colorectal Cancer Study, G.A. Kune, S. Kune, L.F. Watson, *Am. J. Epidemiology* 129(3): 533,1989.

For colorectal cancer, the relative risk was 0.61 for those with one or more children compared with those with no children. The protection against colorectal cancer associated with having children and earlier age of birth of first child, was found to be similar for both males and females. This suggests that a life-style factor, as yet unidentified, is the mediator of these effects.

5.45   Other Cancers

5.45.1   "Reproductive Factors and the Risk of Hepatocellular Carcinoma in Women," C. LaVecchia, E. Negri, S. Franceschi, B. D'Avanzo, *Int'l. J. Cancer* 52: 351, 1992.

A hospital based case-control study in Northern Italy between 1984-91 found that the risk of liver cancer increased with parity. The relative risk for 1 or more induced abortions was 1.6 (0.7-3.6, 95% CD) and for two or more abortions was 2.1 (1.0-4.3, 95% CI) based upon estimates from multiple logistic regression equations.

6   Abortion and Maternal Mortality

6.1   Maternal Death from Abortion

6.1.1   "Legal abortion in the U.S.: trends and mortality," HK Atrash, HW Lawson, JC Smith, *Contemporary OB/GYN* 35:58, Feb. 1990

Abortion-related deaths are defined as deaths (1) resulting from a direct complication; (2) an indirect complication caused by the chain of events initiated by the abortion, or (3) an aggravation of a pre-existing condition by the physiologic or psychologic effects of the abortion. Any death attributable to abortion is considered abortion related regardless of how long it occurred after the abortion. Ed Note: there are a number of definitions of abortion-related deaths or pregnancy related deaths. This is one of them.

6.1.2   *Lime 5. Exploited by Choice,* Mark Crucher, (Denton, Texas: Life Dynamics, Inc., 1996) 135-155

Describes the reporting of flawed data on maternal deaths by the Centers for Disease Control. Examples include: lack of information in medical records, failure to recognize that there was a recent abortion, improper classification, differing definitions of maternal death, confidentiality, lack of cooperation between various government agencies, CDC officials connected to the abortion industry.

6.1.3   "Abortion Mortality. United States, 1972 through 1987," H.W. Lawson et. al. *Am. J. Obstet. Gynecol.* 171: 1365-1372, 1994.

The Centers for Disease Control reported that 240 U.S. women died from legal induced abortion between 1972-1987 with a decreasing overall rate of 4.1 per 100,000 abortions in 1972 to 0.4 per 1000 abortions in 1987. Those at increased risk of death from legal induced abortion included women 40 years old or more, black women and those of the minority races, abortions at 16 weeks gestation or greater and use of general anesthesia.

6.1.4 "Pregnancy-Related Mortality in the United States. 1987-1990." C.J. Berg et. al, *Obstet. Gynecol.* 88: 161-167,1996.

The Centers for Disease Control reported that the pregnancy-related mortality ratio of deaths per 100,000 live births increased from 7.2 in 1987 to 10.0 in 1990. A higher risk of pregnancy-related death was found with increasing maternal age, increasing live birth order, no prenatal care, and among unmarried women. The leading causes of pregnancy-related death were hemorrhage, embolism, and hypertensive disorders of pregnancy. The CDC reported a total of 1453 pregnancy-related deaths during this period including 797 deaths where there was a live birth, 103 deaths with stillbirth, 156 deaths from ectopic pregnancy, 81 deaths from abortion (spontaneous or induced), 6 deaths from molar pregnancy, 112 deaths where the baby was undelivered and 198 deaths where the outcome of the pregnancy was unknown.

6.1.5 "Pregnancy-Related Mortality Surveillance-United States, 1987-1990," LM Koonin et al, *MMWR* 46(SS-4): 17-36 (August 8, 1997).

The causes of pregnancy-related death where there is a live birth are: hemorrhage (21.1%), embolism (23.4%), pregnancy-induced hypertension (23.8%), infection (12.1%), cardiomyopathy (6.1%), anesthesia complications (2.7%) The causes of pregnancy-related deaths where there is an abortion (induced or spontaneous) are: hemorrhage (18.5%), embolism (11.1%), pregnancy-induced hypertension (1.2%), infection (49.4%), anesthesia complications (8.6%).

6.1.6 Communication dated Tune 5. 1987 from Commissioner of Health, *City of New York to All Gynecologists, Anesthesiologists, Administrators and Others Concerned with the Provision of Abortion Services in Victims of Choice,* Kevin Sherlock, (Akron, Ohio: Brennyman Books, 1996)

The New York City Health Department, apparently relying on data likely to have been provided by the Alan Guttmacher Institute, reported that 146 women died from legal abortion between 1981-1984, yet the Centers for Disease Control reported only 42 deaths from legal abortion during that same period. Ed Note: This is a good example of the underreporting of deaths from legal abortion.

6.1.7 *Victims of Choice,* Kevin Sherlock, (Akron, OH: Brennyman Books, 1996)

In an investigation and subsequent analysis of 87 abortion-related deaths of U.S. women between 1980-1989 in 28 states, 47 were classified as unspecified abortion, 33 as legal abortion, and 7 did not include a code classification. Death certificates or coroner reports used 27 different terms or phrases to describe abortion. If the term abortion, septic abortion, induced abortion or incomplete abortion was used on death certificates or coroner/medical examiner reports, deaths were classified as unspecified abortion. Where the term termination of pregnancy or elective abortion was used, about 2/3 were classified as legal abortion deaths. Where the term therapeutic abortion was used, virtually all were classified as legal abortion deaths. Ed Note: It appeared that most, if not all, of these abortion-related deaths were from legal abortion. The wide range of terms used to describe abortion appeared to be a major factor in misclassification.

6.1.8   "Induced Abortion as a Contributing Factor in Maternal Mortality or Pregnancy-Related Death in Women," Thomas Strahan, *Association for Interdisciplinary Research in Values and Social Change* 10(3): 1-8, Nov/Dec, 1996.

Prior induced abortion is a cause of complications in subsequent pregnancies including placenta previa, retained placenta, abrupdo placentae, premature rupture of membranes, and obstetrical infections. Also, induced abortion increases the incidence of suicide compared to other pregnancy outcomes, as well as ruptured ectopic pregnancy. Induced abortion does not provide the protective effect of childbirth and increases the incidence of hypertensive disorders of pregnancy. All of these increase the incidence of maternal mortality.

6.1.9   "An Assessment of the Incidence of Maternal Mortality in the United States," T. Smith, J. Hughes, P. Pekow and R. Rochat, *Am. J. Public Health* 74: 780-783, 1984

The incidence of maternal mortality is higher than vital statistics reports indicate. The person certifying the cause of death may not know that a woman had a recent pregnancy. Also, the definition of maternal death can greatly affect the reported incidence of maternal mortality.

6.1.10   "Legal Abortion Mortality in the United States: 1972 to 1982," H. Atrash, H.T. MacKay, N. Binkin and C. Hogue, *American Journal Obstetrics and Gynecology,* 156(3): 611, March 1987.

Although there is no certainty that all legal abortion-related deaths from 1972 to 1982 were reported to the Center for Disease Control [CDC], it is believed that the use of multiple reporting sources decreases the likelihood that deaths are missed. A study of maternal deaths in the U.S. between 1974-1978, relying only on vital records, identified only 141 abortion-related deaths, 63 of which were related to legal abortion. See "Causes of Maternal Mortality in the U.S." Kaunitz, et al., *Obstet. Gynecol.* 65:605-612, 1985. In comparison, CDC's surveillance of abortion [maternal] mortality identified 188 abortion-related deaths during the same period, 92 of which were related to legal abortion.

6.1.11   "Causes of Maternal Mortality in the United States," A. Kaunitz, J. Hughes, D. Grimes, J. Smith, R. Rochat and M. Kafrissen, *Obstetrics and Gynecology* 65: 605-612, May 1985.

From 1974-1978, the most common causes of maternal deaths, excluding other unspecified causes, were embolism (191), hypertensive disease of pregnancy (421), obstetric hemorrhage (331), ectopic pregnancies (254), obstetric infection (199), cerebro vascular accident (107) and anesthesia/analgesia complications (98). There were 135 deaths from upper genital tract infections among the deaths for obstetric infection. Among deaths due to obstetric hemorrhage 33 were from retained placenta and 19 from placenta previa. Ed. Note - Prior induced abortion may have been

229

an implicating factor in some of these deaths.

6.1.12 "Legal Abortion in the U.S.: Trends and Mortality," H.K. Atrash, H. Lawson and J. Smith, *Contemporary Ob/Gyn* 35(2):58-69 Feb 1990.

According to the Centers for Disease Control the relative risk of death for black women and other minorities increased from 2.4 per 100,000 abortions during 1972-1978 to 2.9 per 100,000 abortions during 1979-1985). (The cause of death from legal abortion during 1979-1985 was hemorrhage (22.2%); infection (13.9%); embolism (15.3%); anesthesia (29.2%) and other (19.4%).

6.1.13 "Fatal Hemorrhage from Legal Abortion in the United States," D. Grimes, et al., *Surgery, Gynecology and Obstetrics,* 157: 461-6, November 1983.

From 1972-1979, hemorrhage was the third most frequent cause of death from legal abortion, accounting for 15% of deaths. If abortions are performed in free-standing clinics, the capability for rapid transportation to a nearby well-equipped hospital must be assured. Inordinate delays while waiting for an ambulance contributed to several deaths. The back-up hospital must have the ability to begin a laparotomy quickly and to transfuse large amounts of blood products.

6.1.14 "Legal Abortion Mortality and General Anesthesia," H. Atrash, *Am. J. Obstet and Gynecol* 158:420-424(1988).

The percentage of deaths from legal abortion caused by general anesthesia complications increased from 7.7% between 1972-75 to 29.4% between 1980-85. At least 23 of the 27 deaths were due to hypoventilation and/or loss of airway resulting in hypoxia.

6.1.15 "Anesthesia or Analgesia Related Deaths of Women from Legal Abortion: The Need for Increased Regulation," Thomas Strahan, *Association for Interdisciplinary Research in Values and Social Change Research Bulletin* 12(1):1-8, Nov/Dec 1997.

6.1.16 "Economic Consequences of Pelvic Inflammatory Disease in the United States," James Curran, *American Journal of Obstetrics and Gynecology*, 138(7):848-851, Part 2, December 1,1980.

Between 1970 and 1975, an average of 897 women hospitalized for PID died each year. Fifty percent of the morbidity and deaths from ectopic pregnancy can be attributed to PID. The extent to which induced abortion may have contributed to these deaths was not stated.

6.1.17 "Abortion Related Maternal Mortality: An In-Depth Analysis," T. Hilgers and D. O'Hare, in *New Perspectives on Human Abortion*, ed. T. Hilgers, D. Horan and D. Mall, (Frederick MD: University Publications of America, 1981).

Analyzes state and national statistics and concludes that the legalization of abortion has had no effect on the already existing downward trend in the maternal mortality rate. Prior maternal deaths for criminal abortion have been replaced by maternal deaths for legal abortion. Maternal mortality rates are generally expressed as the number of maternal deaths which occur during the entire course of pregnancy and the first three to six months following completion of the pregnancy per 100/000 live births.

6.1.18   "Fatal Ectopic Pregnancy After Attempted Legally Induced Abortion," G. Rubin, W. Cates, J. Gold, R. Rochat and C. Tyler, *Journal of the American Medical Association*, 244(15): 1705-1708 October 10, 1980.

Ten cases of death caused by ruptured ectopic pregnancy after attempted legal abortion were identified by the Center for Disease Control [seven blacks, three whites, five nulliparous] from 1973 to 1978. In seven cases tissue obtained at the abortion was sent for outside pathological exam, but results came back too late. The study concluded that an important factor in preventing fatal ectopic pregnancy is the identification of products of conception at the time of the abortion while patient is still available for re-examination. Deaths occurred from one to 44 days following the attempted abortion. See also "Missed Tubal Abortion," Burrows, et al., *American Journal of Obstetrics and Gynecology,* 136(5): 691-92, March 1,1980; "Ectopic Pregnancy and First Trimester Abortion," Schonberg, *Obstet. Gynecol.* (Supp.), 49:73 (1977). Planned Parenthood reported only 11 cases of tubal pregnancy among 41,753 women presented for elective, first-trimester abortions, only two of which were diagnosed prior to rupture.

6.1.19   "Fatal pulmonary embolism during legal induced abortion in the United States from 1972 to 1985," H.W. Lawson, H.K. Atrash, A.L. Franks, *Am.J. Obstetrics and Gynecology*, 162: 986-990,1990.

Of the 213 deaths from legal abortion from 1972-1985, 21 % were due to air, blood clot or amniotic fluid embolism. The risk of death from embolism was higher among minority women and women aged 34-44 years and abortion at later stages of pregnancy.

6.1.20   "Cluster of Abortion Deaths at a Single Facility," M.E. Kafrissen, D.A. Grimes, C.J.R. Hogue, J.J. Sacks, *Obstetrics and Gynecology* 68: 387,1986.

Four abortion related deaths at a single facility were reported from 1979 to 1983. Two abortion deaths occurred when an unlicensed person performed the abortions. It was recommended that prompt treatment of abortion complications and community-based surveillance of serious morbidity should be done.

6.1.21   "Ectopic Pregnancy in the United States. 1970-1986," H. Lawson, H. Atrash, A. Saftlas and E. Finch, Centers for Disease Control, *Morbidity and Mortality Weekly Report*, 38(SS-2) Sept. 1989.

Ectopic pregnancy rose from 17,800 cases in 1970 to 73,700 cases in 1986. Nearly 800,000 women have been hospitalized for ectopic pregnancy since 1970. Thirty-six women reportedly died from ectopic pregnancy in 1986.

6.1.22   "Mortality From Abortion and Childbirth," (letter), M. Lanska D. Lanska and A. Rimm, *JAMA*

250(3): 361-362 July 15, 1983.

Maternal mortality following a cesarean section is approximately 100 per 100,000 births which is roughly 10-20 times greater than the maternal mortality following vaginal delivery. Cesarean sections, while accounting for only 10% of the deliveries, account for 90% of the maternal mortality associated with childbirth. The results suggest that the mortality rate among women who have had abortions (1.9 per 100,000 legal abortions) is almost twice as high as maternal mortality rates for women who have had vaginal deliveries (1.1 per 100,000 live births.

6.1.23   "Trends in the United States cesarean section rate and reasons for the 1980-1985 rise," S. Taffel, P. Placek and T. Liss, *Am. J. Public Health* 77: 955 (1987).

Deliveries by cesarean section in the U.S. increased from 5.5% in 1970 to 16.5% in 1980 and to 27.7% of all deliveries in 1985.

6.1.24   "Maternal Mortality in the United States: Report From the Maternal Mortality Collaborative," R. Rochat, L. Koonin, H. Atrash, J. Jewett, *Obstetrics and Gynecology* 72: 91 1988.

Of the leading causes of direct maternal deaths during 1980-85, 45.5% were known to have been associated with delivery by cesarean section. It was concluded that maternal deaths from childbirth and abortion are under-reported.

6.1.25   "Ectopic pregnancy concurrent with induced abortion: Incidence and mortality," H.K. Atrash, *Am. J. Obstet. Gynecol.* 162(3):726-730, March 1990.

From 1972-1985, 24 women who underwent an induced abortion died as a result of a concurrent ectopic pregnancy. The death-to-case rate was 1.3 times higher in ectopic pregnancy concurrent with induced abortion than for women not undergoing induced abortion. Most of the deaths of women with ectopic pregnancy who underwent abortion were attributed to the failure to diagnose ectopic pregnancy before the women left the facility. Tissue examination to assure there is a product of conception at the time of the abortion is necessary.

6.1.26   "Centers for Disease Control, Abortion Surveillance, 1981," U.S. Dept. of Health and Human Services, Public Health Services, November 1985 p. 9

Between 1972 and 1981 the Centers for Disease Control reported that 21 deaths from ectopic pregnancy occured soon after an attempted legally induced abortion. In the 1978 abortion surveillance report the CDC considered such deaths as abortion-related and included them as a separate subcategory of legal induced abortion. In 1979 the CDC began the independent surveillance of ectopic pregnancy-related mortality and published its first ectopic pregnancy surveillance report in 1982. In the abortion surveillance report of 1981 (and apparently in years following), the CDC excluded all deaths associated with ectopic pregnancies.

6.1.27   "Brief of Amicus Curiae Feminists for Life of America. Women Exploited by Abortion, etc," Christine Smith Torre, Webster v. Reproductive Health Services 88-605 1988 at p. 22

The state of California reported no deaths from abortion during 1982 and 1984, yet there was incontrovertible evidence from death certificates, police reports, coroner's reports and other sources that at least four women and teenage girls died from legal abortions in Los Angeles County alone during 1983 and 1984.

6.1.28   *Aborted Women: Silent No More,* David C. Reardon, (Chicago: Loyola Press, 1987) 109.

In an investigation of four Chicago-based abortion clinics (out of more than 20 in the state), investigative reporters for the Chicago Sun-times uncovered 12 abortion deaths that had never been reported. Even when abortion-related deaths such as these are uncovered, they are not generally included in the "official" total since they were not reported as such on the original death certificates. Citing "The Abortion Profiteers," Pamela Zekeman and Pamela Warrick, *Chicago Sun-Times*, November 12, 1978 (Special Reprint December 3,1978); *Abortion: Questions and Answers* J. Willke and B. Willke (Cincinnati: Hayes Publishing, 1985); "Medical Hazards of Abortion," Thomas Hilgers, in *Abortion and Social Justice.* ed. T. Hilgers and D. Horan, (New York: Sheed and Ward, 1972)

6.1.29   "Before and After Legalization," in *Aborted Women: Silent No More,* David C. Reardon, (Chicago: Loyola Press, 1987) 282-300.

Examines reporting of abortion related deaths before and after legalization. Abortion related deaths were much more likely to be reported when it was still a criminal act. Numerous factors, including the lack of a formal reporting mechanism, render post-legalization assessments of abortion related deaths unreliable.

6.1.30   "The Cover-Up: Why U.S. Abortion Mortality Statistics are Meaningless," David C. Reardon, *The Post-Abortion Review* 8(2):4, April-June 2000. Posted at www.afterabortion.org/PAR/V8.

This article identifies examples of documented abortion related deaths that have been excluded from government figures. The rules regarding coding cause of death using the International Classification of Diseases preclude identifying medical procedures as the cause of death. This coding rule contributes to the lack of good statistics on abortion related deaths.

6.2   Pregnancy-Associated Mortality

There are deaths which occur after pregnancy.. These are referred to as Pregnancy-Associated Deaths and are not counted as a Pregnancy-related Deaths. There is evidence that these deaths occur more frequently after induced abortion than with other pregnancy outcome.

6.2.1   "Pregnancy-associated deaths in Finland 1987-1994-definition problems and benefits of record linkage," M Gissler et al, *Acta Obstet Gynecol Scand* 76:651-657, 1997.

Death certificates of all women of child-bearing age were linked to birth, abortion, and other pregnancies to identify women who had been pregnant during the last year of their life. Only in

22% of the death certificates was pregnancy or its end mentioned. The mortality rate was 27 per 100,000 live births, 48 per 100,000 miscarriages or ectopic pregnancies, and 101 per 100,000 abortions. After abortion, the mortality risk was increased for accidents, suicides, and homicides.

6.2.2   "Suicide Deaths Associated with Pregnancy Outcome: A Record Linkage Study of 173,279 Low Income American Women," DC Reardon et al, *Clinical Medicine & Health Research* 2001030003, April 25, 2001.

A record-linkage study of low income women eligible for state-funded medical insurance in California identified all paid claims for abortion or delivery in 1989. These were linked to the state death registry. Compared to women who delivered, those who aborted had a significantly higher age adjusted risk of dying from all causes (1.62), from suicide (2.54), accidents (1.82), and non-violent causes (1.44), including AIDS (2.18), circulatory diseases (2.87), and cerebrovascular disease (5.46). The results remained significant over an eight year period and over four of six age groups examined.

6.2.3   "Hidden From View: Violent Deaths Among Pregnant Women in the District of Columbia, 1988-1996," CJ Krulewitch et al, *J Midwifery & Women's Health* 46(1): 4, Jan/Feb 2001.

From 1988-1996 the District of Columbia officially reported 21 maternal deaths using standard definitions for pregnancy-related death, but did not include women who died from pregnancy associated but not pregnancy related causes. Thirty additional deaths were identified from autopsy reports , which documented evidence of pregnancy. Of these 30 deaths, homicide was documented as the manner of death in 13 cases (43.3%). Three out of four women with evidence of pregnancy who died from homicide were in their first 20 weeks of pregnancy.

6.2.4   "Enhanced Surveillance for Pregnancy-Associated Mortality- Maryland, 1993-1998," IL Horon and D Cheng, *JAMA* 285(11):1455, March 21, 2001.

A study of pregnancy-associated deaths in Maryland found that among all deaths occurring up to one year after delivery or termination, it was found that homicide (50 deaths) was the most frequent cause of death, with deaths from cardiovascular disorders the second leading cause of death (48 deaths). Death certificates only accounted for 67 out of 247 deaths. Record linkage and medical examiner records provided the balance of the information.

Adolescents and Abortion

Adolescents face many of the same issues and risks as older women, of course. But because of the special legal issues associated with adolescents, the literature related specifically to adolescents is segregated here. Readers are advised to also examine similar headings in the sections above for related information.

7.1 Adolescent Developmental Issues

7.1.1 "Mourning in Adolescence: Normal and Pathological," Benjamin Garber, *Adolescent Psychiatry* 12:371-387(1985).

Adolescents consider it crucial to be part of a group and equally important to conform to the group. They are very conscious of anything that may set them apart from others. Whatever factors set them apart-physical, social or emotional-typically adolescents will try to diminish them.

7.1.2 "Depression in an Adolescent Delinquent Population," J.A. Chiles, M. Millert and G. Cox *Archives of General Psychiatry,* 37: 1179-1184, October 1980,

Depressed adolescents are more likely to be girls; depressive symptoms include cognitive changes. Difficulty concentrating and indecision were significantly elevated in depressed adolescents, as compared with nondepressed adolescents.

7.1.3 "Abortion Counseling: Focus on Adolescent Pregnancy," Carol Nadelson, *Pediatrics* 54(6): 765-769, December 1974,

The adolescent who is making a decision about an abortion, having an abortion, or is in the post-abortion period needs a trusted ally who can help her understand her motivation for pregnancy and abortion, explore her ambivalence and consider alternative solutions. Ambivalence is universal. It is related to the conflict between the positive aspects of conception and pregnancy, and the frustration and sadness over choosing to terminate a pregnancy. Since ambivalence occurs as part of the developmental process of adolescence, it is especially prominent in this age group, and it is more difficult to assess its particular significance. The adolescent who is involved in other critical developmental issues may be desirous of an abortion because her family wants the opposite, or *vice versa.* These issues must be clarified. In addition, the counselor must remember that the adolescent will continue to live with her family, so that helping her with her own decision is not enough. Work with the family is important in order [1] to avoid repetition of the unwanted pregnancy, which is most frequently a distress signal for the adolescent, and [2] to work out problems reflected by the mutual acknowledgment of the adolescent's sexuality.

7.1.4 "Physician Assessed Competitiveness in Adolescent Health Care," R. Blum, *Journal Medical Education* 62:401-407, (1987),

Health care providers described themselves as poorly trained and insufficiently skilled in managing adolescent concerns of social and psychological origins.

7.1.5   "The Contemporary Adolescent Girl," Helene Deutsch, *Seminars in Psychiatry,* 1(1): 99- 112, February 1969.

Illegitimate motherhood occurs not because of a lack of sexual information but because such pregnancies are *compulsive.* Too early involvement in sexual gratification interferes with the development of real tender feelings of love and enchantment. The lack of deeper emotional participation-of longing and wishing, of pain and joy, of hope and despair-constitutes a psychological disaster. The ego ideal of the girl is built, to a large extent, upon the mother-the ideal mother, not the sexually devalued one.

7.1.6   "How Adolescents Approach Decisions: Chances Over Grades Seven to Twelve, and Policy Implications." Catherine Lewis, *Child Development* 52:538-544(1981).

Even when the point of comparison is twelfth graders, rather than adults, seventh, eighth and tenth graders show relative deficiencies in certain aspects of approaching decisions, including imagining risks and future consequences, recognizing the need for independent professional opinions in certain situations, and recognizing the potential vested interests of professionals in providing certain information.

7.1.7   "The Competency of Children and Adolescents to Make Informed Treatment Decisions," L. Weithorn and S. Campbell, *Child Development*, 53:1589-1598(1982).

In general, 14- year-old minors were able to demonstrate a level of competency equivalent to that of adults, according to four standards of competency-evidence of choice, reasonable outcome, rational reasons and understanding-and for four hypothetical dilemmas- diabetes, epilepsy, depression and enuresis.

7.1.8   "Understanding Adolescent Pregnancy and Abortion," Sherry Hatcher, Health Care for Women: 1. Current Social and Behavioral Issues, *Primary Care* 3(3): 407A24, September 1976.

Studies conclude that much of the relevant medical and behavioral research fails to distinguish between the tomboyish early adolescent girl, the oedipally activated and rebellious middle adolescent girl, and the "almost adult" late adolescent. Psychological development models must be based upon individual psychic-social maturity rather than chronological age. Early adolescents tend to deny any responsibility for the pregnancy. A girl's motivation may be to become closer to her mother by becoming a mother herself, or to see if her body really "works." When she admits to herself that she is pregnant she moves to obliterate the pregnancy and seeks abortion as the only way out. The middle adolescent tends to make the male father figure responsible for her situation. The underlying fantasy is one of competition with mother for father; there is a growing desire for autonomy. Ambivalence between moralistic judgment and hedonistic retreat is typical. The man who impregnated her is a means to an end-autonomy and independence from her family. She feels disappointed when her pregnancy does not alter the state of her unresolved dependency needs. The late adolescent is more in touch with her feelings and has the most difficulty deciding to terminate her pregnancy. She is probably the only one of the three groups who will wish to continue her relationship with the responsible boyfriend following her abortion. Following abortion, each group had developmental conflicts at the same stage of psychological maturation.

7.1.9 "Selected Problems of Adolescence," H. Deutsch, *Psychoanalytic Study of the Child,* Monograph No. 3(1967)

Early adolescents try out relationships by play acting them- without the benefit of a solid ego or sense of self. Middle adolescence represents the most egocentric stage. Late adolescents are closest to developing a "motherly ego." See also *The Psychology of Women,* Helene Deutsch, Vols.I and II (1944) (1945).

7.1.10 "Problem Pregnancy and Abortion Counseling with Teenagers. T," Chesler and S. Davis, Social Casework, *The Journal of Contemporary Social Work*, March, 1980 pp. 173-179

Discusses practical approaches to counseling as problem solving using crisis counseling strategies that emphasize both client and paternal assertiveness and the importance of compromise. Demonstrates that relationships and attitudes of adolescents and parents are not fixed but can change over time.

7.1.11 "A Theoretical Framework for Studying Factors that Impact on the Maternal Role," Ramona T. Mercer, *Nursing Research,* 30(2): 73-77, March-April 1981.

A summary of numerous studies on the subject. The maternal role, far from being an intuitive feminine function, is a complex social and integrative process that is learned. Maternal role attainment has been described as occurring in progressive stages through the operations of mimicry, role play, fantasy, introjection-projection-rejection, and grief work over a 12-15 month period including pregnancy and six months afterward. See Reva Rubin, "Attainment of the Maternal Role: Part 1. Processes: Part II, Models and Referents," *Nursing Research* 16:237-245, 342-346, Summer/ Fall 1967; Rubin, "Binding-In in the Post Partum Period" , *Matern. Child Nurs.* 6:67-75, Summer, 1977.

The foundation for the anticipatory stage may be laid as a child observes mothering behaviors in the family context. The formal stage begins with the birth of the infant, as the mother begins identifying her role partner and assumes care-taking tasks. Teenage mothers required from six to ten months postpartum to move to the formal stage. Current research supports that the infant's ability to see, hear and track the human face depict socialization capabilities present at birth. The infant is considered an active partner in the maternal role-making process. The infant initiates approximately 50 percent of the parent-infant interactions. Adaptive maternal behavior is influenced favorably by the mother's perceptions of the amount of positive support she received.

7.1.12 "Early Adolescence. A Time of Transition and Stress," B. Hamburg, *Post Graduate Medicine* 78(1): 158-167, July 1985,

Coming of age in modern America has become increasingly complex, lengthy and, according to many indicators, much more stressful. Early adolescence is probably the most stressful of all developmental transitions. Autonomy in adolescence should not be regarded as requiring rebellion and alienation from parents, but as achieving mature, interdependent relationships. Many early adolescents who engage in sexual relations are actually seeking friendship and approval; sexual activity is not a good way for them to become acquainted.

7.1.13   "Behavioral Considerations in the Health Care of Adolescents," M.E. Felice, *Pediatric Clinics of North America* 29(2): 399-412, April 1982,

The psychological tasks of growth have been described from various perspectives as follows: to establish independence; to become comfortable with one's body; to build new and meaningful relationships; to seek economic and social stability; to develop a workable value system; to verbalize conceptually. See Adams, "The Pregnant Adolescent -A Group Approach," *Adolescence* 11:467-485(1976).

7.1.14   "Pregnancy, Abortion and the Developmental Tasks of Adolescence," C. Schaffer and F. Pine, *Journal of the American Academy of Child Psychiatry* ll(3):511-536 (1972).

Pregnancy followed by therapeutic abortion in adolescent girls heightens, and is experienced in terms of conflicts already present during that developmental period. The conflict most generally aroused was between passive longings for one's own mother and an urge toward active mothering of self, infant and others. There were wide differences in the way the girls handled their abortions. Resolutions included regressive reattachment to their mother; progressive steps toward self-care, in which the abortion serves as an organizing experience; a middle ground where resolutions seem to be highly influenced by external events. Girls who make the more regressive solution are unlikely to use birth control; self-caring will use birth control.

7.1.15   "Adolescent girls and their mothers: Realigning the relationship," Paul Trad, *Am J Family Therapy* 23(1): 11-24, Spring, 1995

A case is presented involving a 14-year old girl who became pregnant impulsively and after having had an abortion, harbored a wish to become pregnant again. The interactional patterns suggested that the mother and daughter were involved in a complex negotiation between developmental progression and regression.

7.1.16   "Normal Adolescent Development," R.E. Kreipe, *New York State Journal of Medicine* 85(5): 214-217, May 1985,

The establishment of an identity is an essential task of adolescence. In the process, there is a consolidation of one's ego, one's self-concept, and one's role in life. According to Erikson's theory of development, if an adolescent fails to attain a stable role or identity, role confusion follows. See Erikson, E. H., *Identity: Youth and Crisis,* (New York:W.W. Norton, 1968). Adolescents who have difficulty establishing an identity do not know who they are, do not know where they are going in life and have trouble establishing long-lasting relationships. Children normally enter adolescence with an unformed sense of identity, but if they enter adulthood without this sense, their further development is impeded. Adolescent mothers often see themselves in shallow terms, in which education, marriage or a career have no relevance. Although intellect does not change dramatically during adolescence, the mode of thinking does change. Inhelder and Piaget proposed the terms "concrete operational thinking" to describe the way adults think. Concrete operations limit one's thinking to literal, here-and-now interpretations of questions. Formal operational thinking, on the other hand, enables one to understand figurative speech. It enables one to think about abstractions, such as future options, or to ask "what if" questions. The transition from one cognitive style to the other occurs during adolescence. Normal adolescents are egocentric; they think about themselves a great deal. Egocentrism is the normal self-centered focus of the adolescent's attention. Often viewed by parents as selfishness or narcissism, egocentrism is a reflection of the adolescent who is appropriately engaged in self-study, self-exploration, and self-determination. See *The Growth of Logical Thinking from Childhood to Adolescence.* B. Inhelder, J. Piaget, (New York: Basic Books, 1958).

7.1.17   "Family Correlates of Female Adolescent's Ego-Identity Development, G," Adams, *Journal of Adolescence* 8:69-82(1985).

Parent-child relations were assessed from both the adolescents, and the parents' perspectives. The findings indicated that parental identity status formation may have an effect on the adolescents' identity formation and that parent-child relations differentiate between less and more mature female adolescent identities. In general, the daughter's perception of her father's and mother's behavior held a very modest association with how the parents viewed their own conduct.

7.1.18   "Coping in Adolescence," J. Shen, *Postgraduate Medicine* 78(1): 153-157, July 1985,

Understanding the "good" foundation stones in personality development is important. Erikson described these as crucial developmental tasks: trust in early infancy, autonomy in late infancy, initiative in early childhood, industry in late childhood, identity in adolescence, intimacy in young adulthood, generativity in adulthood, and integrity in maturity. The "bad" foundation stones are mistrust, shame and doubt in infancy; inferiority and guilt in childhood; and role diffusion in adolescence. The cumulative effect of such desirable or detrimental processes is either growth and development or breakdown. See E. H. Erikson, *Childhood and Society.* New York:W.W. Norton (1950); E. H. Erikson, *Identity: Youth and Crisis,* New York:W.W. Norton (1968).

7.1.19   *The Adolescent and Pregnancy,* Margaret-Ann Corbett and Jerrilyn H. Meyer, (Boston: Blackwell Scientific Publications, 1987), pp. 267-269.

Pregnant adolescents in the Young Mothers Program [YMP] at Yale-New Haven Hospital consented to discuss their feelings about pregnancy and related matters if they could do so anonymously. The staff designed questions to which the adolescents responded. Contraception was viewed with ambivalence and a fluctuating commitment to its use. About a third of the group acknowledged they had considered an abortion because of fears about [1] their capabilities to raise a child by themselves, [2] their being "too young to have a child, " or [3] their capabilities to cope with family/peer reaction to their pregnancy ("I was so frightened I didn't know what to do.") The rest of the group voiced opposition to abortion. While most said they did not believe in abortion, much of their discussion reflected their mothers, opinion on the subject. ("My mother doesn't believe in it and neither do 1.") When asked who helped most during the pregnancy, the girls overwhelmingly indicated mothers or a mother figure such as an aunt. When adolescents were asked what helped most upon learning they were pregnant, they identified love and acceptance. By far the most important source of love was their mothers. Boyfriends were the second most significant group. About 80 percent of the group did not properly predict their mother's reaction. For that group, the negative response they anticipated occurred but later resolved itself in acceptance.

7.1.20   "Self-Destructive Behavior in Children and Adolescents," ed. C. F. Wells and 1. Stuart, *Pregnancies and Abortions,* Lucie Rudd, (New York: Van Nostrand Reinhold, 1981), pp. 208-223.

In our present day mores, many parents do not recognize the great need among children and adolescents for cuddling, physical touching, verbal and physical expressions of parental love. The composite of self, influenced by many inputs, is often one of inadequacy, guilt, self-belittling, and acceptance of the mother's unflattering judgment.

Most of the adolescents who later get into trouble have poor self-images and very often no nurturing to help them change. The need to be petted and admired in a society of peers who are vying with each other to attract and retain the available males will push some adolescents into early sexual activity. When sexual activity satisfies the need for acceptance, and the longing for intimacy, as well as the adolescent need for experimentation, it is very attractive. Pressure occurs not only from the peer group, but also from the mass media. Sex is used to sell everything from toothpaste to cars. The family of the girl plays an essential role. Chaotic families in which the only way to get attention is to act in a negative fashion quite often produce boys who engage in drug abuse and antisocial activities, and girls who experiment in very early sexual activity. HEW deemed in 1975 that adolescent pregnancies were all due to "acting out" a professional term for deviant if not pathological behavior. Some teens become pregnant to improve status, others to defy their families. Some are victims of sex abuse who become pregnant. Even though these pregnancies are not always planned, some of them seem to be linked to deep unconscious needs. It appears almost impossible to prevent them.

7.1.21   "Identification of Women at Risk for Unwanted Pregnancy," V. Abernethy, D. Robbins, G. Abernethy, H. Grunebaum and J. Weiss, *American Journal of Psychiatry* 132 (10): 1027- 1031, October 1975.

There is growing evidence in the psychological and demographic literature that knowledge and availability of modern contraceptive methods is not a sufficient condition for effective birth control. Family life experiences in adolescence appear to be critical in the development of relatively stable attitudes and personality traits that can be implicated in women's predisposition to risk unwanted pregnancy. Both promiscuity and irresponsible use of contraception seem to be common outcomes if [1] the parents' marriage was characterized by distance and hostility; [2] a

240

woman felt alienated from her mother as a young teenager, and [3] the relationship with the father was excessively intimate and excluded the mother. In these situations, there is a redefinition of roles, with the daughter assuming some of the mother's functions as a companion to the husband/father. Low self-esteem in teenage girls motivates a young woman to measure herself primarily on the standard of male approval and attention, which she attempts to win by stereotypic feminine behavior. Unresolved dependency needs and low self-esteem militate against contraceptive behavior.

7.1.22   *The Adolescent and Pregnancy,* Margaret Ann Corbett and Jerrilyn H. Meyer, (Boston: Blackwell Scientific Publications, 1987).

When a pregnancy occurs because of a contraceptive failure or a failure to use contraceptives, the adolescent is often in a predicament. Consequently, she may deny the pregnancy and delay finding professional help. Adolescents frequently fear parental reaction to their pregnancies, let alone a request for an abortion. This is natural and, in cases of parental child abuse, appallingly real. An adolescent who becomes pregnant to escape abuse herself will often, as an adolescent mother, expect unrealistic obedience and what she believes to be correct responses from her child. If her infant fails to meet her expectations, child abuse may result. Therefore, while we promote the quality of care of both the baby and mother in pregnancy, we must do likewise after birth. The clinician who is aware of an abused child's characteristics can identify their presence in pregnancy. If counseling is immediately begun, future child abuse may be successfully averted.

7.1.23   "Emotional Crises of School A- Girls During Pregnancy and Early Motherhood," H. LaBarre, *Journal of the American Academy of Child Psychiatry* 11(3): 537-557(1972).

Describes in detail a separate junior-senior high school for pregnant girls while they carry their babies to term. The sudden loss of the major role and occupation of adolescents, that of student, constitutes a real rejection and punishment of the pregnant girl. To some students, withdrawal from school seemed an overwhelming frustration of hopes and plans and loss of their self-esteem. Pregnancy provides the most profound sisterhood of mutual feelings and experience. The emotional import of belonging to a group of peers, all of whom are involved in the same basic life experience and with whom they can identify, share, learn from and give to, is very significant for pregnant girls.

7.1.24   "Adolescent Morality-A Theologian's Viewpoint," Paul Ramsey, *Post-Graduate Medicine* 72(1): 233-236, July 1982,

Teenage attitudes toward sex are simply a response to the pressures of today's society, a society that almost insists that its young members become sexually active. Loss of virginity and pregnancy are puberty rites devised by our youngsters to fill the void created by a liberalism that hesitates even to pass on its cultural heritage for fear of imposing on individual freedoms. Increasing the number of sex education programs and the availability of contraceptives are not the answer to the current epidemic of teenage pregnancy.

7.1.25 "Current Contradictions in Adolescent Theory," J.C. Coleman, *Journal of Youth and Adolescence* 7(1): 1-11, 1978,

The article points out two contradictions in adolescent theory, i.e., the "classical" point of view and the "empirical', view. One espouses the notion of "storm and stress, " while the other supports a concept of relative calm. One reason for divergence of view is that psychologists responsible for large-scale surveys have tended to overestimate the individual adolescent's ability or willingness to talk about his innermost feelings. Much depends upon the way the study is carried out, but it is important to note how very difficult it often is for anyone-let alone an anxious or resentful teenager-to share fears, worries, or conflicts with a strange interviewer. Those responsible for the empirical view may have underestimated the amount of inner stress experienced by young people.

7.1.26 "Motivational Factors in Abortion Patients," F. Kane, M. Lachenbruch, M. Lipton and D. Baram, *American Journal of Psychiatry* 130(3): 290-293, March 1973,

Forty percent were found to have motivational factors that may have influenced the outcome of the pregnancy, such as guilt over the use of contraception, a severe acting out character disorder or reaction to loss.

7.1.27 "Motivation Factors in Pregnant Adolescents," F. Kane, C. Moan and B. Bolling, *Diseases of the Nervous System* 35:131-134(1974).

Factors such as guilt about the use of contraception, loss of love objects via death of father or mother, and overt wishes for pregnancy by the female or her partner were observed.

7.1.28 "A Comparison of Minor's and Adult's Pregnancy Decisions," Catherine Lewis, *American Journal Orthopsychiatry* 50(3): 446-453, July 1980.

Concludes that minor's decisions were more "externally" based, i.e., what parents thought. Minors more often considered possible deformity of the child.

7.1.29 "Social and Psychological Correlates of Pregnancy Decisions Among Adolescent Women," Lucy Olsen, *American Journal Orthopsychiatry* 50(3), 432-445, July 1980.

Concludes that those who seek and go through an abortion are not a "special" population of unmarried adolescents but are similar to those of the same age in many of their social and psychological characteristics. Pregnancy resolution is a process of "enormous complexity."

7.1.30 "Pregnancy in the Single Adolescent Girl: The Role of Cognitive Functions," W. Godfrey Cobliner, *Journal of Youth and Adolescence,* 3(1): 17-29, (1974),

Three psychological mechanisms were uncovered which virtually block the conversion of birth control knowledge into successful practice. Somatic Area: Only about one fourth of the pregnancies were intended. Sex is mechanistic; a premium is placed on performance to create a desire for repetition. There is a lack of curiosity about one's own body.

7.1.31 "Reasoning in the Personal and Moral Domains: Adolescent and Young Adult Women's Decision-Making Regarding Abortion," Judith G. Smetana, *Journal of Applied Developmental Psychology* 2:211-226(1981).

Subjects treating abortion as a moral issue were more likely to continue their pregnancies, while subjects treating abortion as a personal issue were more likely to obtain an abortion. avoidance and reduced abortion rates in 15- to 17-year olds.

7.1.32 "Impact of the Minnesota Parental Notification Law on Abortion and Birth," J.L. Rogers, R. Boruch, G. Stomsard, D. DeMoya, *American Journal of Public Health* 81 (3):294-298, March 1991.

The impact of the Minnesota Parental Notification Law enacted in 1981 and enjoined in 1986 was examined using linear models and outcome parameters before and after enactment. Data suggested that parental notification facilitated pregnancy old Minnesota women.)

7.1.33 "Pregnancy and Abortion Counseling," American Academy of Pediatrics Committee on Adolescence, *Pediatrics* 63(6) :920-92 I, June 1979.

All options should be explored, including [1] Keeping the pregnancy, marrying the father and raising the child at home. [2] Keeping the pregnancy and relinquishing the infant for adoption. [3] Keeping the pregnancy and raising the child with the help of other family members. [4] Keeping the pregnancy and raising the infant, remaining single. [5] Having an abortion.

7.2 Abortion Decision-Making Among Adolescents

7.2.1 "Developmental Profiles of Adolescents and Young Adults Choosing Abortion: State Sequence, Decalage, and Implications for Policy," V Foster and NA Sprinthall, *Adolescence* 27, No. 107:655, Fall, 1992

The level of reasoning among adolescents and young adults related to abortion was lower than their cognitive reasoning generally. Kohlberg's moral maturity scores on the standard dilemmas for 16-18 year olds was one full stage higher than the abortion scores of the young females in the study. See also "Follow-up After Abortion in Early Adolescence," M Perez-Reyes and R Kalk, *Arch Gen Psychiatry* 28:120, 1973. Many adolescents believed that abortion was not justified but they had rationalized their guilt by considering themselves "exceptions to the rule."

7.2.2 "Psychological Problems of Abortion for the Unwed Teenage Girl," CD Martin, Genetic *Psychology Monographs* 88:23-110, 1973

In-depth interviews found that 60% of girls had strong post-abortion guilt.

7.2.3 "Reasoning in the Personal and Moral Domains: Adolescent and Young Adult Women's

Decision-Making Regarding Abortion," Judith G Smetana, *Journal of Applied Developmental Psychology* 2:211-226, 1981

Subjects treating abortion as a moral issue were more likely to continue their pregnancies, while subjects treating abortion as a personal issue were more likely to obtain an abortion.

7.2.4   "Factors in Pregnancy Decision Making by Teenagers," Thomas Strahan, *Association for Interdisciplinary Research in Values and Social Change* 7(4): 1-8, Jan/Feb, 1995

Major factors in pregnancy decision-making by teenagers include (1) the personality of the teenager; (2) her attitude toward the current pregnancy; (3) previous reproductive history; (4) the attitude and degree of involvement of parents and other family members, the prospective father and peers and (5) the cultural and public policy aspects which may favor or disfavor childbirth.

7.2.5   "Teen Pregnancy in New Orleans: Factors that Differentiate Teens Who Deliver, Abort, and Successfully Contracept," E Landry et al, *Journal of Youth and Adolescence* 15(3): 259, 1986

Among black, never married teenagers age 12-18 who became pregnant, childbearers were more likely to be happy or proud themselves or have parents and boyfriends who were happy and proud of the pregnancy compared to teenagers who had abortions. Teenagers who became pregnant and had abortions were more likely to be angry at the pregnancy or have boyfriends who were angry compared to childbearers. The vast majority knew about birth control and where to get it, but few were using birth control when they became pregnant. Those who had abortions were more likely to try to deny the pregnancy (28.3%) compared to childbearers (18.4%). Those who had abortions were somewhat less likely to tell their parents about the pregnancy than childbearers (83.7% vs. 99.3%).

7.2.6   "Delivery or Abortion in Inner-City Adolescents," Susan H Fischman, *American Journal Orthopsychiatry* 47(1):127, 1977.

A study of unwed black adolescents in Baltimore found that those who delivered were characterized by parents and boyfriends who provided greater support for their decision compared to those who had abortions. The adolescent's relationship with her boyfriend was an important factor. In general, the longer the duration of the relationship, the lower the incidence of abortion. The deliverer's boyfriend was more likely to be working full-time, compared to the aborters' boyfriend who was apt to be attending school full-time or part-time. Deliverers attached greater importance to religion. Those having abortions were more likely to be attending school and at the appropriate grade level compared to deliverers who had a higher probability of having discontinued school. The pregnancy per se was not the primary reason for discontinuance. Pregnancy frequently occurred after the adolescent had left school. Those having abortions came from families with higher socioeconomic status and were less likely to be receiving welfare support (28%) compared to deliverers' families (44%).

7.2.7   "Why Do Women Have Abortions," ? , A Torres and JD Forrest. *Family Planning Perspectives* 20(4):169, 1988.

A 1987 Alan Guttmacher survey of U.S. abortion facilities found that almost two thirds (63%) of teenagers who had abortions at 16 gestational weeks or more attributed the delay to being afraid to tell their partner or parent that they were pregnant.

7.2.8   *Psycho-Social Stress Following Abortion,* Anne Speckhard (Kansas City, MO: Sheed&Ward, 1987).

A study of postabortion women where women frequently had second trimester abortions at a young age reported that abortion was used as a strategy for coping with the pregnancy without ever fully admitting that the pregnancy existed. For possible consequences of denial, see *Integration of Teen Pregnancy and Child Abuse Research: Identifying Mediator Variables for Pregnancy Outcome,* E. Becker-Lausen, A.U. Rickel, J. of Primary Prevention 16(1): 39, 1995 (Dissociation among adolescents was found to be associated with reports of becoming pregnant or of having an abortion in high school. Individuals who detach from reality by dissociation may disregard clues that may otherwise warn them of danger and they become " sitting ducks" for later abuse.

7.2.9   "Factors Discriminating Pregnancy Resolution Decisions: Issues of Unmarried Adolescents," Marvin Eisen, G. Zeilman, A. Leibowitz, W. Chow and J. Davis, *Genetic Psychology Monographs* 108:69(1983).

In a study of 368 white and Mexican-American adolescents from 13-19 years of age, a teenager whose boyfriend, best girlfriend and mother thought she should have an abortion was more likely to abort; when other factors were controlled, her own father's opinion of abortion was not a factor in the adolescent's decision. The most powerful predictor of the teenager's attitude toward abortion for others was her girlfriend's opinion.

7.2.10   "Adolescent Pregnancy: Effects of Family Support, Education, and Religion on the Decision to Carry or Terminate Among Puerto Rican Teenagers," CG Ortiz and EV Nuttall, *Adolescence* Vol XXII. No.88: 897- 917, 1987

Interviews with Puerto Rican teenagers found that those who carried to term were more significantly influenced and supported by family and friends compared to those who had abortions. Fathers were the least influential in both groups, while mothers were the most influential among those to carried to term, and sisters were the most influential among those who had abortions. Contrary to expectations, teenagers in the abortion group had a greater degree of religiosity than those who carried to term. Teenagers who had abortions were more likely to continue their education than those who carried to term.

7.2.11   "Influence of Maternal Attitudes on Urban Black Teens' Decisions About Abortion v. Delivery," E Freeman et al, *The Journal of Reproductive Medicine* 30(10): 731, 1985

A study of black urban, teenagers age 14-17 found that 81% chose the pregnancy outcome that their mothers supported.

7.2.12 "The Significance of Pregnancy Among Adolescents Choosing Abortion as Compared to Those Continuing Pregnancy," M Morin-Gonthier and G Lortie, *The Journal of Reproductive Medicine* 2(4): 255-259, 1984

A French-Canadian study found that family members, girl friends and others were more likely to know about a term pregnancy as compared to abortion. The adolescents wish to be pregnant, wanting someone to love who would love her in return , and opposition to abortion by family, partner and the adolescent was significantly more likely to result in childbirth; If the adolescent believed that she was too young to have a child, or unable to provide for and bring up a child with no one to help her, or if she did not want to prejudice her future was significantly more likely to result in abortion. (Ed Note: The adolescents' perception of her support system appeared to be an important factor.

7.3 Pregnant Teenagers' Reliance on Others to Make Pregnancy Resolution Decisions

7.3.1 "Factors Discriminating Pregnancy Resolution Decisions of Unmarried Adolescents," M Eisen, et al, *Genetic Psychology Monographs* 108:69 (1983)

Peer influence was an important factor among pregnant Mexican-American teenagers. Also, if the teenagers mother or the prospective father favored abortion, one-third of the teenagers who initially favored childbirth had an abortion.

7.3.2 "Adolescent Pregnancy-Decision Making: Are Parents Important?" RH Rosen, *Adolescence,* 15(57):44 (1980)

A Michigan study found that more than half of the adolescents involved their mothers in pregnancy decision making. Male partners also had a major influence, and to a lesser extent, fathers and girlfriends of the adolescent.

7.3.3 "Influence of Maternal Attitudes on Urban, Black Teens Decisions About Abortion v. Delivering," E Freeman, et al *The Journal of Reproductive Medicine* 30(10): 731 (1985)

Among black inner city teenagers, 81% chose the pregnancy outcome that their mothers supported.

7.3.4 "The Significance of Pregnancy among Adolescents Choosing Abortion Compared to Those Continuing Pregnancy," M Morin-Gonthier, and G Lortie, *The Journal of Reproductive Medicine* 29(4):255 (1984)

In a French-Canadian study the attitude of the male partner as well as that of family and friends was important to the outcome.

7.3.5 "To Whom Do Inner-City Minors Talk About their Pregnancies? Adolescents' Communication With Parents and Surrogate Parents," LS Zabin, et al *Family Planning Perspectives* 24(4):148 (1992)

In a study of black, urban teenagers in Baltimore, the probability that an adolescent would consult a parent before deciding what to do about her pregnancy was higher if she was younger, if she lived with the parent, and if she found the parent easy to talk to. Disatisfaction with the pregnancy decision one year after the pregnancy test was most likely if the parent did not support the final outcome, if someone other than the teenager had made the decision, or if the outcome was different from the teenagers preference at the time of the pregnancy test.

Adolescent Abortion and Parental Involvement

7.4 Parental Notice or Consent

7.4.1 "Mandatory Parental Consent to Abortion" Council on Ethical and Judicial Affairs, American Medical Association, *JAMA* 269(1):82 (1993)

Minors may not make considered choices about abortion because of immaturity, inexperience, or poor judgment. Parents are generally in the best position to counsel minors about their reproductive options, and they usually have a deep and respected interest in any significant matter involving their children. However, some minors may, in fact, be physically or emotionally harmed if they were required to involve their parents in the decision to have an abortion. In addition... parental involvement could interfere with the minors need for privacy on matters of sexual intimacy.

7.4.2 "Protecting Adolescents From Harm. Findings From the National Longitudinal Study on Adolescent Health," MD Resnick, et al *JAMA* 278(10):823 (1997)

Parent-family connectedness and school perceived connectedness was protective against every health risk of adolescents except history of pregnancy. Protective effects included less likelihood of emotional distress, suicidality, violence, substance use and cigarette use, alcohol use, marijuana use, and early age at first intercourse.

7.4.3 The Benefits of Legislation Requiring Parental Involvement Prior to Adolescent Abortion, *Values and Public Policy,* EL Worthington, et al (Family Research Council: Washington DC, 1988) 221-243 see also "The Benefits of Legislation Requiring Parental Involvement Prior to Adolescent Abortion," E Worthington, et al (Comment) *American Psychologist,* December, 1989, p. 1542-1545

Parents have a social responsibility and thus a right to be involved in decisions about an adolescent's pregnancy. Adolescent pregnancy should be considered in a social and familial context. (Many teens fear telling their parents about their pregnancy, overestimating the effect of their parents' anger and underestimating the parents' supportiveness.) An adolescent who is afraid to consult her parents prior to an abortion and who is supported by legislation to the extent that she need not consult them probably will not consult them and compounds her dearth of social support.

7.4.4   "Abortion Counseling: Focus on Adolescent Pregnancy," C Nadelson, *Pediatrics* 54(6):765 (1974)

The adolescent who is making a decision about abortion, having an abortion, or is in the post-abortion period needs a trusted ally who can help her understand her motivation for pregnancy and abortion. Ambivalence is especially prominent in this group. The counselor must remember that helping her with her own decision is not enough. Work with the family is important in order to (1) avoid repetition of the unwanted pregnancy, which is most frequently a distress signal for the adolescent, and (2) to work out problems reflected by the mutual acknowledgement of the adolescent's sexuality.

7.4.5   "Predictors of Repeat Pregnancies Among Low-Income Adolescents," M Gispert, et al. *Hospital and Community Psychiatry* 35(7): 719 (1984)

Regular use of contraception following childbirth or induced abortion was associated with a positive relationship between the girls and their mothers and with the presence of the father in the home. The authors concluded that interventions with sexually active adolescents will have little effect if they only focus on changing the adolescents' attitiudes toward contraception. Findings suggest that the mother has an important role and interventions aimed solely at sexually active adolescents that do not include their parents will miss an important part of the picture.

7.4.6   "Teen Pregnancy n New Orleans: Factors that Differentiate Teens Who Deliver, Abort, and Successfully Contracept," E Landry, et al. *Journal of Youth and Adolescence* 15(3): 259 (1986)

Among black, never married teenagers age 12-18 who had abortions, 28.3% tried to deny pregnancy, 88% knew about birth control, 77% knew where to get birth control, but only 22.8% were using a birth control method at the time they became pregnant.

7.5   Effect of Parental Involvement Laws

7.5.1   "The Economic Impact of State Restrictions on Abortion: Parental Consent and Notification Laws and Medicaid Funding Reastrictions," D Haas-Wilson, *Journal of Policy Analysis and Management* 12(3):489-511, 1993

In an analysis of 11 states with parental notification states compared to 40 states without such laws, Minors abortions per 1000 teenage pregnancies in 1985 were 320.8 vs. 382.6; Minors abortions per 1000 women aged 15-19 in 1988 were 9.87 vs. 13.22; Percentage of abortions obtained by minors, 1988 were 9.0% vs. 12.0%)

7.5.2   "Impact of the Minnesota Parental Notification Law on Abortion and Birth," JL Rogers, et al *Am J Public Health* 81(3): 294 (1991)

A decline in abortion rates was observed when the Minnesota parental notification law went into effect while birth rates continued to decline which suggested that the parental notification law facilitated pregnancy avoidance.

7.5.3   "Judging Teenagers: How Minors Fare When They Seek Court-Authorized Abortions," P Donovan, *Family Planning Perspectives* 15(6): 259, Nov/Dec, 1983

In Minnesota between 1980, the last full year without the notification law, and 1982, the first full year during which the law was in effect, the number of abortions obtained by minors decreased by 33 percent, from 2327 to 1565.

7.5.4   "Mandatory Parental Involvement in Minors' Abortions: Effects of the Laws in Minnesota, Missouri, and Indiana," C Ellertson, *Am J Public Health* 87(8): 1367 (1997)

In each state, the in-state abortion rate for minors fell relative to the rate for older women when parental involvement laws went into effect. The laws did not increase the birthrate for minors. The laws appeared to delay minors' abortions past the eighth week but probably not into the second trimester. The impact of out of state abortions was not clear from the data.

7.5.5   "Missouri's Parental Consent Law and Teen Pregnancy Outcomes," VH Pierson, *Women & Health* 22(3): 47 (1995)

Data suggest that since enforcement of the parental consent in 1985, there has been a decrease in selection of abortion as a pregnancy outcome, particularly among white teens. There has been an increase in the percentage of abortions among teens taking place in other states. There has been an increase of births to teenage mothers in the last decade.

7.5.6   "Parental Consent for Abortion: Impact of the Massachusetts Law," VG Cartoff, and LV Klerman, *Am J Public Health* 76(4): 397 (1986)

In the first 20 months after implementation of a parental consent law, only half as many adolescents obtained in-state abortions as had previously done so. More than 1800 minors went to five surrounding states to obtain abortions which accounted for the reduction in in-state abortions. In 1982, an estimated 50-100 minors bore children rather than having abortions , possibly because of the law.

Necessity of Parental Involvement

7.6   Family Estrangement

7.6.1   "Counseling the pregnant adolescent within a family context: Therapeutic Issues and Strategies,"

D Bapiste, *Family Therapy* 13:163 (1986)

Family needs to deal with its pervasive sense of failure precipitated by the pregnancy; family members need to clarify their different views about the pregnancy and unborn baby ; parents and adolescent need to resolve any pre- existing conflict ; it is important to communicate in a crisis situation; parents need to maintain their relationship while they "parent" their daughter through the crisis; parents and adolescents need to resolve developmental independency-dependency issues

7.6.2   "Abortion in teenagers," M Hanson, *Clinical Obstetrics and Gynecology* 21:1175 (1978)

Teenager should enlist the support of a parent or older sibling rather than "go it alone." Parents can help pay for the abortion.

7.6.3   "The genetics of antisocial acting out in children and adults," AM Johnson and SA Szurek, *Psychoanalytic Quarterly* 21:323 (1952)

Unwitting sexual permissiveness by the parent may encourage sexual acting out by the child. Both the parent and the child may need therapy.

7.6.4   "The Impact of a Parental Notification Law on Adolescent Abortion-Decision Making," R Blum et al, *American Journal Public Health* 77(5): 619, May, 1987

In a study of Minnesota teenagers seeking abortion, 70% of those who reported never attending religious services notified at least one parent prior to the abortion vs. 49% of those teenagers who reported attending religious services 10 or more times. (Ed Note: It appears that those parents who may be more likely to object to abortion were less likely to be notified by the teenager.)

7.6.5   "Abortion in Relationship Context," VM Rue, *Int'l Review of Natural Family Planning* 9:95 (1985)

A secret abortion , without disclosure or discussion, creates a psychological burden for the pregnant woman and a barrier to her future relationships with those most significant to her. e.g. Psychosocial Sequelae of Therapeutic Abortion in Young Unmarried Women, JS Wallerstein, et al *Arch Gen Psychiatry* 27:828 (1972)(Keeping the adolescent pregnancy and abortion secret from family caused a burden of guilt which was a continuing source of difficulty.; *Psycho-Social Stress Following Abortion,* A Speckhard, (Sheed & Ward: Kansas City, 1987) 81-82 (Young women from families which were opposed to out of wedlock sex often made the decision to keep the pregnancy and abortion secret to protect the family from stress and to protect their membership in their family of origin. This was often at the cost of increased personal stress and alienation, as well as imitating coping mechanisms both within and outside the family system.

7.6.6   "Parental Influence on the Pregnant Adolescent," A Young, et al, *Social Work* 2:387(1975)

Four-fifths of pregnant adolescents stated that their mother was the most significant person in their lives and social work counseling should include these mothers as well.

7.7 Parental Reaction to Pregnancy Less Negative than Anticipated by Adolescent

7.7.1 "Minor women obtaining abortions: A Study of Parental Notification in a metropolitan area," F Clary, *Am J Public Health* 72:283 (1982)

A Minnesota study found that , among the 37% of mothers notified of adolescent plans for abortion, 67%had a positive reaction, while 13% were neutral and 13% had a negative reaction.

7.7.2 "Adolescent Abortion and Parental Notification: Evidence for the Importance of Family Functioning on the Perceived Quality of Parental Involvement in U.S. Families," MS Griffin-Carlson, and PJ Schwanenflugel, *J Child Psychol Psychiat* 39 (4): 543 (1998)

In a study of 159 adolescents and their parents who accompanied their daughter to seven private abortion facilities in three states, 89.1% of the adolescents said they were glad they told their parents. Negative experiences were reported by 40.9% of the adolescents when they confided in their parents but there were no reports of physical violence. (Most of the adolescents described their parents as permissive.

7.7.3 "Teen Pregnancy in New Orleans: Factors that Differentiate Teens Who Deliver, Abort, and Successfully Contracept," E Landry, et al *Journal of Youth and Adolescence* 15 (3): 259 (1986)

Among black, never married teenagers aged 12-18 who had abortions, 28.3% tried to deny pregnancy, 76% were afraid of their parents reaction and 84% told their parents about the pregnancy. Of the parents who were told about the pregnancy, 6.5% were happy, 80% were surprised, 40.3% were angry, and 2.6% were proud.

7.7.4 *Unplanned parenthood: The social consequences of teenage childbearing,* FF Furstenberg (New York: The Free Press, 1976) 54

Pregnant adolescents often delayed telling their parents and frequently adolescents did not tell their parents at all. Two-thirds of parents stated they were angry when they heard of their daughters pregnancy. The response to the pregnancy was subject to considerable revision by both adolescents and their families during the course of gestation. Both parents and adolescents continually reevaluated their situation as the pregnancy proceeded and, in nearly every instance, their responses became more positive as the pregnancy proceeded.

7.7.5 "Counseling adolescents with problem pregnancies." J Maracek, *American Psychologist* 42:89 (1987)

Parental reactions are often less negative than anticipated, but the anticipation itself is a major source of anxiety.

7.7.6 *The Adolescent and Pregnancy,* M-A Corbett and JH Meyer, (Boston: Blackwell Scientific

Publications, 1987) 267-269

About 80% of pregnant adolescents in a young mothers program did not properly predict their mother's reaction to her pregnancy.The negative response they anticipated occurred but later resolved itself in acceptance.

7.8 Profile of Adolescents Not Disclosing Pregnancy or Abortion to Parents

7.8.1 "Parental Consent: Factors Influencing Adolescent Disclosure Regarding Abortion," MS Griffin-Carlson and KJ Macklin, *Adolescence* 28 (109):1,1993 (1993)

Among women age 12-21 from 5 Atlanta area abortion facilities, 51% confided in their parents, The degree of financial and emotional dependence and the quality and nature of family communication were closely related to the teenagers decision to confide in her parents about the decision to seek an abortion.

7.8.2 "Factors Associated with the Use of Court Bypass by Minors to Obtain Abortions," RW Blum et al *Family Planning Perspectives* 22(4):158 (1990)

A study of minors interviewed at 4 Minnesota abortion facilities found that 43% used the court by-pass option which was part of the state parental notification statute.Minors from the two lowest socioeconomic strata were significantly less likely than wealthier peers to use the court bypass.Minors who reported the most frequent attendance at religious services were significantly less likely than those whose attendance was less frequent to tell both parents of their abortion plans.Perceived maternal supportiveness was the key discriminating factor between those who notified parents and those who went to court. Avoidance of parental notification was only partly due to perceived parental disagreement with the decision. Minors who told neither parent were more likely to live with both parents and to see communication with their mother as less open. Fathers, had the opposite effect; when communication was good and they had been open about sexual matters, their daughters were less likely to discuss the abortion decision with them out of fear that he would be disappointed and hurt.

7.9 Availability of Financial Resources as a Factor

7.9.1 "Why Do Women Have Abortions?" A Torres and JD Forrest, *Family Planning Perspectives* 20(4):169 (1988)

A 1987 Alan Guttmacher study found that 73% of teenage women stated as a contributing reason for having an abortion was that she cannot afford a baby now.

7.9.2 "The Social and Economic Correlates of Pregnancy Resolution among Adolescents in New York

City by Race and Ethnicity: A Miltivariate Analysis" T Joyce, *Am J Public Health* 78(6):626 (1988).

The receipt of Medicaid benefits strongly correlated with decisions for childbirth among unmarried teenagers in New York City in 1984. The likelihood of abortion was only one-half among Puerto Rican teenagers, one-third among Latinos who were non-Puerto Rican, one-sixth for white teenagers, and one-third among black teenagers if they received Medicaid benefits.

7.9.3　"Adolescent Pregnancy in the United States: An Interstate Analysis," S Singh, *Family Planning Perspectives* 18(5):210 (1986)

An Alan Guttmacher study found that the availability of Medicaid funds to pay for abortions was associated with higher abortion rates for pregnant teenagers.

7.10　Differential Psychosocial Impact on Adolescents

7.10.1　"Differential Impact of Abortion on Adolescents and Adults," W Franz and D Reardon, *Adolescence* 105:162 (1992).

Women members of Women Exploited by Abortion who aborted as teenagers compared to women who aborted at 20 years or older were less satisfied with services at the time of the abortion, were more likely to feel forced by circumstances to have the abortion, were more likely to report being misinformed, more often reported severe psychological distress, and more often wanted to give birth and keep the baby.

7.10.2　"Abortion in Adolescence," N Campbell, et al., *Adolescence* 23(92):813 (1988).

Women in a patient led postabortion support group who had poorly assimilated their abortion and who had abortions as adolescents were more likely to report parental marital difficulties, attempt suicide, have severe nightmares, and exhibit immature coping defenses such as retreating into sexual activity or drug and alcohol abuse compared to women who had abortions after the age of 20.

7.10.3　"Family Relationships and Depressive Symptoms Preceding Induced Abortion," D Bluestein and CM Rutledge, *Family Practice Research Journal* 13(2):149-156, 1993.

In a study of pre-abortion depression in a sample of women age 14-43 years, depressive symptoms preceding abortion were moderate to severe in intensity and were more likely to increase as age decreased.

7.10.4　"Pregnancy in the Adolescent Patient," M Polanecyk and K O'Connor, *Pediatric Clinics of North America* 46(4):649 (1999).

Adolescents in general are known to comply with medical regimens more poorly than adults) see "Postabortion Medical Care: Management of Delayed Complications," KA Nichols and SJ

Rasmussen, *Journal of the American Medical Women's Association* 49(5): 165, 1994 Adolescent who had not told her mother prior to abortion, failed to comply with antibiotic regiment and developed a potentially serious postabortion infection.

7.10.5   "Therapeutic Abortion During Adolescence: Psychiatric Observations," P Barglow and S Weinstein, *Journal of Youth and Adolescence* 2(4): 33 (1973)

Two major factors distinguish adolescent emotional response to abortion from those of adult patients: (1) the adolescent decision is more "outer-other"-directed by parents, peer group, or sexual partner and is therefore more difficult and hazardous; (2) developmental immaturity contributes to ambivalence about the decision, to a distorted perception of the procedure, and to a variety of pathological reactions.

7.10.6   "A Comparison of Minors and Adult's Pregnancy Decisions," Catherine Lewis. *American Journal of Orthopsychiatry* 50(3):446-453, July, 1980

This article concludes that minor's decisions were more externally-based compared to adults i.e. what parents thought. Minors more often considered possible deformity of the child.

7.10.7   "Abortion Surveillance-United States, 1996." LM Koonin, et al Centers for Disease Control *MMWR* 48"No.SS4: 1, July 30, 1999

Adolescents are more likely to have a late term abortion i.e. 13 gestational weeks or later compared to older women); Adler, N et al (1990) Psychological responses after abortion, Science 248:41 (A late term abortion is generally acknowledged to be a risk factor for adverse psychological sequelae compared to a first trimester abortion.

7.10.8   "Adolescent Mourning Reactions to Infant and Fetal Loss," NH Horowitz, *Social Casework* 59:551 (1978)

Replacement pregnancies may follow adolescent abortion.

7.10.9   "Adolescent Suicide Attempts Following Elective Abortion: A Special Case of Anniversary Reactions," CL Tishler, *Pediatrics* 68:670 (1981)

Adolescents attempted suicide on the perceived due date of their aborted child.

7.10.10 "Suicides after Pregnancy in Finland: register linkage study,"M Gissler, et al. *British Medical Journal* 313:1431 (1996)

Adolescent suicide during one year following induced abortion was significantly higher than adolescent suicide following childbirth.

7.10.11 "Mediation of Abusive Childhood Experiences: Dissociation and Negative Life Outcomes," E Becker-Lausen, *Am J Orthopsychiatry* 65(4):560 (1995)

Dissociation was significantly related to reports by females of previously becoming pregnant and having an abortion in high school. Individuals who detach from reality by dissociation may disregard clues that may otherwise warn them of danger and become "sitting ducks" for later abuse.

7.10.12 "HIV/AIDS Prevention and Multiple Risk Behaviors of Gay Male and Runaway Adolescents," C Haignere, et al *Int Conf AIDS* 6(3):234. abstract no. S.C. 581, June 20-23, 1990

A study of 75 female runaway adolescents in New York City found that suicide attempts and suicide ideation were found to be significantly related to having had an abortion.

7.10.13 "HIV+ adolescents: factors linked to transmission and prevention," D Futterman et al, *Int Conf AIDS* 9(2):725, abstract no. PO-C19-3049, June 6-11, 1993

Among inner-city adolescents, HIV+ youths were more likely to have STD's and abortion.

7.10.14 "Drug Use Among Adolescent Mothers: Profile of Risk," H Amaro, et al, *Pediatrics,* 84(1):144 (1989)

Drug users among inner city teenage women were significantly more likely to have a prior elective abortion compared to drug non-users. Teenage women with two or more live born children had a much lower incidence of drug use compared to women with a history of elective abortion.

7.10.15 "Drug Use as a Risk Factor for Premartal Teen Pregnancy and Abortion in a National Sample of Young White Women," B Mensch, and DB Kandel, *Demography* 29(3):409 (1992)

Illicit drug use has the strongest effect of any predictor on experiencing an abortion: the odds of an abortion are nearly five times as large for premaritally pregnant white teens who used other illicit drugs compared to those who did not use these drugs.

7.11   Adolescent Violation of Conscience or Belief

7.11.1 "Psychological Problems of Abortion for the Unwed Teenage Girl," CD Martin, *Genetic Psychology Monographs* 88:23 (1973)

Among San Diego teenagers undergoing abortion for mental health reasons, 60% had strong post-abortion guilt. A substantial number changed their moral and religious convictions following pregnancy and abortion including feeling differently about sex, abortions, or killing, changes in formal religious faiths, and changed feelings about their view of God and what was sinful.

7.11.2 "Follow-up After Abortion in Early Adolescence," M Perez-Reyes, and R Falk, *Archives Gen Psychiatry* 28:120 (1973)

In a North Carolina study of adolescents who had abortions, 34% opposed abortion on request, 20% thought abortion was justified only to save the life of the mother, and 29% thought it was permitted only on medical recommendation, yet none of those aborting gave those reasons for doing so. It was concluded that many had rationalized their guilt by considering themselves "exceptions to the rule."

7.11.3   "Developmental Profiles of Adolescents and Young Adults Choosing Abortion: Stage Sequence, Decalage, and Implications for Policy," V Foster and NA Sprinthall, *Adolescence* 27(107): 655 (1992).

Principled moral reasoning was infrequently used as a basis for decision-making among adolescents and young adults.

7.12   Adolescent Long Term Psychological Sequelae

7.12.1   "A disproportionately high percentage of women who had abortions as adolescents have been found in postabortion support or recovery groups." J Vought, *Post-Abortion Trauma* (1991) (39% were teenagers at time of abortion); "Abortion in Adolescence," NB Campbell, et al, *Adolescence* Vol XXIII, No.92, Winter, 1988

49% were between 15-20 at the time of their abortion. Women who had an abortion as adolescents are also more likely to join Women Exploited by Abortion. In a study of 252 WEBA members, 45% reported having had abortions as teenagers, *Aborted Women: Silent No More,* D Reardon, (1987). Women who had abortions as adolescents have been found to be more likely to report chronic long term stress reactions. *The Psycho-Social Aspects of Stress Following Abortion,* AC Speckhard,(1987) 31% of women with long term stress were 14-18 years of age at the time of their abortion.

7.13   Adolescent Demographic Data

7.13.1   "The Social and Economic Correlates of Pregnancy Resolution Among Adolescents in New York City by Race and Ethnicity: A Multivariate Analysis," T Joyce, *Am J Public Health* 78(6):626 (1988)

Teenagers who experienced one prior abortion were approximately four times more likely to terminate a current pregnancy by abortion compared to teenagers with no prior abortion history. Medicaid tended to increase the likelihood of carrying to term. Married adolescents were more likely than unmarried adolescents to carry a pregnancy to term.

7.13.2   "Induced Terminations of Pregnancy: Reporting States, 1988," KD Kochanek, *Monthly Vital Statistics Report* 39(12) Supplement 1-32, April 30, 1991

The National Center for Health Statistics reported that among white teenagers age 18-19 with induced abortions, 22.5% were having their second abortion or more. Among black teenagers age 18-19 with induced abortions, 35.5% were having their second abortion or more.

7.13.3   "Induced Terminations of Pregnancy: Reporting States, 1988," KD Kochenek, *Monthly Vital Statistics Report* 39 (12), Supplement, April 30, 1991, Table 2, Table 11

The National Center for Health Statistics reported detailed abortion statistics for a 14 state area in 1988. Among women under 14 years of age, 28.3% had abortions at 13 gestational weeks or more compared to 24.6% of women age 14, 20.3% of women age 1, 19.0% of women age 16, 16.6% of women age 17, 13.8% of women age 18, 12.2% of women age 19, 11.2% of women age 20-24, 9.1% of women age 25-29, and 7.4% of women age 30-34 years.

7.13.4   "Why Do Women Have Abortions?" A Torres, and JD Forrest, *Family Planning Perspectives* 20:169 (1988)

According to a 1987 Alan Guttmacher survey ,63% of U.S. women who had abortions as teenagers at 16 weeks gestation or more attributed the delay to being afraid to tell their partner or parent that they were pregnant compared to one-third of the women in the overall sample.

7.14   Differential Physical Complications of Adolescent Abortion

7.14.1   "Morbidity Risk Among Young Adolescents Undergoing Elective Abortion," R Burkman et al *Contraception* 30:99 (1984)

Teenagers 17 years old or less were significantly more likely to have postabortion endometritis, cervical lacerations , or hemorrhage greater than 500 ml. following abortion compared to women age 20-29.

7.14.2   "Postabortal pelvic infection associated with chlamydia trachomatis infection and the influence of humoral immunity," S Osser, and K Perrson, *Am J Obstet Gynecol* 150:699 (1984)

Chlamydia positive women age 13-19 were more likely to develop postabortion endometritis (28%) compared to women aged 20-24 (22.7%) or women aged 25-29 (20%). Chlamydia positive women aged 13-19 were more likely to develop postabortion salpingitis (21.9%) compared to women aged 20-24 (13.6%). see Nederlof, KP et al (1990) Ectopic Pregnancy Surveillance United States, 1970-1987, *MMWR* 39, No. SS-4:9 (Ectopic pregnancy is estimated to occur 5-10 times more frequently among women with a prior history of salpingitis. Ectopic pregnancy case-fatality rates are higher in women age 15-19 compared to older women.

7.14.3   "Postabortion Medical Care: Management of Delayed Complications," KA Nichols and SJ Rasmussen, *Journal of the American Medical Women's Assn* 49(8):165 (1994)

A teenager underwent an abortion but did not take her antibiotics as prescribed and developed a low grade fever. She went to an emergency room of a hospital four days after the abortion where she saw a doctor who refused to treat her. Instead, the doctor called the abortion facility and the teenager's mother, who, for personal reasons, the teenager had not told about her pregnancy and abortion. The teenager and her mother then came to the abortion facility where it was determined that the teenager had endometritis. Antibiotics were administered and the infection was cleared up. The article stated that had the teenager not received the appropriate medication, her endometritis could have been quite severe and required hospitalization and intravenous antibiotics and could have resulted in infertility. The state where the abortion occurred did not have any parental notice or consent law. see also Polaneczky, M and O'Connor, K (1999) Pregnancy in the Adolescent Patient, Pediatric Clinics of North America 46(4): 649 Adolescents in general are known to comply with medical regimens more poorly than adults.

7.14.4   "Pain of First Trimester Abortion: A Study of Psychosocial and Medical Predictors," E Belanger, et al. *Pain* 36:339 (1989)

In a Canadian study, pain was more severe in adolescents who underwent first trimester suction abortion under local anesthesia compared with older women. Pre-abortion depression was the principal predictor of pain.

7.15   Adolescent Risk of Breast Cancer

7.15.1   "Age at First Birth and Breast Cancer Risk," B MacMahon, et al, *Bulletin of the World Health Organization* 43:209 (1970)

In a large international study it was found that women having their first birth under age 18 had only about one-third the risk of breast cancer compared to those whose first birth is delayed until age 35 or more. The study also stated that " data suggested an increased risk associated with abortion contrary to the reduction in risk associated with full-term births."

7.15.2   "The Independent Assocations of Parity, Age at First Full Term Pregnancy, and Duration of Breastfeeding with the Risk of Breast Cancer," PM Layde, et al, *J Clin Epidemiol* 42(10):963 (1989)

A Centers for Disease Control study found that increasing number of live born children and duration of breast feeding had a strong protective effect on the risk of breast cancer.

7.15.3   "Effect of Family History, Body-Fat Distribution, and Reproductive Factors on the Risk of Postmenopausal Breast Cancer," TA Sellers, et al, *New England Journal of Medicine* 326:1323 (1992)

The increase in risk of breast cancer associated with low parity or greater age at first pregnancy is more pronounced among women with a family history of breast cancer.

7.15.4   "Familial risk, abortion and their interactive effect on the risk of breast cancer- a combined analysis of six case-control studies," N Andrieu, et al, *Br J Cancer* 72:744 (1995)

The relative risk of breast cancer conferred by a family history of breast cancer increased with the number of abortions.

7.15.5   "Risk of Breast Cancer Among Young Women: Relationship to Induced Abortion," JR Daling et al, *Journal of the National Cancer Institute* 86(21):1584-1592, 1994

Higher risks for breast cancer following induced abortion when the abortion was done at age 18 or younger and particularly if it took place after 8 weeks gestation. see also "Induced Abortion and the Risk of Breast Cancer, M Melbye" et al, *New England Journal of Medicine* 336(2): 81-85, 1997 The relative risk of breast cancer increased with the increasing gestational age of the fetus at the time of the most recent abortion. (Ed Note: Adolescents are more likely to have an abortion at a later gestational age compared to older women.)

7.15.6   "Induced abortion as an independent risk factor for breast cancer: a comprehasive review and analysis," J Brind, et al *Journal of Epidemiology and Community Health* 50:481 (1996).

A meta-analysis of 28 published reports concluded there was an independent increased risk of 30-50% for breast cancer as a result of induced abortion. Higher risks for breast cancer occurred among women with two or more induced abortions compared to women with one induced abortion in seven of ten studies. see also www.abortion cancer.com website for further updates on breast cancer and abortion.

Definition of Terms

Cervical Injury: injury to the neck of the uterus or womb; the lower part of the uterus extending from the isthmus of the uterus into the vagina.

Chlamydia Trachomatis: an infectious organism that is neither a virus nor a bacteria. Some have called it a parasite. Its strains infect humans primarily and often are transmitted directly by close personal contact.

Curettage: Surgical scraping of cleaning by means of a curette, which is a loop-or ring shaped steel knife.

D&C (dilatation and curettage): forcing the enlargement of an opening of the cervix and then inserting a curette into the uterus to cut the developing child (or sometimes a dead child) into pieces and remove the pieces by scraping.

Ectopic Pregnancy: union of the egg and sperm and subsequent development in a location other than in the uterus. It often occurs in the fallopian tube. It is potentially life threatening to the woman and results in the death of the developing child. Sometimes called tubal pregnancy.

Endrometritis: inflammation of the lining of the uterus.

Febrile Morbidity: any infectious complication after induced abortion, including endrometritis, salpingitis, peritonitis or fever.

Febrile Reactions: symptoms indicating fever; sometimes called endrometritis.

Fitz-Hugh-Curtis Syndrome: occurs when the liver capsule becomes involved with inflammatory exudate that later leaves adhesions; a sudden pain in the abdomen, vaginal discharge fever chills are symptoms. Also called perihepatitis.

Incompetent Cervix: insufficiency; incapable of performing the allotted function; unable to retain an intrauterine pregnancy until term because of some deficiency in structure and function.

Induced Abortion: to cause or initiate by artificial means the termination of a pregnancy accompanied by or resulting in the death of the embryo or fetus.

Laminaria: inserting seaweed sticks into the cervix, which then swell and slowly dilate the cervix prior to induced abortion.

Laparoscopy: Examination of the contents of the abdominal cavity with a peritoneoscope passed through the abdominal wall.

Maternal Mortality: the number of maternal deaths which occur during the entire course of pregnancy and during the first three to six months following completion of the pregnancy per 100,000 live births.

Miscarriage: the spontaneous expulsion of a human fetus after the first 12 or 20 weeks gestation, depending upon the definition of spontaneous abortion, without apparent cause.

Pelvic Inflammatory Disease: inflammation of the female genital tract. It starts in the cervix and may spread to any of the female organs and even into the pelvic cavity. It is a major direct cause of sterility.

Prophylaxis: measures designed to preserve health and prevent the spread of disease.

Salpingitis: inflammation of the fallopian tube or the eustachian tube.

Spontaneous Abortion: the spontaneous expulsion of a human fetus during the first 12 weeks of gestation without apparent cause. Some use this term until 20 weeks gestation.

Vacuum Aspiration: induced abortion in the early stages of pregnancy (not usually beyond 12 weeks gestation) by aspiration or suction of the developing child from the uterus through a narrow tube. Approximately 96 % of the induced abortions in the U.S. use this method.

Other Titles Available from Acorn Books

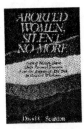

Aborted Women, Silent No More
David C. Reardon

Filled with powerful personal testimonies, this is the most widely-read book in pro-life circles on the detrimental effects of abortion. Conservative Book Club called it "the most powerful book ever published on abortion." *$16.95 / 373 pp.*

Making Abortion Rare: A Healing Strategy for a Divided Nation
David C. Reardon

Lays out a practical plan for ending abortion on demand. Fr. Paul Marx of Human Life International said this book "will accomplish what its title claims—and more." *$14.95 / 204 pp.*

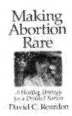

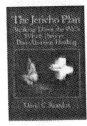

The Jericho Plan: Breaking Down the Walls Which Prevent Post-Abortion Healing
David C. Reardon

Understand the spiritual aspect of abortion and how to foster post-abortion healing within the Church. Makes a great gift for priests and pastors! *$8.95 / 103 pp.*

Victims and Victors: Speaking Out About Their Pregnancies, Abortions and Children Resulting From Sexual Assault
David C. Reardon, Julie Makimaa and Amy Sobie

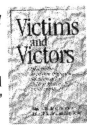

In their own words, women who have experienced sexual assault pregnancies tell why abortion is not the answer. Learn the truth about abortion in the "hard cases." *$11.95 / 187 pp.*

Coming in Spring 2002

Forbidden Grief: The Unspoken Pain of Abortion
Theresa Burke, Ph.D., with David C. Reardon, Ph.D.
Foreword by Dr. Laura Schlessinger

Explores the secret pain carried by many post-abortive women—and the social obstacles that often prevent healing. Learn how to help build a more healing environment for those struggling with a past abortion.

To order, call 1-888-41-ACORN